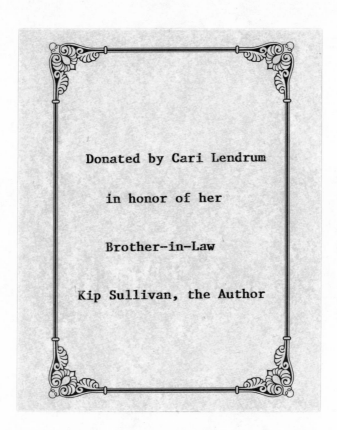

# The Health Care Mess: How We Got Into It and How We'll Get Out of It

## Kip Sullivan

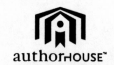

authorHOUSE™

1663 LIBERTY DRIVE, SUITE 200
BLOOMINGTON, INDIANA 47403
(800) 839-8640
WWW.AUTHORHOUSE.COM

First published by AuthorHouse  4/27/2006

ISBN: 1-4208-8551-0 (sc)

Printed in the United States of America
Bloomington, Indiana

This book is printed on acid-free paper.

For my good friend Mike Casper,
who insisted I write this book

# Foreword

When I finally got around to writing the first edition of this book in 2002, I had a long debate with myself about whether to write a book that felt like a textbook or to write a book that felt more like a conversation with a friend. On the one hand, I wanted to write a book that was accurate, well documented, and thorough. That argued for something that resembled a textbook, that is to say, a book written in a formal style and loaded with tables and footnotes. But I also wanted to write a book that was easy for people with no background in health policy to read. For me, that meant writing a book that sounded like me when I talk to audiences. Over the last two decades, I've spoken to thousands of people at hundreds, perhaps thousands, of meetings. Although my speeches are carefully structured to pack the most information I can into the time I've been given, I speak in an informal, conversational style. I've even been known to raise my voice and jab my finger in the air every now and then.

This book is a compromise between those conflicting desires – my desire to write a textbook and my desire to write a book that is easy to read, even somewhat entertaining, God forbid. The book covers every important issue raised by today's health policy debate and it is well documented (maybe even excessively documented). But it is also written in an informal style.

As my work on the first edition of this book came to an end late in 2002, I had a similar debate with myself about what title to give the book. I wanted a title that reflected the content of the book, and I wanted a title that used everyday language that would suggest to potential readers that this book is readable. The title I ultimately selected was rather informal for a book with the ambitions of a textbook and, as you've probably noticed, unusually long. But the more I thought about it, the more I liked it. I settled on this title late in 2002 and never looked back.

Imagine my surprise at learning in September 2005, several weeks after this updated version of the book went into production, that a book with nearly the identical title had been published in the summer of 2005. I discovered that fact by perusing the "books received" section of the July 27, 2005 edition of the *Journal of the American Medical*

*Association.* (Several physician friends of mine pass various medical journals on to me when they're done reading them. I usually don't get around to reading these hand-me-down journals until several months after their publication.) To add to my astonishment, the book with the similar title was written by two single-payer advocates, one of whom I have known about and respected for years.

Because I had worked hard to craft the title of my book, and because finding another title and rewriting portions of my book that referred to the title would delay publication, I decided I would not change the title. But I did feel the need to explain to readers who might be aware of the other book that I did not take my title from the other book.

The simplest proof of this fact is an article I wrote for a magazine called *Social Policy* which appeared early in 2003. The article was entitled, "Understanding the health care reform debate: A primer for the perplexed." The editor of *Social Policy* at that time, Mike Miller, asked me to write an article for *Social Policy* that introduced health policy to beginners. Mike (an organizer with whom I worked in San Francisco in the 1970s) asked me to draft a short list of books and articles that I thought newcomers to the health policy debate might find useful. Because I expected my own book to be published soon, either as a book or as a document on a Web site, I listed the title of my book in the bibliography that appears at the end of the article. Mike published the article in the Winter 2002/2003 edition of *Social Policy*. You can find back issues of *Social Policy* in many libraries. You can also find the article at www.muhcc.org, the Web site of the Minnesota Universal Health Care Coalition.

So how did such a similar title come to grace the front cover of another book? I have no idea. It's possible that the appearance of two books on the same subject at about the same time with nearly the identical title is just a coincidence. I have nothing but respect for scholars brave enough and smart enough to endorse single-payer, as the authors of the other book have done. I have no reason to think they deliberately took my title for their book.

Here's what I do know. In the spring of 2003, I sent the manuscript for the first edition of this book to Physicians for a National Health Program and urged them to post it on their Web site. PNHP did so.

When I decided in the spring of 2005 to update the book and have it published, I asked PNHP to take it off their Web site, which they did in July 2005. In short, the title of my book was available over a two-year period to anyone who used the Internet.

Kip Sullivan
Minneapolis, Minnesota
November 12, 2005

# Table of Contents

# 1

# In the Beginning

## My introduction to the world of health-care reform

In the summer of 1986, John Musick, my boss at Minnesota COACT (Citizen Organizations Acting Together), asked me if I would like to direct a citizen campaign for universal health insurance. At that time, I knew almost nothing about health policy. I couldn't have told you how much the U.S. spent on health care, how many uninsured Americans there were, or what a carotid endarterectomy was. All I was sure of was that the health-care system was complex, the U.S. did not guarantee health insurance to all its citizens, and the opposition to universal coverage by the U.S. health insurance industry and the American Medical Association (AMA) was the main reason why. As I would learn later, the insurance industry and the AMA had thwarted four previous attempts to establish an American universal health insurance program – once just before World War I, again during the Depression, a third time after Harry Truman was elected president in 1948, and again in the early 1970s when Richard Nixon was supporting a universal health insurance plan.

Despite my gross ignorance of health policy, my gut reaction to John's question was excitement. It excited me to think about building an army of people to take on the insurance industry and the AMA. The unaffordability of health insurance and medical care affected all Americans – deeply and personally. It would be three more years before the media began talking about the "health-care crisis," but the staff and members of COACT were already well aware that a crisis was upon us. So too, it turned out, were citizen groups around the country.

COACT's leaders and staff were aware of the problem because we had been organizing low- and middle-income Minnesotans on a variety of economic issues since COACT's formation in Duluth in 1975. By 1980, which is when I went to work for COACT as a community organizer in the southern Minnesota town of Mankato, the problem of unaffordable health insurance was becoming more visible, especially in rural Minnesota where COACT's offices were concentrated. Rural Minnesota had been especially hard hit by the 1980-81 recession. Many farmers, small business owners, and rural citizens were telling us they were coping with hard economic times by, among other things, scaling back the level of insurance coverage they had (for example, they were buying insurance with $500 deductibles for each member of the family), or, worse, dropping insurance altogether.

I had no doubt, then, that a campaign to make health insurance available to all Americans would excite COACT's membership and staff and help us attract even more members. But my excitement at John's question was tempered by what I perceived to be two big obstacles to a successful people's campaign to establish universal insurance in this country.

The first obstacle was the power of our opponents. I did not know at the time that the U.S. health-care system absorbed almost one-eighth of every dollar Americans earn (today we spend almost one-sixth of our income on health care), but I knew the players in that industry, including the insurers, the doctors, the hospitals, and the drug industry, had a lot of money and political power and would use it against any proposal they saw as a threat to their welfare. I assumed that it would take an unusually strong movement – something at least as strong as the civil rights and anti-war movements of the sixties – to beat these guys. Even though COACT represented 20,000 Minnesotans and had an annual budget of about $700,000, we were minnows compared to the whales that dominated the health-care industry.

The second problem I perceived was the complexity of the U.S. health-care system and the difficulty COACT's leaders and staff would have in explaining the problem and the solution to the citizens we would have to mobilize. Within a few years, I would not feel this way. Within a few years I would realize that most people can understand health policy – even enjoy it – if it's introduced to them in bite-sized pieces, free of jargon or, if jargon is unavoidable, with jargon explained.

Despite my concern about the complexity of health policy and the power of our opponents, I told John I would be happy to direct a campaign for universal coverage if the COACT board decided we should undertake it. John agreed that the opposition would be intense and that we would have to work in coalition with other organizations.

Things moved very quickly after that conversation. COACT's board endorsed the health-care campaign that fall, and, in November 1986, officers of Minnesota COACT and the Minnesota Senior Federation (another citizen group representing tens of thousands of citizens) sent a letter to several dozen Minnesota organizations, including religious organizations, farm groups, and unions, inviting them to a meeting to discuss creating a coalition to fight for legislation at the state and federal level to extend health insurance coverage to all citizens. In April 1987, the coalition, subsequently known as the Health Care Campaign of Minnesota (HCCM), was formally created. Within two years, it had grown to 30 groups. I worked closely with HCCM for 11 years, and then, beginning in 2002, with its successor, the Minnesota Universal Health Care Coalition.

## Climbing the learning curve

My knowledge of the health-care system grew in stages that corresponded to the positions that COACT and HCCM adopted. During the last three years of the 1980s, when we were attempting to create new public programs that would make it easier for the uninsured to buy insurance, I learned about the impact the high cost of health insurance was having on people's pocket books and the effect that not having insurance was having on people's health. Between 1990 and 1992, when COACT and HCCM were lobbying state and federal legislators to sponsor legislation creating a "single-payer" health insurance system, I concentrated my studies on why insurance companies are so inefficient compared with Medicare, why the U.S. health-care system is so expensive compared with other countries, and what could be done to reduce America's health-care costs. After 1993, I focused on the consequences of America's ludicrous experiment with "health maintenance organizations" (HMOs). Nineteen-ninety-three was the year politicians, led by Bill and Hillary Clinton, endorsed HMOs as the solution to the health-care crisis. Thanks to that endorsement and to the power of the HMO industry, which by then had taken over most of the health insurance industry, health reform proposals that did not propose a prominent role for HMOs were kept off the American political agenda for the rest of the nineties.

But by the late 1990s, it had become apparent to the entire world that HMOs had failed. They had damaged quality of care without making a dent in inflation. The revolt against HMOs came in two stages – the doctor-patient revolt, which materialized in the mid-1990s, and the employer revolt which was in full swing by about 2000. The doctor-patient revolt focused on the damage HMOs were doing to quality by denying necessary medical services to patients. The "HMO backlash," as the doctor-patient revolt was dubbed by the media, took many forms, most notably legislation introduced in Congress and nearly all state legislatures to protect patients against abuse by HMOs. The employer revolt focused on the high cost of premiums. The HMO industry might have survived the doctor-patient revolt had employers continued to support the cost-control tactics of HMOs. But that was not to be. As annual inflation rates in health insurance premiums rose in the late 1990s, employer support for the experiment with HMOs dissipated. By the year 2000, it was clear HMOs had given us the worst of all worlds – deteriorating quality of medical care and no savings to show for it.

The failure of the HMO industry to function as advertised gave the insurance industry an incentive to cook up yet another awful proposal – insurance policies with very high deductibles. By 2001 these high-deductible policies, which went by a variety of names, including "consumer-driven" policies, "medical savings accounts," and "health savings accounts," had replaced HMOs as the most commonly discussed solution to the health-care crisis, especially among conservatives. (Unlike politicians like Bill Clinton who endorsed HMOs in the early 1990s, politicians like George W. Bush who promote high-deductible policies these days do not propose legislation to achieve universal coverage. They just promote high deductibles.) As the endorsement of HMOs by political and business leaders in the early 1990s forced me to educate myself on HMOs, so the recent endorsement of high-deductible policies by a growing number of politicians (employers have yet to show great excitement about high-deductible policies) has forced me to educate myself about the effect that high deductibles has on cost and quality.

All of these subjects – the causes and consequences of health-care inflation, the promises versus the facts about HMOs and high-deductible policies, the arguments for and against single-payer, and other subjects I have yet to mention – now seem quite understandable to me. I find them easy to explain to others. It is true that these subjects are more complex than others Americans debate today; health policy does have a learning curve. But I've learned the average person can traverse the steepest portion of that curve with no more than ten hours of study.

## Americans will endorse a universal Medicare plan

Although the demise of the HMO project made it easier for advocates of high-deductible policies to be heard, it also opened the door to the single-payer proposal, a proposal that I have worked for since 1989, the year COACT and HCCM endorsed single-payer legislation. A single-payer system is one in which one payer reimburses "providers" – doctors, hospitals, and other individuals and organizations who deliver health care to patients. Because Medicare closely resembles a true single-payer system, single-payer legislation is often called Medicare-for-all legislation.

The fight for a Medicare-for-all plan, and the fight against non-solutions like HMOs and high-deductible policies, is rewarding for several reasons. First, health care is an essential service; its quality and availability can mean the difference between life and death. Second, hundreds of billions of dollars are at stake. Third, and perhaps most important, polls, focus groups and my own experience tell me that a sizable majority of the public share my values and either support Medicare-for-all already or will do so as soon as they are exposed to even a brief presentation of the facts. Knowing that so many people agree with me turns what would be a very interesting fight into a very enjoyable fight as well. I do not labor under the illusion that majority opinion is always right. But in the health policy wars, the public is clearly right and the "experts" – the people who dominate the current debate, including insurance company executives, politicians, big business executives, academicians who take money from the drug and insurance industries, and columnists – are wrong. The experts have lots of theory, money, and access to the media on their side, but the public has facts and common sense on its side.

In Chapter 8, I present the evidence supporting my argument that the public's opinion is consistent with the facts, and conflicts with the opinion of experts. But I can't wait till Chapter 8 to give you a taste of how supportive the public is of a Medicare-for-all system. I'm going to tell you at the outset a true story that indicates that a large majority of Americans will endorse a single-payer system if they are exposed to a fair debate about the causes of the health-care mess and what should be done about it.

The story is about a debate between a single-payer advocate, an HMO advocate, and an advocate of "medical savings accounts" (MSAs). (MSAs are one version of high-deductible policies conservatives began to promote in the mid-1990s. They have deductibles on the order of thousands of dollars.) The debate occurred in front a group of citizens selected to represent all Minnesotans. I was the single-payer advocate. Single-payer won – not by a teeny bit, but by a landslide.

The story begins late in September 1996 when I got a call from a woman named Laurie Sether. She asked if I would be willing to be one of three speakers on health-care reform at a "citizens forum" being convened by the Minneapolis *Star Tribune* and KTCA-TV, the Twin Cities' public television station, on the evening of October 1. Laurie wanted me to present the case for a single-payer health-care system. She said she was still looking for a speaker to advocate "managed competition" (the phrase used to describe proposals built around the HMO industry's mythology), and another to present the case for MSAs.

I didn't ask, but I guessed why Laurie had decided to nail down a single-payer advocate first. People who can speak intelligently about reforming the U.S. health-care system from a consumer's point of view are rare. Conversely, people who can speak in favor of HMOs and high-deductible policies are a dime a dozen. The HMO industry pays lots of people lots of money to peddle HMO propaganda, and the non-HMO wing of the insurance industry pays lots of people to peddle high-deductible policies. But no industry sugar daddy pays consumers or anyone else to advocate for a single-payer system.

Laurie said each speaker would have five minutes to make an opening statement, and then we would take questions for the next three-and-a-half hours from a group of randomly selected Minnesotans. This format concerned me. I saw it as guaranteeing frustration for speakers and audience members alike. Health policy, I said, can be intimidating if basic information isn't presented first. I said I would have preferred to have the *Star Tribune* and KTCA host three different meetings, or failing that, allow each speaker to talk for half an hour. But Laurie said the format was fixed, and the best she could do would be to extend the opening statements to ten minutes. I agreed to participate.

On the morning of October 1, I learned that the managed-competition advocate would be Michael Scandrett, director of what was then called the Minnesota Council of HMOs, and that the proponent of MSAs would be Liz Quam, a woman who had, until recently, been on the staff of the Minnesota Department of Health. Scandrett was an attorney who knew the arguments for managed competition well. Before becoming the director for the Council of HMOs, he had worked as a writer of legislation for the Minnesota Senate. In that capacity, he had written all the major managed-competition bills that the Minnesota legislature enacted in the early 1990s. The HMO industry showed its gratitude by hiring him in 1995 to run the Minnesota Council of HMOs.

At 5:30 on the evening of October 1, the three speakers and the 14 Minnesotans selected to participate assembled around four long tables arranged in a square in a room on the second floor of the *Star Tribune* building in downtown Minneapolis. KTCA-TV put two people – a cameraman and a woman holding a fat microphone at the end of an impossibly long boom – inside this square. Several observers, including Laurie Sether and Glenn Howatt, a *Star Tribune* reporter, sat in chairs along the wall. A woman from the League of Women Voters moderated.

I was the first speaker. I used my ten-minute opening statement to remind people that the other two speakers were promoting proposals supported by the insurance industry – the HMO wing of the industry in the case of managed competition, and the non-HMO wing in the case of MSAs. "Single-payer, on the other hand, isn't getting a dime from the insurance industry," I said. "All the single-payer proposal has is broad public support."

After the other two speakers had made their opening remarks, the citizen panelists started asking questions of the speakers. The first question was a hostile question for Michael from a woman from southern Minnesota who ran a small business. And away we went. Questions from the 14 citizen "jurors" came one after the other. Each of the three speakers offered short comments on most of the questions. As I had predicted to Laurie, the issues posed to Michael, Liz and me arose in no logical order. Throughout the debate, KTCA's cameraman and boom-mike woman darted about within the corral formed by the four tables to record the comments of each speaker.

Three-and-a-half hours later, the moderator brought the discussion to a close and posed a series of questions to the 14 citizens. First she asked them to vote on the three proposals. The vote was eight for single-payer, three for managed competition, one for a hybrid of single-payer and managed competition, zero for MSAs, and two abstentions. The next question the moderator posed was, "Would you be willing to pay more in taxes to cover the uninsured under a single-payer system?" I objected to that question. "A single-payer system will cut total health-care spending at least enough to pay for the uninsured," I argued. "The fair way to pose the question is, 'Assuming your other health-care costs were reduced by $1,000, would you support a tax increase of $1,000 to guarantee universal access under a single-payer?'" The moderator, bless her heart, agreed to this phrasing of the question and put it to the citizen panel. Eleven said yes and three abstained. At that point, Laurie, the woman who had invited me to be part of this debate, stood up and pushed for a vote on a rephrased version of the question: She wanted people to consider whether their employers would pass on the savings to them in the form of higher wages if a single-payer relieved employers of the burden of paying for insurance. I was annoyed at this effort by a non-participant to influence the outcome of the debate, but I said nothing. The moderator let that question be put to a vote. But the vote remained the same. I was pleased to see these citizens turn down an appeal to their selfishness. Finally, the moderator asked the citizens if they thought Congress had failed to give single-payer a fair hearing. Eleven said yes, three said no.[1]

I couldn't have been happier with the outcome of this forum. The lopsided votes in favor of single-payer was strong evidence that single-payer will win any reasonably fair debate, even a relatively short debate that skitters from topic to topic as this one had. The outcome of this debate, and other evidence that a large majority of Americans like the single-payer proposal once they understand it, is the single most important reason why I believe America will, sooner or later, solve the health-care crisis by enacting a Medicare-for-all system or something very similar to it.

## Mapping our journey

Enacting a Medicare-for-all system will happen sooner rather than later if ordinary citizens, reporters, and politicians comprehend the main issues in the debate about the health-care crisis. But comprehending those issues is very time-consuming for people who are new to the health-care reform debate and who have no guide to introduce them to the jargon and the main issues. This book is designed to be that guide. It is the book I wish I had had when I leaped into the health policy debate in 1986.

This book is divided into 12 chapters. Chapter 2 presents a short history of the U.S. health-care system. I learned early in my career that people are more likely to understand my comments about the health policy debate if they have been exposed to the jargon that permeates health policy, and that the easiest way to make people comfortable with that jargon is to tell the story of how the health-care system came to be. This story itself is fascinating, and it doesn't take long to tell. But once you've heard it, you know not only all the important jargon, you know the logic – the good logic and the crazy logic – that motivated the movers and shakers (the insurers, the doctors, the hospitals, the drug companies, the employers, and the politicians) who created the system we live with today.

Once you've heard the history of the U.S. system, you're ready for Chapter 3 – a review of the data showing that the current system is failing badly. I start with data demonstrating that the U.S. system is the most expensive in the world, even though our system has the "advantage" of leaving millions of Americans with no health insurance. Because we have a few people in our midst who labor under the illusion that it's no big deal to be uninsured, I spend some time in Chapter 3 going over the data that demonstrate that being uninsured is a threat to your health. Of course, being *insured* is no bowl of cherries either. For millions of employers and individuals, health insurance premiums are a huge financial burden.

Chapters 4 and 5 examine explanations offered by defenders of the U.S. system for why our system is so expensive. When you read about some guy saying somewhere that the U.S. system is expensive because Americans are "over-insured" or sue too often, what's the answer to those arguments? Chapters 4 and 5 evaluate these and other excuses for our incredibly expensive system.

When you're done with Chapters 4 and 5, you're left with only one possible explanation for why the U.S. system is so expensive, namely, it's *wasteful*. Chapters 6 and 7 present the evidence supporting this explanation. In Chapter 8, I present the evidence that the public agrees with my argument that the system, not patient behavior, is the primary cause of the health-care crisis. Chapters 9 and 10 present the evidence that "market" solutions – managed competition, high deductibles, and tax credits – are incapable of eliminating the waste in the system.

In Chapter 11, and to some extent in Chapters 6 and 7, I examine the evidence that a single-payer system is the best solution to the health-care crisis. I explain that Medicare, our national program for the elderly and disabled, is a rough approximation of a single-payer system. Unlike the nation's nonelderly, who are insured by more than a thousand insurance companies, Medicare is the sole payer for clinics and hospitals which treat the elderly. Hence, calling Medicare a single-payer for the elderly and disabled is roughly accurate. If we plugged some of the coverage holes in Medicare (prescription drugs remains a big one even after the enactment of the so-called Medicare Prescription Drug, Improvement and Modernization Act of 2003), kicked the HMOs out of Medicare, and then reduced the Medicare eligibility age from 65 to zero, we'd have a Medicare-for-all (single-payer) system.

In Chapter 12, I attempt to predict where the health policy debate will take us in the foreseeable future. I predict that it will focus primarily on Medicare for the next several years and avoid dealing with the system-wide causes of health-care inflation. The delay in address-ing the real causes of inflation will be facilitated in part by right-wing claims that high-deductible policies will solve the health-care crisis if Americans will just be patient and let high deductibles work their magic. But high-deductible policies will fail as badly as HMOs did. When the failure of big-deductible policies becomes obvious, Congress, the White House, and state legislatures and governors will no longer be able to ignore effective system reform. The public won't tolerate rising health-care costs and rising numbers of uninsured forever.

A collision between the tectonic plate of health-care inflation and the tectonic plate of public opinion has already begun. A political earthquake, or, more likely, a series of quakes, will erupt sooner or later, and this quake or quakes will lead to real reform. We may not create a Medicare-for-all style system overnight (we are more likely to build the new system in stages over a decade or two), and the final product may not look exactly like Medicare (we might, for example, administer the new system through regional or state agencies, not a single national agency). But I am confident we will build a new health care system, and I am confident it will look a lot like Medicare.

---

## Endnotes

[1] Glenn Howatt, "Canadian-style care starting to look more attractive to panel-ists," Minneapolis *Star Tribune*, October 9, 1996, A15.

# 2

# How We Got Into This Mess: A History of the U.S. Health Insurance System

## Origins of the U.S. health insurance system

So how did the U.S. come to be the only industrialized country in the world without a national health insurance system? How did employers get hornswoggled into paying for health insurance? Where did HMOs come from and why did anyone think they were a good idea? Is it true, as conservatives argue, that Medicare "is going bankrupt" and can only be "saved" if we turn the nation's elderly over to HMOs? Why is health care in the U.S. so expensive? These and other questions about our system are easier to answer once you understand the history of the U.S. system.

The U.S. health insurance industry is only about 75 years old. Prior to the 1930s, health insurance was virtually nonexistent in the U.S.* Health insurance companies had not yet been formed, and government health insurance programs (such as Medicare) did not yet exist. You

---

* The only people who had anything resembling health insurance prior to the 1930s were a handful of workers in a few industries with high injury rates operating in remote areas, notably, railroads, lumber, and mining, and the few Americans who obtained medical coverage from a variety of "mutual aid associ-

could buy life insurance, burial insurance, insurance against being disabled, and "sickness" insurance (which would pay you a certain portion of your wages, not your medical bills, if you got sick). But very few people could buy health insurance.

The main reason the insurance industry wasn't selling health insurance prior to the 1930s was that the costs of illness were so unpredictable compared with the costs of other types of misfortune the industry insured against. If I sell you a policy guaranteeing you two-thirds of your current wages for up to six months if you get sick, I have a pretty good idea of how much money I should charge you in order to have the revenues to meet your claims and make a profit. Similarly, if I sell you disability, life, and burial insurance, my costs are relatively predictable. But the true cost of insuring you for medical bills is tougher to predict because the types of illness which afflict humanity are so numerous and varied.

In Europe, however, health insurance was available to large segments of society in the 50 years preceding the Depression. During this period, beginning with the German government in 1883, European governments established prototypes of the national health insurance programs that exist today in every industrialized nation except the U.S. These programs are not what we think of today when we hear the phrase "national health insurance." They were limited to working people, and they often emphasized sickness insurance over health insurance.

When the Depression hit the industrialized world in 1929, large numbers of U.S. patients were unable to pay for medical care, and, as a result, physician and hospital income plummeted. In California, for example, physician income fell by 45 percent between 1929 and 1933.[1] Hospitals and doctors responded by forming the nation's first successful health insurance companies. Baylor University Hospital in Dallas, Texas, established the first health insurance company in 1929. The

---

ations," sometimes called "lodges" and "fraternal orders." Lodges and fraternal orders were more common among immigrant communities, and were virtually nonexistent in rural America. The railroads and other companies that provided medical care directly to their workers typically did so by contracting with doctors to treat all company employees who might need medical attention. These arrangements were the predecessors of today's HMOs (see discussion of the early HMOs in Chapter 9.)

hospital agreed to provide 1,400 teachers in the Dallas school system with up to 21 days of hospital coverage in exchange for the princely sum of $6 per year per teacher, due in monthly installments of 50 cents. The coverage took effect on December 20, 1929, just two months after the stock market crash of 1929. The first teacher to have her bills paid under this new form of insurance was Alma Dickson. She slipped on an icy sidewalk a few days after her coverage took effect, broke an ankle, and spent the Christmas holidays at Baylor University Hospital.[2]

Encouraged by Baylor University Hospital's success, hospitals throughout the country began setting up their own insurance companies. An insurance company formed by eight hospitals in St. Paul, Minnesota, in 1933 used a blue cross in its advertisements. The company eventually assumed the name Blue Cross. Like Baylor's insurance company, the St. Paul Blue Cross company marketed itself to larger employers. Employees of the St. Paul Union Stockyards Company were the first to sign up at 75 cents a month. The Blue Cross name and the familiar Blue Cross insignia were quickly adopted by similar hospital-sponsored insurance companies all over the country. By 1949, more than 6 million Americans were enrolled in 39 Blue Cross plans.[3] Doctors, seeing that hospitals were succeeding in the insurance business, soon established their own insurance companies under the name Blue *Shield*. The first Blue Shield was established by the California Medical Association in 1939.[4]

Until recently, all Blue Cross and Blue Shield companies were nonprofit, which means, among other things, that they couldn't pay exorbitant salaries and they couldn't issue stock (and, therefore, they didn't have to respond to stockholder demands for high profits). The reason for this is that the states, not the federal government, have historically regulated the insurance industry, and when hospitals first approached state legislatures asking for permission to set up their own insurance companies, the legislatures gave them permission but only on the condition that the insurance companies be nonprofit, just as the vast majority of hospitals were. Legislators didn't want for-profit insurers milking the nonprofit hospitals and, conversely, they didn't want nonprofit hospitals getting around the prohibition against excessive profits by siphoning off huge profits from for-profit insurance companies.

When established life insurance companies like Metropolitan Life and Prudential (most of which were for-profit) saw that the Blue Cross and Blue Shield companies were surviving, they too began to offer health insurance. The first health insurance policies offered by private insurers other than Blue Cross and Blue Shield appeared in 1934. By the end of the 1940s, the number of for-profit insurers competing with the Blues was in the hundreds.[5] To compete with the Blues, for-profits used a method of premium-setting known as "experience rating," which means the insurer offers low rates for healthy groups and individuals and high rates for less healthy people. This practice, which became widespread by the early 1950s, posed a serious threat to the Blues. If they didn't abandon their practice of charging the same price to every customer, a practice known as "community rating," and take up experience rating, they would be left with sicker and sicker enrollees, and they would eventually have to price themselves out of the market.* By the late 1950s, most Blues had switched to experience rating, and by the 1980s, community rating was rare.

The number of people who could afford to buy health insurance rose rapidly in the late 1930s and early 1940s as government expenditures on the armed forces pushed the economy out of the Depression. The fortunes of the young health insurance industry were further boosted by the federal government's decision to impose wage and price controls during World War II, but to exempt health insurance.† The extremely tight labor market created by World War II put great pressure on employers to offer high wages and benefits to retain employees. The

---

* Despite their gradual abandonment of experience rating, Blue Cross and Blue Shield companies lost market share during the 1950s to the for-profits. Between 1948 and 1958, Blue Cross plans' share of the market fell slightly from 51 to 50 percent, and Blue Shield plans' share fell from 49 to 44 percent (Robert Cunningham III and Robert M. Cunningham, Jr., *The Blues: A History of the Blue Cross and Blue Shield System*, Northern Illinois University Press, DeKalb, IL, 1997, 97).

† Wage and price controls were imposed in 1942; the exemption for employee fringe benefits, including health insurance, was created in 1943. The exemption was not unlimited; employers could raise employee fringe benefits only up to 5 percent of total payroll. Note that *offering* health insurance is not the same as *paying* for it. During the 1940s, the large majority of employees paid for all of the cost of their employer-sponsored health insurance (Robert Cunningham,

loophole in the wage-and-price controls created for health insurance caused many firms that had not previously offered health insurance to begin doing so. After the war, unions began to bargain aggressively for health insurance. By 1954, over 60 percent of Americans had hospital insurance, 50 percent had surgical insurance, and 25 percent had some form of insurance for non-surgical medical services (mainly physician services in hospitals).[6]

Most of these insured Americans got their insurance through their employer, primarily because employer-sponsored health insurance was less expensive than insurance purchased by individuals. That is still the case today. Employer-sponsored insurance is less expensive because it costs the insurance companies less to sell insurance to groups than to individuals. The administrative cost to insurers of selling a single policy to one employer with 200 employees, for example, is much less than the cost of selling 200 separate policies to 200 individuals.

Broadly speaking, two classes of people were left out of America's emerging employer-based health insurance system: the retired and the unemployed. In 1965, Congress enacted Medicare for the elderly and Medicaid for the very poor.* Medicare, which was operated at the federal level by what was then called the Department of Health, Education and Welfare,[†] began to enroll seniors on July 1, 1966. By 1970, 97 percent of elderly Americans were enrolled in Medicare; that proportion remains the same today.[7] Although Medic*aid* is partially financed by the federal government, it is administered by the states, and partly for that reason enrollment in Medicaid grew more slowly than did enrollment in Medicare.

---

"Joint custody: Bipartisan interest expands scope of tax-credit proposals," *Health Affairs*, Web Exclusives, 2002:W290-W298, footnote 29, W298). Nevertheless, working for an employer who offered health insurance was a draw for workers because insurance was so much less costly when purchased as part of a group than as an individual.

* In 1972, Medicare was extended to the disabled of any age and those with end stage renal (kidney) disease of any age. For the sake of brevity, I will some times refer to Medicare enrollees as "seniors" or "the elderly." Readers should not forget that that is shorthand for "the elderly *and* nonelderly disabled *and* kidney-disease patients."

† The Department of Health, Education, and Welfare is now called the Department of Health and Human Services.

## Table 2-1: Government programs cut the number of uninsured: The uninsured in the U.S., selected years, 1953-2003

| Year | Uninsured | Percent |
|------|-----------|---------|
| 1953: | 71 million | 44 |
| 1958: | 64 million | 37 |
| 1963: | 63 million | 33 |
| 1965: | Medicare and Medicaid enacted | |
| 1970: | 49 million | 24 |
| 1976: | 23 million | 11 |
| 1980: | 30 million | 13 |
| 1985: | 37 million | 15 |
| 1990: | 34.7 million | 13.9 |
| 1995: | 40.6 million | 15.4 |
| 1996: | 41.7 million | 15.6 |
| 1997: | 43.4 million | 16.1 |
| 1998: | 44.3 million | 16.3 |
| 1999: | 42.6 million | 15.5 |
| 2000: | 38.7 million | 14.0 |
| 2001: | 41.2 million | 14.6 |
| 2002: | 43.6 million | 15.2 |
| 2003: | 45.0 million | 15.6 |
| 2014 (projected): | | 18.7 |

Sources: Estimates for 1976 and earlier are based on studies by various researchers. The estimates for the years after 1976 are based upon annual surveys by the U.S. Census Bureau, usually reported each August or September. The Census Bureau began conducting annual surveys on the number of uninsured in 1979. The source for the 1980 and 1985 statistics is http://www.census.gov/hhes/hlthins/historic/hihisttl. html, accessed October 1, 2003. The source for statistics for 1990 through 2003 is http://www.census.gov/hhes/hlthins/historic/hihisttl.html. The Census Bureau's survey questions changed in 1988 and again in 1999, lowering the number of uninsured both times. The source for the 2014 projection is Stephen Heffler et al., "Trends: U.S. health spending projections for 2004-2014," *Health Affairs*, Web Exclusives, 2005, http://content.healthaffairs.org/cgi/content/abstract/hlthaff.w5.74v1, accessed May 28, 2005.

## Table 2-2: Minorities are the hardest hit: Uninsured rates by race, 2002

| | |
|---|---|
| Hispanics | 32% |
| Blacks | 20% |
| National average | 15% |
| Whites | 11% |

Source: Robert Pear, "Big increase seen in people lacking health insurance," *New York Times*, September 30, 2003, A1.

Medicare and Medicaid had a huge impact on the uninsured rate. The rate fell from about 33 percent in 1963 to 11 percent in 1976 (see Table 2-1). The 1976 figure was probably the lowest uninsured rate America ever recorded. The percentage of Americans without health insurance climbed every year after that until 1999. The rate dipped in 1999 (due in part to a change in the way the Census bureau phrased its questions) and again in 2000; it has been rising since 2001. Table 2-2 indicates that minorities had uninsured rates above the 15-percent national average rate for 2002, while the uninsured rate among whites was slightly below the national average.

## The origins of HMOs and the modern U.S. health-care system

Health-care inflation in the U.S. worsened in the late 1960s, largely because Medicare and Medicaid permitted many more Americans to buy health care. Inflation was to be expected. Any time additional buyers flood a market in great numbers, prices will rise unless government sets limits on those prices. Medicare and Medicaid permitted millions of the nation's elderly and poor to buy medical services that had previously been out of their reach. With all those new patients seeking health care, with no immediate increase in the supply of doctors and hospitals, and with no price controls, total expenditures on health care were bound to rise.

In 1929, the year when Baylor University Hospital was forming the first Blue Cross company, Americans were spending 4 cents of every dollar earned on health care. We were still spending about 4 cents per dollar earned in 1948 when Harry Truman campaigned on a promise to promote national health insurance if he were elected president. By 1970 that number had risen to 7 cents.[8] Today we spend more than 15 cents of every dollar of income on health care (see Table 2-3).

Although the 7 cents we were spending on health care in 1970 looks low today, it seemed high in 1970. In January 1970, both *Fortune* and *Business Week* ran cover stories on "the health-care crisis," and Senator Ted Kennedy introduced a national health insurance bill that would be called a single-payer bill today. President Richard Nixon was looking for a way to control health-care inflation that did not rely on the price controls all other industrialized nations used. A Minnesota physician named Paul Ellwood came up with a proposal that appealed to Nixon, a proposal Ellwood called "the health maintenance strategy." On February 5, 1970, Ellwood met with Nixon's advisors at the DuPont Plaza Hotel in Washington, DC, to discuss this strategy. He argued that the cause of health-care inflation was the way insurance companies paid doctors, and that the solution was a new type of health insurance company that he called the "health maintenance organization."*

You can think of an HMO as an insurance company and a doctor's office under one roof. Traditionally, insurance companies and doctors' offices were separate entities. In other words, doctors didn't work for insurance companies, either as contractors or as salaried employees; doctors were independent agents. They or their patients submitted bills to insurance companies for each service the doctor provided, and the insurance company paid the doctor's fee, no questions asked. This arrangement is commonly called "fee-for-service" medicine, because doctors are paid a fee for each service they render to patients.

---

* According to Joseph Falkson, the phrase "health maintenance organization" was invented by Ellwood and Nixon's advisors at the February 5, 1970 meeting. Ellwood contributed the phrase "health maintenance," and the group as a whole settled on "organization" because it was a neutral term (as opposed to "corporation," "group practice," and "partnership," which were apparently also considered) (Joseph L. Falkson, *HMOs and the Politics of Health System Reform*, American Hospital Association, Chicago, IL, 1980, 32). According to Ellwood, he invented the phrase "health maintenance organization" in May 1970 ("An interview with Paul Ellwood, Jr., MD," *Managed Care*, November 1997, http://www.managed-caremag.com/archives/9711/9711.qnaellwood.shtml, accessed October 6, 2002).

## Table 2-3: From billions to trillions: Total spending on health care in the U.S., selected years, 1960 to 2003

| | Total health expenditures | |
| | Billions of dollars | Percent of GDP* |
|---|---|---|
| 1960 | 27 | 5.1 |
| 1970 | 73 | 7.0 |
| 1980 | 246 | 8.0 |
| 1990 | 696 | 12.0 |
| 1991 | 762 | 12.7 |
| 1992 | 827 | 13.0 |
| 1993 | 888 | 13.3 |
| 1994 | 937 | 13.3 |
| 1995 | 990 | 13.4 |
| 1996 | 1,040 | 13.3 |
| 1997 | 1,093 | 13.2 |
| 1998 | 1,151 | 13.2 |
| 1999 | 1,222 | 13.2 |
| 2000 | 1,310 | 13.3 |
| 2001 | 1,426 | 14.1 |
| 2002 | 1,559 | 14.9 |
| 2003 | 1,679 | 15.3 |

* GDP stands for gross domestic product. It is a measure of total income earned by all Americans.

Source: Kaiser Family Foundation, *Trends and Indicators in the Changing Health Care Marketplace 2002*, Exhibit 1.1, http://www.kff.org/insurance/7031/ti2004-1-set.cfm, accessed May 25, 2005.

There was a kernel of truth to Ellwood's argument. If doctors are paid a fee for every service they provide, and if doctors know that no one will challenge their decisions to order services, some doctors will order too many services. But in concentrating so intently on the *volume* of medical services sold, Ellwood gave little attention to another very obvious cause of medical inflation – *price*. You don't have to have a PhD in economics to know that total spending on anything, be it health care or pineapple juice, depends on two numbers – the *volume* of the good or service sold, and the *price* at which the good or service is sold. All other industrialized countries have treated the *price* of medical care as the primary problem. For three decades, the U.S. has treated *volume* of medical services as the primary problem. It's not an exaggeration to say we can thank Paul Ellwood for that. Because of his influence on Nixon, Ellwood played a very important role in the HMO revolution.

Ellwood told Nixon's staff that his proposal would control health-care inflation by giving doctors financial incentives to deny medical services to their patients.[*] In other words, Ellwood proposed to turn the fee-for-service incentive upside down. The incentive could be turned upside down, said Ellwood, by letting HMOs pay doctors a set fee per person per year. This method of payment is called "capitation" ("capita" is Latin for "head"). Under the capitation payment method, the doctor cannot make more money by ordering more tests and services. In fact, it's the other way around. Under capitation, the doctor makes more money the fewer services the doctor orders. That's because the doctor is being paid a fee per patient per year that doesn't change to reflect the number of services the doctor orders. If the doctor's patients wind up costing, on average, a lot less than the capitation fee, the doctor pockets the difference.

Ellwood argued that capitation would cause HMOs to be unusually good at keeping people healthy. If patients were healthy, they would not need medical services and, therefore, would not be draining HMOs of their profits. Ellwood's belief that the profit motive would drive HMOs to keep their patients healthy led him to think that the name "health maintenance organization" was an appropriate label for this newfangled type of insurance company.

---

[*] For a summary of Ellwood's pro-HMO arguments to Nixon, see Paul M. Ellwood et al., "Health maintenance strategy," *Medical Care* 1971;9:291-298.

In addition to capitation, the other distinguishing feature of the early HMOs was their limited choice of doctors. (Today, only the latter feature – a limited choice of doctors – distinguishes HMOs from other types of health insurance companies. Capitation is now used by non-HMO insurers as well.) If you are insured by a traditional insurance company, you can see any doctor you choose. But if you are insured by an HMO, you must choose from among the doctors available in the HMO's "network." Why do HMOs insist on limiting the doctors you can choose from? HMOs argue that limiting the doctors you can see permits the HMO to select only the best doctors. But there is no scientific evidence to support the claim that doctors who work for HMOs are better than doctors who do not. A more compelling explanation is that limiting your choices gives the HMO more influence over its doctors. An HMO that provides a clinic with 50 percent of its patients is more likely to get cooperation from that clinic than it will from a clinic that gets just 5 percent of its patients from the HMO.[9] A clinic that is heavily dependent upon HMO patients is more likely to deny services.

HMOs did not rely solely on capitation to ensure that their doctors cut costs. HMOs also pioneered a cost-control technique known as "utilization review." Utilization review means someone other than the doctor and the patient decides whether a medical service is necessary. Utilization review can occur before, during, or after a medical service is provided. Prior authorization of surgery is an example of utilization review that occurs *prior* to a service being provided. A review of a doctor's decision to keep a patient in the hospital after the patient has been hospitalized is an example of *concurrent* utilization review. A decision by an insurer to deny payment for an emergency room visit after the patient has gone to the emergency room is an example of utilization review *following* provision of a service.

We can think of drug "formularies" as a form of utilization review or, more precisely, of prior utilization review. Formularies are lists of drugs insurers will pay for. Some HMOs, for example, will pay for the antidepressant Zoloft but not Prozac. HMOs claim they make these drug decisions on both quality and cost grounds, but cost is the main criterion. (Even if HMOs wanted to make quality their main criterion in selecting drugs for inclusion in formularies, they couldn't because so little research has been done comparing the efficacy of one drug with another.) If an

HMO can tell the manufacturer of Zoloft that it will buy a large volume, the manufacturer will offer the HMO a big discount. An HMO that forces its doctors to prescribe only Zoloft and never Prozac is more likely to meet its minimum volume requirement and get the discount. And, to repeat, an HMO is in a better position to force its doctors to prescribe Zoloft if it insures a high proportion of the doctor's patients. Which, to repeat, is why HMOs limit your choice of doctor.

An obvious question should occur to anyone at this point: Why won't capitation and utilization review cause HMOs to damage health instead of maintain it? Ellwood had an answer for this question. He said somebody (he didn't say who) would be responsible for publishing "performance reports" on HMOs. These performance reports, he said, would scare HMOs into making sure their doctors did not offer inferior medical care in response to the pressure of financial incentives and utilization reviewers. For a variety of reasons, primarily expense, this idea of "performance reports" was doomed from the beginning. Documents which accurately tell consumers which HMO is better than another have yet to appear.

Despite the glaring flaws in Ellwood's HMO proposal, his logic persuaded Nixon. The following statement to Congress in 1972 by Elliot Richardson, Nixon's Secretary for the Department of Health, Education, and Welfare, indicates the Nixon administration had bought Ellwood's logic lock, stock and barrel: "HMOs have a strong financial interest in preventing illness, or failing that, in treating it in its early stages, promoting a full recovery, and preventing any recurrences; they are motivated to function efficiently because they must stay within pre-determined budgets."[10] At Nixon's request, Congress passed the Health Maintenance Organization Act of 1973. This law subsidized the formation of the planet's first HMO industry. As Table 2-4 indicates, the number of Americans enrolled in HMOs grew slowly during the 1970s, then soared in the 1980s. HMO enrollment peaked at 30.1 percent of the American population in 1999, then fell back to 30.0 percent in 2000 on its way to 26.4 percent in 2002.

Why would people enroll in HMOs if HMOs restricted their choice of doctor and encouraged doctors to deny services? Answer: People saved money, either for themselves or their employers. For the last 20 to 25 years, HMO premiums have tended to be 5 to 10 percent lower

## Table 2-4: Enrollment in HMOs grew rapidly after 1985: Enrollment in HMOs, selected years, 1976 to 2002

| | 1976 | 1980 | 1990 | 1995 | 1999 | 2000 | 2001 | 2002 |
|---|---|---|---|---|---|---|---|---|
| Number (millions of people) | 6.0 | 9.1 | 33.0 | 50.9 | 81.3 | 80.9 | 79.5 | 76.1 |
| As percent of US population | 3 | 4 | 13 | 19 | 30.1 | 30.0 | 28.3 | 26.4 |

Source: Centers for Disease Control and Prevention, http://www.cdc.gov/nchs/data/hus/tables/2003/03hus132.pdf, accessed April 1, 2004.

than the premiums of traditional insurance companies. Why? Because HMOs enrolled healthier people, they provided fewer services, they shifted costs onto the taxpayer, and they extracted discounts from hospitals and drug companies that traditional insurers could not get (see Chapter 9 for further discussion).

The vast majority of those who enrolled in HMOs were people who used to have insurance from a traditional insurance company. As traditional insurers like Prudential and Blue Cross Blue Shield watched their customers leave for HMOs, they began to adopt utilization review so that they could cut services as HMOs had. Some traditional insurers even set up their own HMOs. In Minnesota, for example, Blue Cross Blue Shield created an HMO called Blue Plus. Traditional insurers also began to experiment with bonuses. Bonuses would go to doctors who kept health-care use under certain levels.

By the mid-1980s, the cost-control techniques pioneered by HMOs – financial incentives for doctors (capitation and bonuses) and utilization review – had come to be known collectively as "managed care."* As

---

* Jacob Hacker and Ted Marmor report that the phrase "managed care" does not appear in either of two widely read histories of the U.S. health care system published in the early 1980s – Paul Starr's lengthy 1982 history of the U.S. health-care system, *The Social Transformation of American Medicine*, and Lawrence Brown's 1983 book, *Politics and Health Care Organizations*. According to Hacker and Marmor, the phrase "managed care" first appeared in the *New York Times* in 1985, but was not used frequently until the early 1990s; the *Times* mentioned the phrase 27 times in 1990, 287 in 1994, and 587 times in 1998 ("The misleading language of managed care," *Journal of Health Policy, Politics, and Law* 1999;24:1033-1043).

traditional insurers began to adopt managed-care tactics, health policy experts began referring to health insurance companies that used any form of managed care, including HMOs, as "managed-care insurers" or "managed-care plans" (MCPs). (For reasons I never understood, the word "plan" gradually replaced the words "policy" and "company" during the 1970s and 1980s.) Experts reserved the phrase HMO for MCPs that restricted the patient's choice of doctor to a finite list of doctors. An HMO was defined as an MCP that told its enrollees which doctors it could see and which they couldn't see; patients insured by an HMO were not free to pay a little more and see any doctor they wanted. Non-HMO MCPs, on the other hand, either gave their enrollees complete freedom to pick their doctors, or, more commonly, they gave their enrollees financial incentives to stay within a particular network of doctors. However, even in those non-HMO MCPs which use financial incentives to keep patients within a limited panel of doctors, enrollees were free to see any doctor they want if they were willing to pay more out-of-pocket.

By the 1990s, meaningful differences between HMOs and non-HMO MCPs, other than restrictions on choice of doctor, seemed to be non-existent. I say "seemed to be" because finding out exactly what MCPs do to "manage care" is extremely difficult, even for health policy experts. Judging from both media reports and the professional literature, non-HMO MCPs were just as likely to use utilization review and financial incentives to induce doctors to cut services as HMOs were, and just as likely to use the ultimate threat – refusing to include a doctor within their networks – as HMOs were. Blue Cross and Blue Shield of Minnesota (BCBSM), for example, has never been classified as an HMO, but it has been as brutal in its use of managed-care tactics as any HMO. In an agreement reached with Minnesota Attorney General Mike Hatch in 2001, BCBSM admitted to instructing its staff to use a variety of tactics to deny mental health services to children. These tactics included not returning phone calls, putting doctors on hold for 15 minutes, rejecting any claim for which information such as a Social Security number was missing even if BCBSM already had the information in its computers, telling parents anorexia and other diseases never required hospitalization, and telling parents to ask juvenile courts and foster-care programs for help so that BCBSM would not have to pay for treatment.[11]

The enthusiastic adoption of managed-care techniques by traditional insurers such as the Blues so muddied the distinction between HMOs and non-HMO MCPs that reporters and the public long ago abandoned any effort to distinguish between them. For the media and the public, any insurance company that uses managed care is an HMO. Because the differences between HMOs and non-HMO MCPs are now so minor, I have no problem with this broader use of the term "HMO." But MCPs classified as HMOs continue to charge premiums slightly below those of non-HMO MCPs (although this is not true in all parts of the country), which suggests that the HMOs' tighter restrictions on choice of doctor does something to permit HMOs to cut costs a little more effectively than non-HMO MCPs. Limited choice of doctor probably facilitates lower premiums for HMOs in two ways – inhibiting sicker patients from enrolling in HMOs, and giving HMOs greater leverage over doctors in their networks. Because HMOs appear to have an advantage of some sort over non-HMO MCPs, however slight, and because experts and the insurance industry continue to make the HMO-non-HMO distinction, I will use the experts' definition of "HMO" (an MCP that limits choice to a panel of doctors) throughout this book.

In the late 1980s, enrollment in all types of MCPs soared. "In 1990, only 5 percent of people with employment-based health insurance were in unmanaged fee-for-service plans," reported the Congressional Budget Office.[12] In January 1993, Ellwood announced the victory of the MCP juggernaut. "Indemnity insurance is essentially dead," he said, "and it was HMOs that did it."[13]* Today, nearly all Americans who are privately insured are insured by an MCP. Very few have traditional insurance.† Among Americans over 64 insured by Medicare (which is 97 percent of all elderly), 13 percent were enrolled in MCPs (nearly all of them HMOs) as of 2005.

---

* "Indemnity insurer" is often used to describe the old-fashioned health insurance company that MCPs have virtually eliminated. These insurers would reimburse patients after patients had paid their medical bills. The formal term for reimbursing people who have incurred a cost or suffered a loss for which they are insured is to "indemnify" them.

† Citing data from the Health Insurance Association of America (the former trade group for non-HMO MCPs), Jacob Hacker and Ted Marmor wrote, "Only 2 percent of private health plans in 1997 conformed to the traditional model of fee-for-service indemnity insurance. Another 16 percent used fee-for-service payment but employed some form of utilization review. Thus between 80 and

In addition to financial incentives and utilization review, HMOs and other types of MCPs have relied heavily on extracting discounts from doctors, hospitals, and drug companies. However, many, perhaps most, observers who use the phrase "managed care" do not include discounting in their definition of "managed care." If there were a category known as "managed *cost*," perhaps discounting would fall into it.

## The ascent of managed competition

Despite the rapid spread of MCPs in the 1980s, health insurance premiums rose at double-digit rates annually in the late 1980s and early 1990s. And as inflation rose, so did the number of uninsured. These developments called the entire HMO project into question, and placed national health insurance and price controls back on the national agenda. In Minnesota, the Health Care Campaign of Minnesota was organized in April 1987 and I was hired as its first half-time organizer. In January 1989, David Himmelstein and Steffie Woolhandler, doctors at Harvard Medical School, published a call for a single-payer system in the *New England Journal of Medicine*.[14] In December 1989, COACT and HCCM were among the first citizen groups in the country to endorse the single-payer proposal. In 1990, the Coalition for Universal Health Insurance in Ohio introduced the first single-payer bill into a state legislature.[15] By 1991, single-payer legislation had been introduced in several states and the U.S. House of Representatives. By 1992, Senator Paul Wellstone had introduced a single-payer bill in the Senate. By 1994, according to *USA Today*, single-payer bills had been introduced in "more than a dozen" states.[16]

The burgeoning single-payer movement worried HMO advocates. As Michael Scandrett, the director of Minnesota's HMO industry trade group, observed, single-payer "was the demon in the closet"[17] – the bogeyman legislators and managed-care advocates feared they would have to deal with if they didn't find a market-based solution to health-care inflation. As Jacob Hacker noted in his fascinating book about the demise of the Clinton plan, "By 1990 [managed-care advocates Alain]

---

98 percent of today's private health insurers appear to fall into the general category of managed care" ("The misleading language of managed care," *Journal of Health Politics, Policy and Law* 1999;24:1033-1043, 1036-1037).

Enthoven and Paul Ellwood were worried. Both men were committed to a private-sector approach to health-care reform, and both feared that the government was on the verge of assuming broad regulatory authority over the medical system."[18]

Managed-care advocates thought they found a solution in a theory called "managed competition." Economists and MCP proponents Alain Enthoven, who invented the phrase "managed competition,"[19] and Richard Kronick presented the theory in a two-part article published in the *New England Journal of Medicine* in 1989. The theory was a more elaborate version of Ellwood's "health maintenance strategy." Like Ellwood, Enthoven and Kronick subscribed to the unproven belief that insurers that adopted managed-care tactics were more efficient than insurers that did not. Like Ellwood, they endorsed "performance reports," or "report cards" as MCP advocates began to call them in the early 1990s. But they went beyond Ellwood by arguing that the mere presence of MCPs and report cards was not enough to provoke the rigorous competition among insurers necessary to make the entire health-care industry – the insurer sector and the provider sector – more efficient. According to Enthoven and Kronick, the rapid spread of MCPs hadn't reduced inflation because competition among insurers, especially between MCPs and traditional insurers, was not vigorous enough.

Competition could be invigorated, they said, if it were "managed." Specifically, they recommended that Congress eliminate tax subsidies for the purchase of health insurance in order to make consumers more "cost conscious," and they recommended the formation of large purchasing coalitions so that consumers would have more negotiating clout with insurers. (I will discuss managed competition in more detail in Chapter 9.)

In 1990, the year after the Enthoven-Kronick articles appeared, Enthoven and Ellwood began to meet regularly in Ellwood's home in Jackson Hole, Wyoming (where Ellwood had moved in the early 1970s) along with four dozen conservative experts, corporate executives, health professionals, and politicians. By the end of the year the group was calling itself the Jackson Hole Group.* The group added a few wrinkles to the Enthoven-Kronick managed-competition proposal and published

---

* In appendix B of his book, *The Road to Nowhere*, Jacob Hacker lists 51 participants in meetings of what came to be called the Jackson Hole Group held between 1990 and 1992 (*The Road to Nowhere: The Genesis of President Clinton's Plan for*

it in 1992. The Jackson Hole Group's version of managed competition formed the template for dozens of market-based bills introduced in Congress and state legislatures in 1993 and 1994, and for Republican proposals after 1994 to "reform" Medicare.

The development of the Jackson Hole plan began in earnest at a four-day meeting at Ellwood's mansion in February 1990. His guests discussed what Ellwood called "the crisis in the health-care delivery system." The guests included executives of Aetna, Cigna, Travelers, Metropolitan Life, and Prudential (five large insurance companies that had begun to morph into MCPs); Bernard Tresnowski, the head of the Blue Cross and Blue Shield Association (which represented all the state-level Blues plans, many of which had also transformed themselves into MCPs); Senator Dave Durenberger (R-MN); and Enthoven.[20] According to Hacker, who based his account of these and other Ellwood-hosted meetings on interviews with participants in these meetings, "All of [the participants] agreed with Enthoven and Ellwood's grim assessment of the situation, and all recognized that their interests were on the line. By the end of the four-day conference, the group had tentatively agreed to work with Enthoven and Ellwood to come up with a serious reform proposal."[21]

Over the next 18 months, Ellwood, Enthoven, and a health policy consultant named Lynn Etheredge, who had been asked to join the group by Blue Cross's Tresnowski, wrote several drafts of a managed competition proposal. After getting endorsement from the members of the group, the three men gave the paper the grandiose title, "The Jackson Hole initiatives for a Twenty-First Century American health-care system," and submitted it to an economics journal. It was published in 1992.[22]

Critics and supporters alike saw managed competition as an attempt to save the health insurance industry. Ellwood et al. warned that a government-financed and regulated system (read: single-payer) would result if readers did not endorse managed competition. "At stake is whether

---

*Health Security*, Princeton University Press, Princeton, NJ, 1997). The *New York Times* said the total number of participants over the same time period was "about 100" (Robin Toner, "Hillary Clinton's potent brain trust," February 28, 1993, A1). Thirty-two people were listed as "Jackson Hole participants" at the end of the Jackson Hole Group's 1992 paper in *Health Economics*.

the Twenty-First Century American health system will be built around competitive markets," they said.[23] Dr. Steffie Woolhandler, a leader of the U.S. single-payer movement, took a different view. "Managed competition is a last-ditch effort to preserve a role for the insurance industry in health care," she said.[24]

The publication of the Jackson Hole Group's paper in the first issue of an obscure journal of economics did not make headlines. What catapulted managed competition into the headlines was the endorsement of the theory by presidential candidate Bill Clinton in the fall of 1992. The Clinton-Gore campaign used the phrase "managed competition" in a press release issued on October 8, 1992, the *New York Times* endorsed the concept on October 10, 1992, and Clinton uttered the phrase in the first presidential debate with George Bush and Ross Perot on October 12, 1992.

For roughly the next two years, managed competition was praised effusively by the small handful of Americans – mainly politicians, corporate executives, professors, and pundits – who dominated the health-care reform debate. The *New York Times'* editorial page led the cheer-leading. "The debate over health-care reform is over," said the *Times* in an editorial published on October 10, 1992. "Managed competition has won. That outcome is … wondrous.…"[25] In 1993, state legislatures all over the country debated managed competition, and in the spring of 1993 the Minnesota and Washington legislatures enacted legislation based on the theory. In September 1993, President Clinton introduced his Health Security Act, a bill his advisors called "managed competition with a budget." It included all the components of managed competition plus an "employer mandate" (a phrase which means employers would be required to pay for insurance for their employees), but it also required the health-care system to operate within a budget, which, in practice, meant premiums would be subjected to price controls.

Just as managed competition was gathering steam among politicians, enrollment in MCPs, the centerpiece of all managed-competition proposals, shot up, primarily because small employers began to push their employees into MCPs as large employers had in the 1980s. Best of all, from the point of view of managed-care advocates, premium inflation began to drop rapidly in 1992 and didn't stop dropping until 1996 (it fell from 10.9 percent in 1992 to 0.5 percent in 1996).[26] Managed-care advocates crowed that this reduction in premium inflation, coming concurrently with the unusually rapid increase in enrollment in MCPs in the early 1990s, was proof that MCPs were finally working as advertised and that managed competition would save the nation from its health-care crisis. Politicians, health policy experts, and reporters universally agreed. Managed-competition advocates that I knew in Minnesota were in seventh heaven during 1993 and 1994.

## The fall of managed competition and managed care

But the establishment's infatuation with managed competition changed to ambivalence during the mid-1990s. For the elite, managed competition first began to lose its luster with the death of Bill Clinton's Health Security Act in the fall of 1994. The bill, which had been greeted with so much enthusiasm by health policy experts, large employers, and politicians in 1993, was on life support by the spring of 1994, and pronounced dead by Senate Majority Leader George Mitchell (D-ME) on September 26, 1994. In 1995, the legislatures of Washington and Minnesota repealed substantial chunks of the managed-competition bills they had enacted just two years earlier. During 1995, the theory of managed competition rapidly disappeared from the media's radar.

To make matters worse, *public* opinion about MCPs deteriorated rapidly beginning in approximately 1995. Public opinion of managed care had never been good – polls taken in the late 1980s and early 1990s indicated a majority of the public opposed managed-care cost-control tactics (see Chapter 8). After 1995, public opinion became even more hostile. By 1996, consumers and doctors were in open revolt against the new MCP-dominated system. The revolt, dubbed the "HMO backlash" by the media, was manifested not just in polling data, but in a blizzard of "HMO horror stories" in the media, legislation introduced in state legislatures and Congress to protect patients from MCPs, lawsuits by doctors and patients against MCPs, and an endless stream of popular invective against "HMOs" in the media, late-night comedy routines, cartoons, movies, novels, and everyday conversation.

The great MCP juggernaut might have survived these stormy seas if it had been able to keep premium inflation low. After all, it was the HMO advocates' promise of cost reduction, not their promises of "health maintenance," that sold the HMO project to the business community,

Congress, and Nixon in the first place. As I have just noted, health-care inflation cooled between 1992 and 1996, and managed-care advocates claimed that managed care deserved all the credit. Enthoven, for example, announced in 1997 that "there is no explanation [for the drop in inflation] except competitive markets and managed care."[27] The *New York Times'* editors, who had so eagerly promoted managed competition in 1992 and 1993, also attributed the inflation lull to managed-care companies. "The rise of managed care has brought … a surprisingly swift deceleration of health-care inflation," they declared in October 1997.[28] By early 1998, *U.S. News and World Report* was still under the illusion that MCPs saved money. "The mounting complaints about HMOs have tended to obscure the genuine gains that have occurred in the managed-care era … ," wrote reporter Susan Brink. "Thanks to managed care, most Americans have more money in their pockets [and] more companies can afford to provide health benefits to employees."[29] (This quote illustrates the tendency of the media and the public to define HMOs broadly to mean all insurers that use managed-care tactics.)

But by 1997, it was clear to more perceptive observers that "competitive markets and managed care" were losing the war against inflation. "Health care costs edging up and a bigger surge is feared," announced a *New York Times* headline in January 1997.[30] "Price surge on the way," said a headline in *Modern Healthcare* in June 1997.[31] By 1999, even the unperceptive could read the writing on the wall: Premium inflation had returned and relief was nowhere in sight. "[I]f the system of managed care no longer manages costs, what sort of future does it have?" asked the *Wall Street Journal* in 1999. By 2000, premium inflation had returned to double-digit levels. Because underlying inflation remained very low, real premium inflation levels approximated the real premium inflation levels of the late 1980s and early 1990s that preceded the 1992-96 inflation lull. By 2000, a substantial portion of the experts – the politicians, large employer representatives, academicians, and pundits – who had so enthusiastically promoted managed competition eight years earlier were discussing what sort of system would replace the MCP-dominated system.

Although the insular health policy community (the professors and think-tank experts who write for journals like *Health Affairs* and *Health Services Research*) continued to assert that tinkering with the MCP industry would fix it (the most common tinkering suggested was the ever-popular and ever-elusive MCP and provider report card), and although Republicans persisted in promoting managed competition as the solution to the alleged "crisis" in the Medicare program, Democrats and most employers and pundits had, by 2000, ceased promoting managed competition. "I'm not as sure as everybody else is about managed care any longer," said Donna Shalala, Clinton's Secretary of Health and Human Services at the end of Clinton's term. "And I started out as their biggest fan."[32] "The protagonists of managed care now are in full retreat," wrote managed-care advocate James Robinson in an article entitled, "The end of managed care," in the *Journal of the American Medical Association* in 2001.[33] In an interview with the *Los Angeles Times* in 2001, George Lundberg, the former editor of the *Journal of the American Medical Association* who as recently as 1996 had co-authored an article with Paul Ellwood defending managed care, offered this caustic assessment of managed care:

> Managed care is basically over. People hate it, and it's no longer controlling costs. Health-care inflation is now back in the double digits. So if it's not saving money, then why should we have it? But like an unembalmed corpse decomposing, dismantling managed care is going to be very messy and very smelly, and take awhile.[34]

As 2001 came to a close, Art Caplan, the director of the Center for Bioethics at the University of Pennsylvania and, in the early 1990s, an advisor to Hillary Clinton, observed, "Events of the past year demonstrate beyond a doubt that managed care has failed – and failed dismally. The greatest single ethical crisis facing American health care as we move into the new year is what to do about it."[35]

The most astonishing condemnation of the new system came from Paul Ellwood himself. On May 2, 1999, the *Boston Globe* published an article describing some scathing remarks Ellwood made at a conference at Harvard University the previous day. Ellwood hammered the quality of medical care provided in America – he called it a "national disgrace" – and repudiated his long-held belief that competition between HMOs and other MCPs would maintain or improve quality (the *Globe* paraphrased Ellwood saying that would "never" happen). "We thought in proposing the HMO idea that they would respond to both price and quality demands," Ellwood was quoted as saying. They didn't, he said; they responded only to price and, he implied, they let quality deteriorate. "Ultimately, this thing is going to require government intervention," said Ellwood. "The question is what form government intervention will take." Ellwood told the audience his change of heart stemmed from personal experience. He said he had fallen off a horse recently and crushed a vertebra in his neck. The article continued:

> The fact that Ellwood is not paralyzed today, he said, is no thanks to the care he received. He recounted a series of near-miss medical adventures that could well have left him paralyzed. Encountering a young neuro-surgical resident, Ellwood was immediately commanded to stand up – a potentially disastrous maneuver. '"But I did it," he said. "I was sedated – and he was a doctor. When you're a patient you're vulnerable and the power slips away from you." That night, the protective collar he was wearing came off, "and the nurses didn't know how to put it back on." The next day, the surgeon said he didn't need a special surgically installed brace to im-mobilize his head and refused to install it when Ellwood insisted.

Ellwood reached this conclusion: "Patients can get just atrocious care and can do very little about it."[36]* When I read these words, I shook my head and wondered, Why do some guys literally have to fall on their heads before they understand how the world works?

---

* The *Globe* reported that Ellwood said he had been treated by "fee-for-service doctors working in an institution that was part of a national for-profit hospital chain," but that Ellwood also said "care is no better in prepaid health plans, or HMOs, and that the idea that such plans would compete on quality has not worked as he thought it would." To imply, as the *Globe* and Ellwood did, that a fee-for-service sector, free of MCP influence, existed in the U.S. in the late 1990s was misleading. By then, true fee-for-service medicine was virtually nonexistent in the U.S. The accurate description of Ellwood's doctors and nurses is, almost certainly, that they were working in a hospital which, like hospitals all over the country, had gutted its RN staff and put pressure on its doctors to deny care in order to look good to MCPs it sought contracts with.

In 1996, Ellwood had told a similar story to Lisa Belkin, a reporter with the *New York Times Magazine*. He said he required surgery "some time ago" (the article did not indicate what type of surgery), and he was surprised to learn that his surgeon intended to perform the procedure on an outpatient basis, that is, without hospitalizing him overnight after the surgery. He said his doctor sent him home while he was still under the effects of anesthesia and suffering the pain homo sapiens feel when they have been cut with a sharp knife. On the way home in a car driven by a friend, Ellwood began to experience nausea, dizziness and vomiting, all of which are common side effects of surgery and which, in days of yore, were considered common enough to hospitalize patients who had undergone surgery. "I had to decide whether to go back to the hospital to die or to go on home to die," Ellwood joked, "so I decided to come on home to die." When he returned to see his surgeon for a checkup, he told the surgeon what had happened to him. "The guy got this little smile on his face," Ellwood said. "Then he leaned in real close and looked me right in the eye [and said], 'Ellwood ... it's ... your ... own ... damn ... fault.'"[37]

---

## Table 2-5: Our taxes pay for 60 percent of health-care spending: Percent of national health-care spending paid for by taxes, 1965 and 1999

|  | 1965 | 1999 |
|---|---|---|
| Medicare | 0% | 18% |
| Medicaid | 0 | 15 |
| Other health programs | 25 | 12 |
| Public employee health benefits | 1 | 5 |
| Tax subsidies | 4 | 9 |
| Total tax-financed * | 31 | 60 |

\* Total percent figures do not equal the sum of the columns due to rounding.

Source: Steffie Woolhandler and David U. Himmelstein, "Paying for national health insurance – and not getting it," *Health Affairs* 2002;21(4):88-98, Exhibit 2.

## How the system is financed

While the managed-care revolution was transforming the U.S. health-care system, another significant but less visible change was occurring: The government was paying for a larger and larger portion of the U.S. health-care bill. As Table 2-5 indicates, taxes financed 60 percent of total health-care spending in the U.S. in 1999, up from 31 percent in 1965, the year Congress enacted the Medicare and Medicaid programs. Not surprisingly, the table indicates the most important reason for this change was the enactment of the Medicare and Medicaid programs.

The fact that taxes pay for 60 percent of our health-care bill surprises most people. Our health-care system is usually described as an "employer-based system," and statistics indicate that a majority of Americans have been insured through employer-sponsored health insurance for about the last half-century. As of 2003, 54 percent of Americans got their health insurance through an employer.[38] So how can taxes account for 60 percent of total health-care spending? There are several answers.

First, government programs insure sicker people than American employers do. Medicare, the largest government health insurance program in the country, is an obvious example. Medicare insures the most expensive sectors of the population, namely, the elderly and the disabled. Ninety-seven percent of all Americans age 65 and over are insured through Medicare. Unlike the private sector, Medicare cannot pick and choose who it will insure.

Second, one-fifth of all workers are employed in the public sector and, therefore, have their insurance paid for by taxes.[39] If, for some reason, you wanted to treat public employees as part of the pool of Americans who receive "employer-sponsored" insurance rather than tax-financed insurance, the proportion of the total U.S. health-care bill paid for by taxes would drop from 60 percent to 55 percent.

Finally, employers who offer insurance, and employees who accept it, get tax breaks.*

---

* Employer-sponsored insurance, and employer contributions to "health savings accounts," are exempt from income and payroll taxes; employees whose employers offer them "flexible spending accounts" (accounts that employees use to pay for medical expenditures not covered by their insurance) don't pay taxes

The 40 percent of health-care spending not financed by taxes is paid for by employers and individuals. If you add up what individuals pay in the form of out-of-pocket expenditures (money spent on medical services not covered by health insurance) and in premiums (including not only the premiums individuals pay when they buy individual insurance, but the 20 to 30 percent of employer-sponsored premiums that employees pay), individuals pay roughly half of the 40 percent that taxes don't pay for, and employers pay the other half.

## History review and a peek at the future

So there you have it. As of 2003, 16 percent of us had no insurance, and the huge majority of the other 84 percent had insurance through an HMO or other type of MCP. Our jerry-built health insurance system is only 75 years old, but during its short life the system has undergone rapid, at times even tumultuous, change. To recapitulate, here are the major phases our system has gone through.

- Blue Cross (hospital) and Blue Shield (physician) companies sprang up during the 1930s.
- For-profit insurance companies, seeing the Blue Crosses and Blue Shields succeed, started selling health insurance in the late 1930s.
- Employers started offering health insurance as a fringe benefit during the 1940s, which accelerated the spread of health insurance. By the 1950s two-thirds of Americans had basic hospital and physician coverage.
- But the poor and elderly were not served by the new insurance industry, so Congress enacted Medicare and Medicaid in 1965. While Medicare and Medicaid made huge reductions in the percentage of Americans with no health insurance, they added, temporarily, to the medical inflation rate.
- In response to the increase in health-care inflation, Nixon and Congress subsidized the world's first HMO industry, and

---

on the money they put into those accounts; and individuals, employed or not, can deduct medical costs in excess of 7.5 percent of their adjusted gross income.

HMOs began taking market share from traditional insurers, slowly in the 1970s and rapidly in the 1980s.

- The spread of HMOs caused both the nonprofit (Blue Cross and Blue Shield) and for-profit sectors of the traditional insurance industry to adopt HMO cost-control tactics and change into managed-care plans. Between roughly 1985 and 1995, MCPs took over the insurance industry.

- Between 1989 and 1993, managed competition was transformed from an obscure theory into the nation's de facto health policy.

- But the death of Clinton's managed-competition bill in 1994, the rise of the consumer backlash against managed care in 1996, and the return of intolerable premium inflation in the late 1990s spelled the end for managed competition, and dealt a body blow to the MCP industry.

At the dawn of the new millennium, the American health-care system was unstable. Even experts who had vigorously defended MCPs against the backlash were acknowledging that the tension between patients, doctors and employers on the one hand and MCPs on the other could not go unresolved forever – that change in the system was inevitable. But there is nothing resembling a consensus among experts on how substantial that change will be or what, if anything, should replace MCPs. There is a consensus among experts, and substantial agreement among even health-care professionals, that we can't go back to the old system of traditional insurance that MCPs replaced because that system, like today's MCP system, was too expensive.

I believe expenditure controls on doctors, hospitals, and drug companies are inevitable, and that odds are high that America will adopt a national health insurance program based on the single-payer, Medicare-for-all model, especially if meaningful campaign finance reform is enacted. Before we implement price controls and a single-payer system, however, the U.S. will go through a phase in which we experiment with tax credits and Health Savings Accounts (or other types of insurance policies with big deductibles). I predict the entire process will take somewhere in the range of one to two decades. I think two decades is the outer limit because of the large number of baby boomers who will be needing health care by then. The elderly cost a lot more to take care of than the nonelderly. If this nation hasn't figured out how to provide health care efficiently before the boomers turn gray, the pressure for price controls and a Medicare-for-all system will be at an all-time high, and the credibility of those who said managed care or large deductibles would solve the problem will be at an all-time low.

## Endnotes

[1] Author's calculation based on figures reported in Paul Starr, *The Social Transformation of American Medicine: The Rise of a Sovereign Profession and the Making of a Vast Industry*, Basic Books, New York, 1982, 270.

[2] Robert Cunningham III and Robert M. Cunningham, Jr., *The Blues: A History of the Blue Cross and Blue Shield System*, Northern Illinois University Press, DeKalb, IL, 1997.

[3] Thomas Bodenheimer and Kevin Grumbach, "Paying for health care," *Journal of the American Medical Association* 1994;272:634-639.

[4] Ibid.

[5] Cunningham and Cunningham, Jr., op cit., 81.

[6] Paul Starr, *The Social Transformation of American Medicine: The Rise of a Sovereign Profession and the Making of a Vast Industry*, Basic Books, New York, 1982, 313.

[7] Marilyn Moon, "Medicare matters: Building on a record of accomplishments," *Health Care Financing Review* 2000;22(1):9-22.

[8] All three statistics are from Starr, op cit. The 1929 figure is at p. 262. Starr reports that the percent of GNP spent on health care in 1945 was 4 percent (p. 281), and 4.5 percent in 1950 (p. 335). The figure for 1970 is also at p. 335.

[9] J. A. Alexander et al., "Risk assumption and physician alignment with health care organizations," *Medical Care* 2001;39(7 Suppl 1):I46-61.

[10] Testimony by Elliot Richardson before the Subcommittee on Public Health and Environment, 1972, quoted in Harold Luft, "Why do HMOs seem to provide more health maintenance services?" *Milbank Memorial Fund Quarterly* 1978;56(2):140-168, 140.

[11] Josephine Marcotty and Glenn Howatt, "Blue Cross denials had high cost, Hatch says," Minneapolis *Star Tribune*, February 1, 2001, B1; and Josephine Marcotty, "Blue Cross, state reach settlement," Minneapolis *Star Tribune*, June 19, 2001, A1.

[12] Congressional Budget Office, *Effects of Managed Care: An Update*, March 1994, 9, citing E.W. Hoy et al., "Change and growth in managed care," Health Affairs 1991;10(4).

[13] Kenneth M. Coughlin, "After 20 years, HMOs are still challenged to deliver quality," *Business and Health*, January 1993, 17-23, 17.

[14] David U. Himmelstein and Steffie Woolhandler, "A national health program for the United States: A physicians' proposal," *New England Journal of Medicine* 1989;320:102-108.

[15] Marie Gottschalk, "The missing millions: Organized labor, and the defeat of Clinton's Health Security Act," *Journal of Health Policy, Politics and Law* 1999;24:489-529.

[16] Judi Hasson, "Single-payer system picks up momentum," *USA Today*, April 28, 1994, 10A.

[17] Pamela A. Paul-Shaheen, "The states and health care reform: The road traveled and lessons learned from seven that took the lead," *Journal of Health Politics, Policy and Law* 1998;23:319-361, 351.

[18] Jacob S. Hacker, *The Road to Nowhere: The Genesis of President Clinton's Plan for Health Security*, Princeton University Press, Princeton, NJ, 1997, 52-53.

[19] Alain Enthoven, "Managed competition in health care and the unfinished agenda," *Health Care Financing Review*, Supplement, 1986:105-119.

[20] Hacker, op cit., 52-53.

[21] Ibid., 53.

[22] Paul M. Ellwood et al., "The Jackson Hole initiatives for a Twenty-first Century American health care system," *Health Economics* 1992;1:149-168.

[23] Ibid., 152.

[24] Robin Toner, "Hillary Clinton's potent brain trust on health reform," *New York Times*, February 28, 1993, A1.

[25] "The Bush-Clinton health reform," *New York Times*, October 10, 1992, A20.

[26] Paul B. Ginsburg and Jon R. Gabel, "Tracking health care costs: What's new in 1998," *Health Affairs* 1998:17(5):141-146.

[27] Alain Enthoven and Sara J. Singer, "Markets and collective action in regulating managed care," *Health Affairs* 1997;16(6):26-32, 27.

[28] "Smart rules for health plans," *New York Times*, October 27, 1997, A18.

[29] Susan Brink, "HMOs were the right Rx: Americans get lower medical costs – but also more worries," *U.S. News and World Report*, March 9, 1998, 47-50, 47.

[30] Milt Freudenheim, "Health care costs edging up and a bigger surge is feared," *New York Times*, January 21, 1997, A1.

[31] Ron Shinkman, "Price surge on the way: Study says healthcare costs will jump in next five years," *Modern Healthcare*, June 9, 1997, 8.

[32] Robin Toner, "Before leaving health agency, Shalala offers a little advice on a big job," *New York Times*, January 16, 2001, A16.

[33] James C. Robinson, "The end of managed care," *Journal of the American Medical Association* 2001;285:2622-2628, 2622.

[34] Linda Marsa, "Former JAMA editor laments the state of medical care," *Los Angeles Times*, March 26, 2001, http://www.latimes.com/print/health/20010326/t000026016.html, accessed March 28, 2001.

[35] Arthur Caplan, "In 2001, managed care our No. 1 health crisis," MSNBC, December 21, 2001, http://www.msnbc.com/news/671464.asp, accessed December 23, 2001.

[36] Richard A. Knox, "HMOs' creator urges reform in quality of care," *Boston Globe*, May 2, 1999, A1.

[37] Lisa Belkin, "But what about quality?" *New York Times Magazine*, December 8, 1996, 68, 106.

[38] Kaiser Family Foundation, *Statehealthfacts.org*, http://www.statehealthfacts.org/cgi-bin/healthfacts.cgi?action=compare&category=Health+Coverage+%26+Uninsured&subcategory=Insurance+Status&topic=Distribution+by+Insurance+Status, accessed July 21, 2005.

[39] Steffie Woolhandler and David U. Himmelstein, "Paying for national health insurance – and not getting it," *Health Affairs* 2002;21(4):88-98.

# 3

# Evidence That the U.S. Health-Care System Is Failing

## Evaluating health-care systems

If you were asked to come up with a list of criteria with which to evaluate a nation's health-care system, what would they be? When I first started studying the U.S. system two decades ago, I had three simple criteria: cost (Are costs excessive?), access (Does everyone have access to necessary health services?), and quality (Are the services we're getting high quality?). In the course of resisting the takeover of our health-care system by managed-care plans (MCPs) during the 1990s, I adopted two more criteria: privacy (Are patient medical records available to third parties without patient consent?), and democracy (Have insurance companies, hospital chains, and pharmaceutical manufacturers become so powerful that a thorough debate about health-care reform is impossible?).

By any of these measures, the U.S. health-care system is a mess. Costs are extremely high, the number of uninsured is high and growing, quality is declining, medical privacy is a thing of the past, and democracy has been corrupted thanks to the huge companies that have taken over our health-care system and the money they have rained on Congress, state legislatures, state and federal regulators, and colleges and universities. In this chapter I will focus on the first two criteria – cost and access. I'll deal with the quality issue at more length in

Chapters 5 and 9. I'll discuss the destruction of privacy and the corruption of democracy briefly in Chapter 11.

## The U.S. health-care system costs a bundle

The first thing most people think of when you ask them whether they think health care is affordable is the high cost of health insurance premiums. The average premium for employer-sponsored family coverage in the country was just under $5,000 for family coverage and just under $2,000 for single coverage as recently as 1996. ("Family coverage" refers to an insurance policy for an employee plus dependents, typically two or three dependents, while "single" coverage refers to coverage for just the employee). Less than a decade later, premiums were double the 1996 level. In 2004, premiums for family coverage hit $10,000 a year and single coverage reached $3,700 a year.[1] Table 3-1 shows how much employer-sponsored coverage cost in 2003 for the U.S. and nine states. All these figures include both the employer's and the employee's contributions to the premiums (for the past decade, employees have been paying about 25 to 30 percent of family premiums and 15 to 20 percent of single premiums).[2] Don't forget, premiums for people who buy insurance on their own (that is, separate from a group of employees) are usually much higher than the premiums employers pay. When we discuss the futility of tax credits in Chapter 10, we will encounter some outrageous premiums for people buying individual policies.

But money that employers and individuals pay to insurance companies in the form of premiums is not the only way Americans pay for health care. As we saw in the last chapter, we also pay two other ways: We pay

## Table 3-1: Health insurance is expensive: Premiums for employer-sponsored health insurance in selected states, and U.S. average, 2003, $s

|  | CO | FL | MA | MN | NY | OK | OR | SC | WA | US |
|---|---|---|---|---|---|---|---|---|---|---|
| Family | 9,522 | 9,331 | 9,867 | 10,066 | 9,439 | 8,739 | 8,861 | 8,918 | 9,212 | 9,249 |
| Single | 3,645 | 3,592 | 3,496 | 3,679 | 3,592 | 3,285 | 3,362 | 3,371 | 3,520 | 3,481 |

Source: Kaiser Family Foundation, http://www.statehealthfacts.org/cgi-bin/healthfacts.cgi, accessed August 11, 2005.

taxes to support government insurance programs (such as Medicare and Medicaid), and we pay "out of pocket," that is, we pay out of our own wallets and bank accounts for medical care that is not covered by insurance. A medical expenditure can be uncovered and, therefore, require an out-of-pocket payment (a) because we don't have insurance, (b) because we have insurance but it doesn't cover what we need (for example, we need a prescription drug but our insurance doesn't cover drugs), or (c) because we have insurance that covers what we need but we have to pay a "co-payment" (for example, the first $15 of a prescription refill) or a "deductible" (for example, the first $500 of our medical expenses per year).

When we add up these three types of expenditures – premiums, taxes, and out-of-pocket payments – over the course of a year, we find that the U.S. spent about $1.7 trillion annually on health care in 2003 (see Tables 2-3 and 3-2). As Table 3-2 indicates, 53 percent of this sum goes to hospitals (31 percent) and doctors (22 percent). Expenditures on prescription drugs (11 percent) and nursing homes (7 percent) constitute the third and fourth largest types of expenditures.

Most people have little occasion to think in terms of trillions of dollars. So, to make this more manageable, let's break this gargantuan national health-care bill down into costs per American. In 2001, the U.S. spent $4,887 per person on health care. How high is that? As Table 3-3 indicates, that's extremely high by world standards. You see that Switzerland, the nation with the world's second-most-expensive health-care system, spent just $3,222 in 2001, a third less than the U.S. did. Norway, the nation with the third-most-expensive system, spent only $2,920 which is 60 percent of the U.S. figure. Fourth-place Germany and fifth-place Canada each spent 57 percent of the U.S. amount, and sixth-place Luxembourg spent 56 percent. Most of the 24 countries listed spent less than half what the U.S. spent.*

Another way to measure health spending is as a percent of Gross Domestic Product. GDP is a measure of the total income of a nation. We have already encountered this measure. Recall that in Chapter 2 I

---

* The 24 countries listed in Table 3-3 are all members of the Organization for Economic Cooperation and Development headquartered in Paris. The OECD, which collects and publishes economic and demographic data on member nations, currently consists of 24 industrialized nations and six developing nations with close ties to the West.

## Table 3-2: Hospitals and doctors account for half of all health expenditures: National health expenditures, 1970 and 2003, billions of dollars

| Category of expenditure | 1970 | 2003 |
|---|---|---|
| Personal health care | | |
| Hospital care | 27.6 (38%) | 515.9 (31%) |
| Physician services | 14.0 (19%) | 369.7 (22%) |
| Prescription drugs | 5.5 (8%) | 179.2 (11%) |
| Nursing home care[a] | 4.2 (6%) | 110.8 (7%) |
| Dental services | 4.7 | 74.3 |
| Other personal health care | 1.3 | 49.5 |
| Other professional services | 0.7 | 48.5 |
| Home health care | 0.2 | 40.0 |
| Nondurable medical equipment | 3.3 | 32.5 |
| Durable medical equipment | 1.6 | 20.4 |
| Subtotal | 63.2 | 1,440.8 |
| Insurance overhead (gov. and private)[b] | 2.8 | 119.7 |
| Public health activities (gov.) | 1.4 | 53.8 |
| Research[c] | 2.0 | 40.2 |
| Construction | 3.8 | 24.5 |
| Total | $73.1 | $1,678.9 |

(a) This category is for long-term care services in nursing homes only. Long-term care services provided in hospital-based facilities are counted as hospital care.

(b) These numbers are for insurance overhead (or administrative costs) only. They do not include the overhead costs of hospitals, doctors and other providers.

(c) Research expenditures on drugs are excluded from "research" and instead are included in the "prescription drug" category.

Source: Cynthia Smith et al., "Health spending growth slows in 2003," *Health Affairs* 2004;23(1):147-159, Exhibit 1.

## Table 3-3: U.S. costs are the highest in the world: Spending on health care by 24 industrialized nations, 2001

| Country | Percent of GDP spent on health | Per capita spending (in U.S. dollars) |
|---|---|---|
| United States | 13.9 | 4,887 |
| Switzerland | 11.1 | 3,322 |
| Norway | 8.0 | 2,920 |
| Germany | 10.7 | 2,808 |
| Canada | 9.7 | 2,792 |
| Luxembourg | 5.6 | 2,719 |
| Iceland | 9.2 | 2,643 |
| Netherlands | 8.9 | 2,626 |
| France | 9.5 | 2,561 |
| Australia | 9.2 | 2,513 |
| Denmark | 8.6 | 2,503 |
| Belgium | 9.0 | 2,490 |
| Sweden | 8.7 | 2,270 |
| Italy | 8.4 | 2,212 |
| Austria | 9.2 | 2,191 |
| Japan | 8.0 | 2,131 |
| United Kingdom | 7.6 | 1,992 |
| Ireland | 6.5 | 1,935 |
| Finland | 7.0 | 1,841 |
| New Zealand | 8.1 | 1,710 |
| Portugal | 9.2 | 1,613 |
| Spain | 7.5 | 1,600 |
| Greece | 9.4 | 1,511 |
| Czech Republic | 7.3 | 1,106 |

Source: Organization for Economic Cooperation and Development, reported in Uwe Reinhardt et al., "U.S. health care spending in an international context," *Health Affairs* 2004;23(3):10-25, Exhibit 1.

said the U.S. spent 4 percent of its total income on health care in 1929, about 4 percent in 1948 when Harry Truman campaigned for national health insurance, 7 percent in 1970, and 15 percent today. Table 3-3 indicates that the U.S. ratio of health spending to income is very high. Only two other nations listed in the table spent more than 10 percent of their incomes on health care.

## Access: Tens of millions are uninsured and underinsured

The extraordinarily high cost of the U.S. system looks even worse when you consider that the U.S. is the only nation in the industrialized world that permits large numbers of its citizens to go without health insurance. If the roles were reversed, you might understand how the U.S. could spend twice what the rest of the First World spends on health care per person. But the roles are not reversed. It's the U.S. that insures only 84 percent of its citizens; it's the rest of the industrialized world that insures virtually 100 percent of its citizens.

In the course of my public speaking and lobbying, I have heard opponents of universal coverage claim that there is no need for a universal health insurance plan because the uninsured get medical care whenever they need it. Those who make this claim never offer any proof of it. If they offer any justification at all, they cite the fact that most doctors

---

**Table 3-4: The uninsured see doctors less often: Doctor visits per person per year by insured and uninsured nonelderly, chronically ill, 1996**

|                                  | Insured | Uninsured |
|----------------------------------|---------|-----------|
| People with heart disease        | 9.0     | 2.9       |
| People with hypertension         | 10.0    | 7.4       |
| People with arthritis            | 10.7    | 7.9       |
| People with chronic back pain    | 10.2    | 8.3       |

Source: Families USA, *Getting Less Care: The Uninsured with Chronic Health Conditions*, 2001, Washington, DC.

and hospitals offer some "charity care" to poor patients. The unspoken assumption is that charity care is available to anyone who needs it, and charity care is the equivalent of "good care." I want to take a minute to address these assumptions because, if they're true, then what I just said about the U.S. looking even more expensive if you take the uninsured into account isn't true. Is it true that uninsured people get adequate medical care when they need it?

The research indicates unequivocally that uninsured people get fewer medical services than insured people, and when they do get care, it is often delayed. "Not having health insurance does make a difference," wrote Dr. Steven A. Schroeder in the pages of the *New England Journal of Medicine*. "Those who have it are likely to receive more and better health care. Those who do not have it are more likely to delay obtaining necessary, even lifesaving care."[3] Studies indicate that total spending per uninsured person is somewhere in the neighborhood of 55 to 60 percent of total spending per insured person.*

Data from one of the latest and best studies on this issue are shown in Table 3-4. This table indicates that uninsured people with chronic illnesses see doctors less often than do insured people with chronic diseases. The huge differences in visit rates for people with heart disease are especially disturbing. Table 3-5 confirms Table 3-4's findings on doctor visits, and also indicates that the uninsured are more likely to delay getting care and are slightly more likely to use emergency room services. Table 3-6 presents data from another study indicating the uninsured are more likely to delay getting care.

So research has demonstrated that the uninsured get fewer services, but does that difference mean uninsured people suffer worse health outcomes? Studies of this question are a lot fewer than studies that

---

* In a report to Congress which, among other things, estimated the cost of insuring the uninsured, the U.S. General Accounting Office stated that per capita health expenditures on the uninsured were about 60 percent of the expenditures on the insured (U.S. General Accounting Office, *Canadian Health Insurance: Estimating Costs and Savings for the United States*, Washington, DC, April 1992, 13). A more current study puts the percentage at 55 percent (Kaiser Family Foundation, "Treating uninsured will cost $125 billion by 2004, including $41 billion in uncompensated care, study says," May 11, 2004, http://www.Kaisernetwork.org /daily_reports/rep_index.cfm?DR_ID=23645, accessed May 11, 2004).

**Table 3-5: The uninsured see doctors less often, go to ERs a little more often, and delay care more often: Differences in access to health care between Minnesota's insured and uninsured, 1995**

|  | Group* | Individual* | Uninsured |
|---|---|---|---|
| Percent delayed getting care in last 12 months | 11.5 | 11.8 | 38.5 |
| Percent with doctor visit in last 3 months | 54.2 | 42.7 | 28.8 |
| Percent with emergency room visit in past 12 months | 14.8 | 10.3 | 15.9 |

* "Group" means insured as part of a group, typically at a place of employment. "Individual" means insured through a policy purchased by an individual.

Source: Kathleen Thiede Call et al., *Minnesota Health Care Insurance and Access Survey, 1995,* Institute for Health Services Research, University of Minnesota, Minneapolis, MN, August 1996.

**Table 3-6: The uninsured delay seeking care more often: Percentage of insured and uninsured hospitalized patients who delayed* obtaining care**

| | |
|---|---|
| Uninsured poor | 33.3% |
| All uninsured | 23.9 |
| Medicaid | 22.7 |
| HMO | 18.2 |
| Traditional insurance | 15.7 |

* Delay was defined by the patients. They were asked, "[D]o you feel that you delayed seeing a doctor or other medical person longer than you should have?" Patients who delayed getting medical attention were in the hospital about 9 percent longer than patients who said they did not delay.

Source: Joel S. Weissman et al., "Delayed access to health care: Risk factors, reasons, and consequences," *Annals of Internal Medicine* 1991;114:325-331.

simply asked whether uninsured people get fewer services, but they all point in the expected direction: Lack of insurance is a health risk. One of the most recent reviews of the literature on this subject was published in 2002 by the Institute of Medicine (IOM), an agency created by Congress in 1970 to advise the federal government on health matters. The IOM concluded: "The strongest research studies consistently show that working-age Americans ... who do not have health insurance have poorer health and die prematurely.... Being uninsured is associated with a variety of worse health-related outcomes...."[4] The IOM estimated that 18,000 Americans died in 2000 because they had no health insurance.[5] The author of another lengthy 2003 literature review agreed: "[H]ealth insurance improves health," he wrote.[6]

Here is one example of the studies the IOM reviewed. Researchers at Harvard reported that breast cancer in uninsured women is more advanced at the time it is first diagnosed than it is in insured women, and that uninsured women with breast cancer die sooner.[7] Another study reviewed by the IOM examined differences in health status among insured and uninsured adults aged 51 to 61. The study found that the uninsured adults were 1.6 times more likely to suffer a "major decline" in health between 1992 and 1996 than the insured were.[8]

But you don't have to be completely uninsured to forgo necessary health care for financial reasons. A large body of research indicates that even co-payments and deductibles will cause many people to delay or forgo needed services, including services needed for serious symptoms.[9] And, of course, pre-existing condition exclusions and the failure of an insurance policy to cover a certain type of health-care service are even more inhibiting than deductibles or co-payments. Drugs and mental health services are examples of services often left out of insurance policies; long-term care is virtually never covered by health insurance. The effect of a drug coverage gap on patient behavior is significant. Medicare beneficiaries with prescription drug coverage bought 24.35 prescriptions in 1998 compared with 16.65 purchased by beneficiaries without drug coverage.[10]

Those without drug and mental health coverage are an example of the "underinsured." I have never seen a study that attempted to measure the *total* number of underinsured in the U.S. The few studies I have seen measured the number of *nonelderly* underinsured. The most widely cited of these studies used a rather conservative definition of underinsurance and concluded that 29 million nonelderly Americans were underinsured in 1994, or about 11 percent of the entire population. The authors defined "underinsured" to mean having insurance that exposed the insured person to "out-of-pocket expenditures in excess of 10 percent of family income in the event of a catastrophic illness."[11] They noted that the percent of underinsured among the nonelderly had increased substantially since 1977 because the value of typical catastrophic coverage had not kept up with the cost of health care.

If we define long-term care as a form of health care to which all Americans should have access, the proportion of us who are underinsured is far greater than 11 percent. Long-term care is not covered by a typical health insurance policy. Long-term care coverage is sold in separate policies, and only 5 percent of Americans have such policies. Medicare, contrary to many people's impression, covers very little nursing home care. Medic*aid* is the nation's primary financier of long-term care services. But Medicaid is not insurance because you have to impoverish yourself to become eligible. If we include long-term care in our definition of health insurance, we may say 95 percent of us are underinsured.

The figures in Table 3-7 suggest that a substantial portion of the elderly are among the underinsured even though 97 percent of them are

## Table 3-7: Out-of-pocket health costs for the elderly, selected years

|  | 1965 | 1968 | 1977 | 1980 | 1984 | 1988 | 1998 | 2002 |
|---|---|---|---|---|---|---|---|---|
| Percent of income paid for health care | 19 | 11 | 12.3 | 12.7 | 13.7 | 18.1 | 18.6 | 19 |

Sources: Marilyn Moon, "Health policy 2001: Medicare," *New England Journal of Medicine* 2001;344:928-931 (for years 1965 and 1968); U.S. Senate Special Committee on Aging, cited in David U. Himmelstein and Steffie Woolhandler, *The National Health Program Book*, 1994, 35 (for years 1977 through 1988); Marilyn Moon, *Growth in Medicare Spending: What Will Beneficiaries Pay?* Washington, DC, Urban Institute, 1999, Chart ES-1, vii (for 1998); and Kaiser Family Foundation, *Medicare Chart Book 2005*, Section 4, http://www.kff.org/medicare/upload/Medicare-Chart-Book-3rd-Edition-Summer-2005-Section-4.pdf, accessed July 27, 2005 (for 2002).

covered by Medicare. The table indicates that the elderly were paying 19 percent of their total incomes for health care (not counting long-term care) in 1965, the year before Medicare began, and that this percentage fell to 11 percent in 1968. But at the turn of the millennium it was at 19 percent once again. Recall that the estimate of 29 million *non*elderly underinsured in 1994 defined underinsured to be those exposed to a risk of having to pay out more than 10 percent of their income in the event of a serious illness. The figures in Table 3-7 indicate the average elderly American has been incurring out-of-pocket medical expenses in excess of 10 percent of his or her income ever since Medicare was enacted. That means that the number of underinsured *of all ages* was considerably higher in 1994 than 29 million. Even if we exclude long-term care from the definition of health insurance, the number of *under*insured of all ages may exceed the number of *un*insured. It is a safe bet that the un- and underinsured constitute at least a third of the U.S. population.

## Why our system is so expensive

The fundamental cause of the health-care mess is the high cost of health care. The high cost of health care is the cause of the growing number of uninsured and underinsured. It is the reason why out-of-pocket expenses are rising for the elderly. It is the reason why President Nixon, Congress and large employers pushed the country into a doomed experiment with managed care. It is the reason George W. Bush, Republican legislators at the state and federal level, and the insurance industry are now promoting high-deductible policies. It is a significant cause of our inability to find the political will to set up a national health insurance program to guarantee coverage to all Americans.

To prescribe a solution to any problem, one must first have an accurate diagnosis. In this case, we have to have an accurate diagnosis of the causes of the high cost of American health care. We shall derive such a diagnosis in the next four chapters. In the next two chapters (Chapters 4 and 5), I review common explanations for America's high costs that are either misleading or flat wrong. In Chapters 6 and 7 I lay out the evidence supporting my argument that waste in the health-care system is the real cause of the high cost of our system.

Let me begin my diagnosis by observing again that total expenditures on anything, be it health care, pianos or Tiddly Winks, is a product of two numbers – volume and price. In the case of health care, the $2 trillion the U.S. spends annually is a product of the *volume* of medical goods and services sold times the *price* at which those goods and services are sold. Thus, the most basic question we can ask at the outset of our investigation is, Is *volume* of services the primary problem, or is *price* the main problem? To put it another way, Is the problem primarily that too many medical services are being ordered (either because ignorant patients demand them or greedy doctors promote them), or is the problem primarily that the price at which medical goods and services are sold is unnecessarily high?

Think for a moment about what's at stake here. If *volume* is the problem, that's a strong argument either for "managing" health care with the managed-care tools we talked about in Chapter 2 – financial incentives and utilization review, strengthened with limitations on choice of doctor – or imposing large deductibles on patients. If, however, *price* is the primary problem, that's a strong argument for not attempting to ratchet down volume (that is, leaving doctors and patients alone), and instead concentrating on price reductions, that is, subjecting doctors, drug companies and insurers to price ceilings, and hospitals to either price ceilings or, preferably, budgets.

If your primary identification is with patients (which should be the case for the vast majority of Americans who are not in the upper echelons of the health-care industry), your self-interest should lead you to prefer the price-is-the-problem diagnosis. If *volume* turns out to be the primary problem, then you must be prepared to accept (a) limits on your freedom to choose the medical services you and your doctor think you need and/or (b) huge deductibles. However, if *price* turns out to be the primary problem, it's the supply side – the MCPs, clinics, hospitals, and drug companies – that must suffer limitations on their freedoms, in this case, their freedom to buy and charge whatever they want. Conversely, if you're a hospital manager, drug company executive, or insurance company executive, your self-interest, narrowly defined, should lead you to prefer the volume-is-the-problem diagnosis.[*]

---

[*] Doctors have conflicting interests in this volume-versus-price debate. As professionals with an interest in being able to make decisions with some independence, and as advisors to and decision makers for patients, doctors should oppose the limitations on doctor-patient authority that the volume-is-the-problem

Given the greater firepower of the insurers, doctors, hospitals, and drug companies, it is no surprise that conventional wisdom in this country is that volume is the main problem. It was this conventional wisdom that led to the disastrous managed-care experiment. The volume-is-the-problem claim is the most fundamental premise underlying managed-care theology. It is also the fundamental premise underlying the right wing's endorsement of high-deductible policies. The only difference between managed-care theology and large-deductible theology is that managed-care adherents believe volume is excessive because *doctors* are greedy, while large-deductible advocates believe volume is excessive because *patients* are "overinsured."

The greater firepower of the health-care industry also explains why price is not talked about as the main problem and why system-wide price controls have never been on the table for discussion. As we will see in Chapter 8, the average American opposes managed care and, depending on the poll you read, either supports price controls or perceives prices to be excessive. But despite the public's position *against* managed care and *for* a solution that addresses excessive prices, the power of the health-care industry guaranteed that American policy makers would blame patients and doctors for driving up volume and avoid a discussion of price controls.

The disproportionate influence the health-care industry has over the health-care reform debate can be seen in a listing of the most common explanations for high U.S. health-care costs. In the course of speaking to thousands of people about what's wrong with the U.S. system, and in the course of reading about health policy for two decades, I've heard every explanation imaginable for the high cost of our system compared to the cost of other nation's systems. In Table 3-8, I've listed the six categories into which these explanations fall. They are: Americans get too many medical services; we are getting older; we have more slovenly lifestyles; we sue for malpractice too often; we're more violent; and quality of care is better in the U.S.

What is most interesting about the list in Table 3-8 is that the first five excuses (the excessive services, age, lifestyle, malpractice, and violence

---

diagnosis calls for. But as business people interested in freedom to set their own fees, they should oppose the price-is-the-problem diagnosis because it calls for government-enforced limits on fees.

excuses) blame consumers, while the sixth (superior quality) praises the health-care industry. With the exception of excuse number 1(a) (the MCP industry's favorite excuse, the one which blames doctors for the alleged overuse of the system), none of these six excuses places any blame on the supply side of the health-care market – on insurers, drug manufacturers, hospitals, and clinics. In Chapters 6 and 7, we'll discuss a seventh explanation for high American health-care costs for which there is abundant evidence and with which most Americans agree: The U.S. system is expensive because the supply side is extraordinarily wasteful.

I call these explanations "excuses" because they are misleading or just plain bogus. It is misleading, for example, for the experts who dominate the health-care debate, and the reporters who pass on the experts' opinions as fact, to blame America's high costs on the aging of the population. Yes, it's unquestionably true that health-care costs rise slowly as the proportion of a nation's population over 65 rises. But it is grossly misleading to suggest that America's health-care costs are twice those of other countries because Americans are older than people of other nations. The malpractice excuse (number 4 on the list in Table 3-8) is an example of an excuse that is just flat out false. The cost of frivolous malpractice suits is just too small to play anything resembling an important role in driving up U.S. health-care costs. I'll examine all six excuses in more detail in the next two chapters.

## Table 3-8: Six excuses for the high cost of America's health-care system

(1) Americans get too many medical services
    (a) because doctors order too many services
    (b) because patients demand too many services
(2) Americans are older
(3) Americans have worse lifestyles
(4) Americans sue for malpractice too often
(5) Americans are more violent
(6) US quality is superior

# Endnotes

[1] Kaiser Family Foundation, *Trends and Indicators in the Changing Marketplace*, Exhibit 3.1, http://www.kff.org/insurance/7031/ti2004-3-set.cfm, accessed May 28, 2005.

[2] Ibid., Exhibit 3.5, http://www.kff.org/insurance/7031/ti2004-3-5.cfm, accessed May 28, 2005.

[3] Steven A. Schroeder, "Health policy 2001: Prospects for expanding health insurance coverage," *New England Journal of Medicine* 2001;344:847-852, 847.

[4] Institute of Medicine, *Care Without Coverage: Too Little, Too Late*, National Academy Press, Washington, DC, 2002, 4. Among the studies IOM cited were these: Paul D. Sorlie et al., "Mortality in the uninsured compared with that in persons with public and private health insurance," *Archives of Internal Medicine* 1994;154:2409-2416; Peter Franks et al., "Health insurance and mortality: Evidence from a national cohort," *Journal of the American Medical Association* 1993;270-737-741; Nicole Lurie et al., "Termination from Medi-Cal – Does it affect health?" *New England Journal of Medicine* 1984;311:480-484; and Nicole Lurie et al., "Termination of Medi-Cal benefits: A follow-up study one year later," *New England Journal of Medicine* 1986;314:1266-1268.

[5] Institute of Medicine, op cit., Table D.1, 163.

[6] Jack Hadley, "Sicker and poorer – the consequences of being uninsured: A review of the research on the relationship between health insurance, Medicare care use, health, work, and income," *Medical Care Research and Review* 2003;60 (Supplement):3S-75S.

[7] John Z. Ayanian et al., "The relation between health insurance coverage and clinical outcomes among women with breast cancer," *New England Journal of Medicine* 1993;329:326-331.

[8] David W. Baker et al., "Lack of health insurance and decline in overall health in late middle age," *New England Journal of Medicine* 2001;345:1106-1112.

[9] J. Grana and B. Stuart, "The impact of insurance on access to physician services for elderly people with arthritis," *Inquiry* 1996/97;33:326-338; Julie Hudman and Molly O'Malley, *Health Insurance Premiums and Cost-Sharing: Findings from the Research on Low-Income Populations*, Kaiser Commission on Medicaid and the Uninsured, http://www.kff.org/medicaid/4071-index.cfm, accessed April 5, 2004; J. V. Selby et al., "Effect of copayment on use of the emergency department in a health maintenance organization," *New England Journal of Medicine* 1996;334:657-658; and M. F. Shapiro et al., "Effects of cost sharing on seeking care for serious and minor symptoms: Results of a randomized controlled trial," *Annals of Internal Medicine* 1986;104:246-251.

[10] John A. Poisal and Lauren Murray, "Growing differences between Medicare beneficiaries with and without drug coverage," *Health Affairs* 2001;20(2):74-85.

[11] Pamela Farley and Jessica S. Banthin, "New estimates of the underinsured younger than 65 years," *Journal of the American Medical Association* 1995;274:1302-1306.

# 4

# Excuses for the High Cost of American Health Care: The Overuse Excuse

## Overview

In this chapter, I review the first of the six excuses for America's high costs listed in Table 3-8. This explanation – that Americans get too many medical services – has been the most common explanation for America's high health-care costs for the last four decades.

Prior to the takeover of the health-care system by managed-care plans (MCPs), the alleged overuse of the system was blamed primarily on the traditional fee-for-service method of paying doctors. Managed-care advocates, you recall, argued that Americans were grossly overusing the system because fee-for-service payment gave doctors an incentive to order too many services. Managed-care advocates were still selling this notion years after managed care had clearly failed. In a 1998 essay, the CEO of Blue Cross and Blue Shield of Minnesota summarized the MCP version of the overuse excuse this way:

> In the 1970s and early 1980s, ... [m]edical journals were loaded with studies, and the popular press carried tales about, unnecessary tests and procedures.... Managed care emerged to curb health care's financial excesses....

> Managed care achieved cost control largely by reversing
> the financial incentives of fee-for-service medicine.[1]

In an interview with the *Washington Post* published in February
2001, William Donaldson, CEO of Aetna, explained the giant MCP's
mission as "trying to bring some discipline to ... doctors ... who send
out for 25 tests or who do things that are unnecessary." Donaldson,
who developed his expertise in supervising doctors by co-founding the
Wall Street investment firm of Donaldson, Lufkin and Jenrette and
serving as undersecretary of state under Henry Kissinger, went on to
explain how it is that America's doctors have become so profligate. They
got that way at medical school, he said. "The medical profession has
been taught in school that everything is okay," Donaldson opined. "I
mean: 'Send out for 1,000 tests. Do it.' You know, with no attention
to price control. No attention to the efficient and effective practice of
medicine."[2]

But by the late 1990s, HMO and managed-care advocates were in
retreat and advocates of high-deductible policies, including executives
of insurance companies such as Golden Rule, leaders of the American
Medical Association, representatives of conservative think tanks like the
Cato Institute, and politicians like Rep. Newt Gingrich (R-GA) and
Sen. Phil Gramm (R-TX), were getting lots of attention in the media.
Almost overnight, it became less fashionable to say doctors and the
fee-for-service method caused unnecessary services. Now it was fashionable to blame "overinsured" patients.* The following statement by
a reporter in a 2002 story in the *Washington Post* is typical of the new
version of the overuse excuse: "But if there is one overarching cause of
soaring health-care expenditures, it is Americans' insatiable appetite for
each and every medical test and treatment available, the experts agree."[3]
Here are other examples.

> By shielding consumers from the consequences of their
> health-care purchasing decisions, the third-party pay-
> ment system encourages excessive use of medical services

---

* This has been less true of medical and health policy journals. These journals continue to devote much attention to inappropriate ordering of services by
doctors.

and drives up health-care costs." (Michael Tanner, Cato Institute, 1999)[4]

"The people to blame in the end ... are consumers," says senior economist Christopher Thornberg of UCLA's Anderson Forecast, a national survey of businesses. "People don't adequately take into account the true costs of the services they're consuming." (*USA Today*, 2002)[5]

Carl Mercurio, a researcher who tracks managed care, doesn't blame the HMOs, though.... Mercurio says, "As Americans, we want the best health care in the world and we want unlimited access to health care and we don't want to pay for it." (CBS Evening News, 2002)[6]

Notice how effortlessly the villains got switched. In the worldview of managed-care advocates, the problem was that *doctors* had the wrong incentives, not patients. In the worldview of large-deductible advocates, the problem is that *patients* have the wrong incentives – they demand too many medical services because their insurance pays for "everything." This disagreement over who is causing the alleged overuse of the system is your first clue that neither camp has much data to support its position.

Overuse of the system in fact occurs. But so does *under*use. As we shall see in a moment, underuse is far more prevalent than overuse. If politicians and the media permit managed-care and high-deductible advocates to bray about overuse and ignore underuse, we run the risk that employers (our de facto health policy makers) and legislators will (a) do little about underuse or, worse, adopt mechanisms that worsen the underuse problem in an effort to fix the overuse problem, and (b) ignore waste generated by the health-care industry. Exposing Americans, especially low-income Americans, to deductibles of $2,000 to $4,000 per person (and more for families) is an example of the trouble we could cause ourselves if we diagnose overuse and ignore underuse. A huge deductible may well cause some patients to stop overusing the system, but it will also cause other patients to forgo necessary medical services.

(I'll discuss the damage big deductibles inflict on quality of care at greater length in Chapter 10.)

We must focus on overuse *and* underuse, not overuse alone. Moreover, we must acknowledge that underuse is much more common than overuse, which means that if we solve both problems simultaneously we will probably raise costs, not lower them. Only if we make the unethical decision to ignore underuse can we define overuse as primarily a cost issue. In short, we must think of over- and underuse as a single problem of "inappropriate use," and we should think of this problem as a quality problem, not a cost problem.

To illustrate how misleading the overuse argument is, let me offer this analogy. Imagine that your local high school has just been informed that its heating costs are twice those of surrounding high schools. Imagine moreover that the causes of the problem are primarily "supply-side" problems – price-gouging by the gas utility, poor construction by the company that built the school, and faulty thermostats – not problems created by teachers and students, problems we could label "demand-side" problems. But the supply-side culprits – the gas company, the construction company, and the manufacturer of the thermostats – decide to distort the community debate about high heating bills by propagating the claim that students are the problem. These corporations accuse the students of overusing heat by opening windows in the winter and by turning up the thermostats in their rooms rather than dressing warmly. To buttress this misleading claim, the supply-side culprits send researchers into the school and discover that in fact about 10 percent of the rooms are overheated and that some of the overheating is due to student behavior such as opening windows. But they also discover that about half the rooms are *under*heated. When they calculate the cost of the overuse and underuse of heat they have documented, they find that if both the overheating and underheating problems were solved, the school's heating bill would rise, not fall (because underuse is so much worse than overuse). But they leave out all mention of the underheated rooms in their report to the school board, their press releases, and their other public comments. And, of course, they say nothing at all about their own contributions to the problem – excessively high gas prices, poor construction of the school, and defective thermostats.

If no one came forward to rebut the supply-side culprits' arguments, you can see how distorted the public debate within this community about the "heating crisis" would be. And, in such an environment, you can see how the school board might be persuaded to adopt bad policy. If the school board hears only about the overheated rooms and nothing about the underheated rooms and, moreover, nothing about the supply-side problems, it is much more likely to assume the heating crisis is a demand-side problem – a problem caused by irresponsible, selfish students – and to look no further. Once it has made this flawed diagnosis, the school board will then be prone to make a bad or, at best, inadequate prescription, such as turning down thermostats throughout the entire school (which aggravates underuse in the underheated rooms) or making students in overheated rooms pay a portion of the heating bill. Worst of all, lacking any information on the supply-side causes – the real causes – of the heating crisis, the school board is likely to take no action to address those causes.

The shriveled debate about health policy in the U.S. resembles this hypothetical debate about one school's heating crisis. *Under*use of medical care, even by insured people, is more common than overuse, yet the debate about the U.S. health-care crisis has been primarily about overuse. Meanwhile, the real causes of the health-care crisis go unexamined. The primary causes of the crisis lie on the supply side – insurance companies and providers devote enormous portions of their revenues to administrative costs, hospitals and clinics buy more equipment than they need, physicians (especially specialists) charge more than they should, drug companies set drug prices far higher than necessary, and fraud (nearly all of it on the supply side) sucks up as much as 10 percent of our health-care dollar. Yet, thanks to the power of the suppliers of health insurance and medical care, the debate about health-care reform focuses on what to do about overuse. And, because of that one-eyed focus, we've had to endure a nationwide experiment with managed care, and now that that has failed, we're about to suffer through another doomed experiment premised on overuse, this one dreamed up by the high-deductible wing of the health insurance industry. It is very important, therefore, that Americans understand the truth about the overuse diagnosis.

I turn now to a review of the evidence that both overuse and underuse are problems, and that underuse is the more serious problem.
I begin with an examination of the published studies on over- and
underuse in the U.S. I devote the next 24 pages to an examination of
the literature on this question. I think you'll find this discussion quite
interesting. The discussion will demonstrate that determining what is
and is not necessary medical care is usually difficult to do. We will see
that Americans are not crybabies and hypochondriacs who rush to the
doctor at the first sign of illness. We will see, for example, that one-
fourth of all *insured* patients who should have heart surgery refuse to
have it done.

However, for those who do not want to immerse themselves in the
details of the debate about overuse and underuse, let me summarize the
next 24 pages in two sentences: *The best and latest evidence indicates
Americans underuse health care about 46 percent of the time and overuse
it about 11 percent of the time.* In other words, contrary to decades of
insurance industry propaganda, the average American significantly
*underuses* health care.

After I've examined the literature on over- and underuse, I'll review
utilization rates of hospital and physician care in the U.S. and other
countries. We will see that the U.S. utilization rates are actually lower
than utilization rates in other countries, which means overuse in the
U.S., however bad it may be, explains little of the huge difference between the health-care costs of the U.S. and other countries.

## The evidence that some medical services are overused

America's grand experiment with managed care required that a critical mass of politicians and business leaders accept two propositions: (1)
that American doctors frequently order unnecessary medical goods and
services, and (2) that MCPs were capable of distinguishing necessary
from unnecessary care and would only cut back on the unnecessary
care. A substantial body of evidence indicates proposition 1 is true; but
there is no evidence that proposition 2 is true.

As we saw in Chapter 2, Paul Ellwood and other early proponents
of HMOs did not argue that the primary cause of health-care inflation
was the excessive *price* at which medical services were sold. The HMO
advocates had nary a discouraging word to say, for example, about the

high prices and the enormous profits of the pharmaceutical industry. You can scour the pro-managed-care literature and never find a discussion of why the incomes of U.S. specialists are so high compared to those of specialists who practice in England, France, or Australia, to take another example. No, Ellwood and his disciples were fixated on *volume.* They argued that the primary problem was an excessive volume of services, and that the fee-for-service system was to blame. The fee-for-service system, they said, gave doctors an incentive to provide services even if the services weren't necessary, and to ignore preventive services because doctors make more money under a fee-for-service system when patients get sick.*

In the early 1970s when Ellwood began promoting his overuse thesis, he had little scientific evidence to support it. Since that time, however, studies have been published which suggest, and in some cases demonstrate, that America is paying for a substantial number of unnecessary medical services. These studies fall into two categories: variation-in-rate-of-treatment studies (studies which demonstrate that the rate at which certain types of services are provided varies greatly, even within small geographic areas); and "appropriateness" studies (those in which doctors are asked to examine the files of patients who received certain treatments and to indicate whether they think the patient was an appropriate candidate for that treatment). The best known and most influential author of variation studies is John Wennberg, a doctor currently on the faculty of Dartmouth Medical School. The best known and most influential source of studies of appropriate use of medical services is the Rand Corporation, a think tank in Santa Monica, California.

---

* As it turned out, HMOs saved money both ways – by cutting volume *and* price (they cut prices by extracting discounts from clinics, hospitals and drug companies). But the statements made, and papers published, by the leading HMO and managed-care advocates such as Paul Ellwood, Walter McClure, Alain Enthoven, and the Jackson Hole Group did not claim that MCPs would reduce health-care inflation by becoming huge and using their clout to extract discounts from providers and drug companies. After all, if that was all there was to managed care, who needed it? Medicare was already much larger than any HMO could ever be and, by the 1980s, had clearly demonstrated its ability to induce providers to treat patients for fees considerably below those charged by private-sector insurers.

The first variation-in-rate-of-treatment studies were published in the early 1970s, about 15 years prior to the publication of the first appropriateness studies. The early variation studies were called "small-area studies" because they examined differences in rates of surgery between communities that were near one another. The first of these studies appeared in 1973 (the year the federal HMO Act was enacted) in *Science*. The study, authored by John Wennberg and one of his colleagues, demonstrated that the rate at which doctors performed surgery varied greatly among New England communities separated by no more than a few miles. Tonsillectomy rates in Vermont communities, for example, ranged from 3 to 15 per 1,000 residents.[7] In subsequent studies, Wennberg reported that the probability that a woman in Maine would have a hysterectomy by the time she was 70 ranged from a low of 20 percent to a high of 70 percent,[8] and that the rate of back surgery varied tenfold among Maine communities.[9] (Interestingly, Wennberg and his colleagues also found that small-area variations were as large in Norway and Britain as they were in New England.)[10] These and other variation studies indicated that variation was greatest for surgeries such as tonsillectomy, hysterectomy, prostatectomy, and coronary artery bypass where the indications for surgery were less precisely defined. For procedures such as appendectomy, gall bladder surgery, and hip fracture repair, where the indications are more clearly defined, variation tended to be a lot less.

Mark Chassin, Robert Brook and other scholars at the Rand Corporation demonstrated that variations in rates are just as large among states as they are among neighboring communities. In 1986, they published an analysis of the rate at which 123 procedures were used in states (and in the case of some large states, *regions* of those states) across the country. "We found large and significant differences in the use of services provided by all medical and surgical specialties," they wrote. "Of 123 procedures studied, 67 showed at least threefold differences between sites with the highest and lowest rates of use."[11] Interestingly, they noted that states that had high use rates of one medical service had low rates of other services.

A few studies documented that the rates of some types of surgery vary greatly by country. For example, one study reported that Cesarean-section rates varied among 13 industrialized nations in 1980 from a high of 17 per 100 deliveries (the American rate) to a low of 4

(Czechoslovakia). (Canada ranked right behind the U.S. with 16 per 100 deliveries.)[12] In 2001, the variation in C-section rates had narrowed somewhat. The highest rate that year among 22 industrialized nations examined was 40 per 100 deliveries (South Korea) and the lowest was 15 (Norway). (That year the U.S. did 24 C-sections per 100 deliveries.)[13]

In 1989, Wennberg organized the Center for the Evaluative Clinical Sciences at Dartmouth Medical School. In 1996 this institution published *The Dartmouth Atlas of Health Care*. According to the 2000 edition of this atlas, heart patients in Elyria, Ohio, get angioplasty seven times more often than heart patients in York, Pennsylvania, 360 miles away, and men in Baton Rouge, Louisiana, undergo prostate surgery at a rate more than eight times higher than those in Tuscaloosa, Alabama.[14]

As provocative as the variation studies are, they do not demonstrate that surgeons in the high-rate areas are doing unnecessary surgeries, or that the surgeons in the low-rate areas are denying necessary care to their patients. Mark Chassin and his Rand colleagues made this point explicitly in their national study of 123 procedures:

> [T]he available data do not allow us to explain the wide variations we have observed.... [W]e cannot establish the "correct" use rates from these data. For any given procedure, geographic differences may reflect substantial inappropriate overuse in the high-use areas with very little inappropriate use in the low-use areas. On the other hand, the variations may have occurred because physicians in the low-use areas were not providing enough services to those who needed them, whereas those in the high-use areas were meeting legitimate medical needs in an appropriate manner.[15]

The authors speculated that differences in the "incidence of disease" might explain these variations.

However, the inconclusiveness of variation studies did not prevent Wennberg (who later became an advocate of managed competition)* and

---

* Wennberg became a member of the Jackson Hole Group, the exclusive club of health policy experts, insurance company executives, big business ex-

other managed-care advocates from implying or stating that variation in rates of medical services is in fact proof of overuse, not underuse. This testimony by Wennberg before the Senate Appropriations Committee in 1985 is an example:

> [I]f the low-cost patterns of care were the norm, we would not be faced with the pending bankruptcy of the Medicare Trust Fund, nor would we now be concerned with the specter that medical care must be rationed. For many medical and surgical conditions, the variations suggest opportunities to reduce expenditures under the Medicare and Medicaid programs without reducing the benefits of medical care.[16]

Other participants in the health policy wars not only cited Wennberg's studies as proof of rampant overuse, but leaped to yet another unfounded conclusion – that the alleged overuse was the fault of doctors. For example, the Pepper Commission (a federal commission on health care), citing Wennberg, stated in its 1990 report, "The most important factor [causing variations] seems to be differences in the practice styles of physicians."[17] AARP, a group which supported managed competition in the early 1990s, had this to say about Wennberg's work in a 1992 article in its newsletter entitled, "Unnecessary operations raise costs":

> "What's the reason for these differences in rates of surgery?" asks Howard A. Fishbein, MD, an epidemiologist at the Center for Medical Effectiveness Research at the Agency for Health Care Policy and Research [a federal

ecutives, and politicians we met in Chapter 2. This group promoted managed care and managed competition. However, Wennberg apparently reversed position some time between 1993 (the year the *New York Times* described him as a member of the Jackson Hole Group) and 1996. In the latter year, he authored an article for *Health Affairs* in which he stated he did not approve of "strategies that micromanage the doctor-patient relationship...." (John E. Wennberg, "On the appropriateness of small-area analysis for cost containment," *Health Affairs* 1996;15(4):164-167, 165).

agency established in 1989 that Wennberg lobbied to create]. "Most of the variation can probably be explained by differences in the practice styles of physicians...." When surgeons with a fervent belief in the value of surgery are carefully educated, though, Fishbein says they tend to slow down their use of surgery.[18]

The implication of Fishbein's statement is that medical scientists have determined (a) that the lower rates of surgery are the correct ones, (b) that the doctors who perform higher rates of surgery do so because they bring more fervor than science to their jobs, and (c) these excessively enthusiastic doctors can be induced to do less surgery when they are "educated" by their better informed colleagues or by MCPs. All of these implications were unproven and grossly misleading in 1992, and they remain unproven and grossly misleading today.

Dr. Fishbein's assertion that "most of the variation" can be attributed to differences in physician "practice styles" was not merely unsupported by science, it actually contradicted at least one very good scientific study published in 1987 by Chassin and his Rand colleagues. That study was designed to answer the question, Do high-use areas also have high rates of inappropriate use? The results appeared in the first of three "appropriateness" studies (the second type of overuse study we are examining here) that Rand scholars published in 1987 and 1988. This study had a three-part design. First, the authors calculated utilization rates for 153 procedures in eight states. They found that rates of use of these 153 procedures varied greatly among the states. Then they asked a panel of doctors to judge whether three of these procedures were given only to appropriate candidates for these procedures. Then they compared the rate of inappropriate use of these three procedures with the overall utilization rates in the eight states to see if they could find a correlation between inappropriate use of these three procedures and above-average utilization rates for all 153 services.

The three procedures they selected for analysis of appropriate use were coronary angiography (a test done to look for blockages in coronary arteries), upper gastrointestinal tract endoscopy, and carotid endarterectomy (a procedure that cleans plaque out of the arteries that run up the sides of the neck). They asked a panel of nine doctors – one panel for each of the three procedures – to agree on a set of criteria with which to judge the appropriateness of the procedure, and then to review the medical records of patients who had undergone that procedure and to indicate whether they thought the procedure was appropriate, inappropriate, or of uncertain value. These physician panels concluded that 17 percent of the angiographies, 17 percent of upper gastrointestinal tract endoscopies, and 32 percent of carotid endarterectomies were inappropriate.[19]

However, when Chassin et al. looked for a correlation between high rates of inappropriate use of these three procedures and high overall rates of use of the 153 procedures, they found none. "[I]n no case can differences in appropriateness explain the large differences in overall rates," they concluded. "Thus, we did not find evidence to support the hypothesis that areas with high use of medical and surgical procedures show these high rates primarily or to any meaningful extent because physicians in these areas perform procedures more often for inappropriate indications than their counterparts in areas of lower use."[20] Other experts agree with this conclusion. "The practice variations literature has not led to the expected conclusion that variations result from overuse," wrote one expert in a 1998 book on the subject.[21]

In the decade after Rand scholars published the first appropriateness studies in 1987, a handful of other appropriateness studies were published. Until the late 1990s, these studies focused almost exclusively on overuse. In view of the small number of these studies, and given their limitations, it was impossible to state what portion of the thousands of treatments available in the U.S. were overused and how extensive the overuse of these treatments was.

To give you some idea of how limited the evidence of overuse was even as late as 1998, nearly three decades after Ellwood began peddling the overuse diagnosis, take a look at Table 4-1. You see there descriptions of the results of just 16 studies of "inappropriate use" (that is, overuse) discussed in a 1998 literature review in the *Milbank Quarterly*.* The 16 studies examined a total of 13 treatments for acute

---

* A literature review is based on a search of the scientific literature to find all the good studies on a given subject. The authors of the *Milbank Quarterly* article actually found 48 articles that were good enough to be included in their review. Only 16 of these studies identified the percentage of patients who received unnecessary acute or chronic care. The others either dealt with preventive care,

and chronic conditions.* Five of these studies examined treatments of acute conditions (all but one were respiratory conditions) and 11 dealt with chronic conditions. The authors observed that it is difficult to "provide a numerical summary" of the studies' findings. However, they calculated a "simple average" (which means they didn't weight the studies according to the prevalence of the disease examined) and reported that "30 percent [of acute-care patients] received contraindicated ... care" and "20 percent of [patients with chronic conditions] received contraindicated care."[22]†

It is not wise to extrapolate from the studies described in Table 4-1 to the entire U.S. health-care system. First, the 13 treatments examined in the 16 studies described in the table constitute a very tiny portion of all treatments offered in this country. There are now 8,000 treatments listed in *Current Procedural Terminology*, the thick book of codes published by the American Medical Association that doctors use to determine which code they should use on claim forms[23] (up from about 7,200 a decade ago).[24]

The second reason why it is unwise to extrapolate from the simple averages of overuse shown in Table 4-1 is that the guidelines used to determine appropriateness are controversial. Consider, for example, the issues raised by the study that claimed to find a 23-percent overuse of ear tubes for otitis media (infection of the inner ear, a condition suffered by three out of four kids under age six) (this study is referred to in Table 4-1). The study, done by Rand researcher Robert Brook and three others,[25] drew withering criticism from physicians, which is some indication that the guideline used in the study to determine what constitutes appropriate use of ear tubes is not universally supported. As one expert put it, "In view of the low degree of agreement on the optimal management of glue ear [another phrase for otitis media], it is not surprising that the conclusions of this appropriateness study were challenged...."[26]

---

or underuse of acute and chronic care.

* Table 4-1 lists 18 conditions studied. However, two of the studies examined more than one condition, which is why the total number of studies – published papers – comes to 16.

† By my calculation, the simple average for chronic patients was 12 percent, not 20, but in view of how crude this methodology is, we needn't tarry long on this difference.

# Table 4-1: Examples of studies reporting the provision of unnecessary services, 1987 to 1997

| Type of treatment | Year of study | Study findings |
|---|---|---|
| **Acute conditions** | | |
| Antibiotics | 1996 | 60% of patients with colds given antibiotics |
| | 1995 | 16% of patients with upper respiratory infections given antibiotics |
| | 1996 | Antibiotics given to more than 70% of patients with pharyngitis, 50% with rhinitis, and 30% with upper respiratory infections |
| Hospitalization | 1995 | 9% of hospital admissions for pneumonia, and 4% of admissions for bronchitis/asthma inappropriate |
| Ear tubes for otitis media | 1994 | 23% percent inappropriate |
| **Chronic conditions** | | |
| Depression | 1993 | 7% of hospital admissions inappropriate |
| Hysterectomy | 1993 | 16% inappropriate |
| Angiography | 1993 | 4% inappropriate |
| | 1987 | 17% inappropriate |
| Coronary artery bypass graft | 1988 | 14% inappropriate |
| | 1993 | 2% inappropriate |
| | 1996 | 2% inappropriate |
| Angioplasty | 1993 | 4% inappropriate |

(Table 4-1 continued)

| | | |
|---|---|---|
| Calcium channel blockers for heart attack patients | 1993 | 21% inappropriate |
| Pacemakers for heart attack patients | 1988 | 20% inappropriate |
| Carotid endarterectomy | 1987 | 32% inappropriate |
| Upper gastroendoscopy | 1987 | 17% inappropriate |
| Cataract extraction | 1996 | 2% inappropriate |

Source: Mark A. Schuster et al., "How good is the quality of health care in the United States?" *Milbank Quarterly* 1998;76:517-563.

---

The decision about when to treat otitis media with ear tubes is complex because it is impossible to predict with certainty all the benefits and adverse reactions that will result from the insertion of ear tubes. The issue is not whether the tubes will permit the inner ear to drain and thereby relieve pressure and pain in the short run; that happens quite predictably. The issue is whether this short-term benefit is augmented further by longer-term improvements in the child's IQ and his ability to hear and speak, and whether these benefits outweigh the possible side-effects, which include adverse reactions to general anesthesia, recurrent infection around the tube, permanent perforation of the ear drum, and hearing loss due to recurrent infections. The research on whether prolonged ear infections do long-term damage to IQ, for example, is inconclusive. One study concluded that children who have otitis media for more than 130 days by the time they are seven are more likely to have a slightly lower IQ than kids who suffered less than 30 days of otitis media. Other studies have not confirmed this association.[27]

Because there are several benefits and risks associated with ear tubes that must be weighed, and because there is scant and/or conflicting scientific evidence about most of them, totaling up all benefits and subtracting all risks, and thereby deriving an unambiguous guideline applicable to all patients, is very difficult to do. But that's precisely what "appropriateness" researchers have to do. The ear tube study defined "appropriate tube placements" to mean "those for which the expected health benefits exceed the expected negative health consequences by a sufficiently wide margin that the procedure is worth doing" (financial costs were not a factor).[28] Moreover, the guideline used in the study was developed by a private-sector, for-profit, utilization review firm called Value Health Sciences (VHS) that did utilization review for MCPs. According to a report in *Medical Economics*, "The VHS company brochure claimed that [it] saved clients $67.5 million from treatment denials in 1995...."[29] Two of the four authors of the Rand ear tube study worked for and held stock in VHS. Is it any wonder that the study's conclusion that 23 percent of tube placements are inappropriate drew a lot of criticism?

A report accompanying another guideline on ear tubes, this one developed by the federal Agency for Health Care Policy and Research, conceded explicitly that the process of determining when ear tubes are appropriate is somewhat subjective. "Of note," said the report, "is that the final recommendations are at least partially subjective; judgments about the quality of the science could not be fully objective...."[30] Other experts have observed that subjectivity arises not only in judging the quality of "the science" of a study (that is, the strength of its methodology), but also in the process of assigning weights to the benefits and harms caused by a treatment.

Just as the variation studies were misused, so too were the appropriateness studies. Beginning in the late 1980s, big business executives, politicians, and scholars sympathetic to managed care developed the habit of indicting the entire U.S. health-care system based on the handful of appropriateness studies available. By roughly 1990, it was conventional wisdom among those who dominated the American health-policy debate that America was wasting one-fourth of its health-care dollar on unnecessary medical services. As reporter Julie Kosterlitz put it in a 1991 article for the *National Journal*, "Somewhere along the line, an assertion of uncertain origin – that perhaps 25 percent of all care delivered in this country was most likely unnecessary – gained currency in federal health policy circles."[31]

The Rand studies, and remarks about these studies by Rand scholars, were unquestionably the origin of this claim. Based on the small number of appropriateness studies available in 1989, Rand's Robert Brook wrote in the *Journal of the American Medical Association* that year, "If one could extrapolate from the available literature, then perhaps one-fourth of hospital days, one-fourth of procedures, and two-fifths of medications could be done without."[32] Brook's extrapolation was broadcast widely by the media. *Financial World*, for example, reprinted Brook's estimate that a fourth of all services are unnecessary in a breathless article entitled, "How doctors have ruined health care."[33] Brook was quoted in AARP's newsletter saying, "Our best guess is that one-quarter of the things we do to people – not only surgery but all medical procedures – we could get rid of without having any impact on health."[34] As the following statement by *Consumer Reports* indicates, the magazine decided the percentage of the health-care dollar wasted on unnecessary services was 20 percent, not 25 percent: "For a wide range of clinical procedures, on average, roughly 20 percent of the money we now spend could be saved with no loss in quality of care."[35]

The claim by Brook and others that the small body of appropriateness studies supported the conclusion that overuse of medical services was rampant was repeated by many other health policy experts. President Clinton also endorsed the 25-percent figure. In his September 22, 1993 speech to the nation introducing his managed-competition bill to Congress, Clinton claimed his bill would cut total health-care spending by $200 billion, or about a fourth of total spending that year.[*] Big business groups all over the country asserted that unnecessary care was costing the nation dearly and that MCPs, armed with appropriateness studies, could solve the problem. "If utilization management and reimbursement were based on quality standards of scientific literature, we would see the costs level out considerably," intoned John M. Burns, MD, vice president of health management for Honeywell, Inc.[36] The increasingly MCP-dominated health insurance industry was, of course, quite eager to promote the notion that "science" had determined once and for all that most medical services were overused.

---

[*] In his 1993 speech, Clinton didn't explain how he thought $200 billion would be saved. But the arguments he and others in his administration made for his bill made it clear they thought the savings would come from reduced services. In 1994, the Congressional Budget Office announced Clinton's plan would save only $37 billion over six years (which amounted to less than a 1 percent cut in total spending per year, far below Clinton's 25-percent figure) (Tom Hamburger, "CBO puts high price on managed competition," Minneapolis *Star Tribune*, May 5, 1994, 7A).

## The evidence that underuse is rampant

Sad to say, health policy researchers are unduly influenced by the opinions of those who have political and economic power. Thus it was that during the heyday of managed care – roughly the last three decades of the 20th Century – researchers like Wennberg and the scholars at the Rand Corporation focused their attention on overuse. It was not until managed care's reputation began to fade in the latter half of the 1990s that the American health policy community began to turn its attention to the problem of underuse. Two Rand Corporation experts took note of this bias in a 1997 article. "Most health services research to date has been directed at identifying and reducing excessive utilization," they wrote. "Little attention has been given to underuse of care."[37] Interestingly, it would be the Rand Corporation, the think tank that had done so much to promote the misperception that the average American overused medical care, that would do more than any other organization to correct that misperception.

There are, broadly speaking, two types of underuse. The first is underuse caused by the failure of patients to get necessary medical services even though they visited a doctor or other health-care professional. Studies that seek to identify this type of underuse face the same difficulties that studies of overuse face, the most significant of which is determining when a service is necessary. The second type of underuse is due to the inability or unwillingness of patients to seek medical care in the first place. This type of underuse is even more difficult to identify. As Mark Chassin put it, "Studying this problem requires searching for events that should have happened but didn't. Identifying patient populations who should have received a particular health service is a difficult and expensive task."[38] It is an expensive task because it requires interviewing a randomly selected group of individuals and, depending on the medical service in question, examining them (for example, taking their blood pressure or checking their teeth for decay).

Studies of underuse of both types were reviewed by Schuster et al. in the 1998 *Milbank Quarterly* literature review of overuse that I cited in my discussion of Table 4-1. Because the results of these studies are much harder to reduce to a few summary statements in a table, I do not present the results in table form as I did for the overuse studies in Table 4-1. Here are some examples of their findings:

- Between 10 and 48 percent of pneumonia patients received appropriate care (for example, blood pressure readings and oxygen therapy);
- Between 6 and 33 percent of hip fracture patients failed to receive appropriate components of care (for example, a serum potassium test and an electrocardiogram);
- 44 percent of pregnant women failed to get all necessary tests during their first or second visit to a physician;
- 45 percent of diabetics did not receive a blood cholesterol screening during the previous year;
- 45 percent of people with high blood pressure did not have it under control;
- 33 percent of women over age 69 with breast cancer failed to receive appropriate treatment;
- 30 percent of heart attack patients who should have received thrombolytics did not;
- 14 percent of deaths in a hospital from stroke, pneumonia, or heart attack could have been prevented with appropriate care.[39]

After surveying the studies of underuse, Schuster et al. did the same simple calculation of underuse rates they had done for overuse and concluded that "about 50 percent" of patients failed to receive necessary *preventive* care, 30 percent of *acute care* patients failed to get necessary care, and 40 percent of *chronically ill* patients failed to receive necessary care. Table 4-2 compares these figures with the *over*use figures reported by Schuster et al. You can see that the overuse and underuse rates were even for acute care, but that underuse was much worse in the preventive and chronic care categories. This is a crude method of comparing overuse and underuse rates, so readers should not view them as precise. Nevertheless, they do suggest underuse is the more prevalent problem.

Schuster et al. made it clear their literature review was not "exhaustive." It was limited to studies published in peer-reviewed journals between 1987 and June 1997. In Table 4-3, I list more data on underuse derived from studies that fell outside the time frame used by Shuster et al. With one exception, these studies appeared around or after June

---

## Table 4-2: Underuse of health-care services is more prevalent than overuse: Results from the 1998 review by Schuster et al.*

| Type of service | Extent of overuse | Extent of underuse |
|---|---|---|
| Prevention | 0% | 50% |
| Acute care | 30% | 30% |
| Chronic care | 20% | 40% |

* The authors of this study examined a total of 48 articles published between 1987 and June 1997. These articles covered a wide array of services, ranging from heart surgery to antibiotics to ear tubes to prenatal care to immunizations. The authors divided the articles into three categories – preventive services, acute care services, and chronic care services – and calculated the "simple averages" of the amount of over- and underuse for each category.

Source: Mark A. Schuster et al., "How good is the quality of health care in the United States?" *Milbank Quarterly* 1998;76:517-563, 521.

---

1997. As was the case with the underuse studies reviewed by Schuster et al., the list in Table 4-3 includes examples of both types of underuse – underuse by patients who actually visited a doctor and underuse by people who never sought care in the first place. These studies reveal substantial rates of underuse, some as high as 80 and 90 percent, for a wide variety of common illnesses and conditions.

In Table 4-3, I list a pre-1987 study because it was one of the most rigorous studies of health-care utilization ever done, and because its discovery of gross underuse was so surprising and so little noted. The study I am referring to, the Rand Health Insurance Experiment, is well known to health policy experts. The study, conducted between 1974 and 1981, looked at how health-care utilization rates and health are affected by out-of-pocket payments. It spawned more than a dozen papers published over the course of the 1980s and early 1990s. One of those papers reported that only 22 percent of patients who were insured with first-dollar coverage, that is, insurance with no co-payments or deductibles, bothered to visit a doctor after suffering from one of five "serious symptoms." The "serious symptoms" were "chest pain when

# Table 4-3: Underuse of health care is widespread: Other studies on underuse not included in the review by Schuster et al.

- Nine of ten nursing homes have staff levels below "minimally necessary" levels.[a]
- Eight of ten Americans *insured with first-dollar coverage* do not seek treatment for serious symptoms such as loss of consciousness or unexplained bleeding.[b]
- Two-thirds of all Americans with mental disorders do not seek treatment.[c]
- Three-fifths of elderly Medicare beneficiaries diagnosed with gall stones plus inflammation of the gall bladder, inflammation of one or several bile ducts, or inflammation of the pancreas, or more than one of these inflammatory conditions, failed to have a cholecystectomy (surgery to remove the gall bladder).[d]
- Half of all *insured* Americans suffering from high blood pressure are not getting treated for it.[e]
- Half of *insured* patients who should have an angiogram do not get it.[f]
- Half of all Americans suffering from depression do not get treatment for it, and four-fifths do not get adequate treatment.[g]
- Half of newborns are discharged early, and two-thirds of those receive delayed follow-up care.[h]
- A third of Americans do not see a dentist at least once a year.[i]
- Three-tenths of the nation's diabetics do not know they have diabetes.[j]
- One-fourth of *insured* patients who should have either bypass surgery or angioplasty get neither.[k]
- One-seventh of those with disabilities who have a prescription fail to take their drugs as prescribed.[l]
- One-eighth of insured adult Americans either do not get medical care they need or they delay getting it.[m]

(a) Robert Pear, "U.S. recommending strict new rules at nursing homes," *New York Times*, July 23, 2000, A1; Robert Pear, "Nine of ten nursing homes lack adequate staff, study finds," *New York Times*, February 18, 2002, http://www.health-

(Table 4-3 continued)

coalition.ca/nyt.html, accessed April 11, 2003. Problems created by staff shortages include preventable conditions such as severe bedsores, malnutrition, dehydration, abnormal weight loss, severe infections, and congestive heart failure. The report estimated that adequate staffing of nursing homes would require an 8 percent increase in total spending (or $7.6 billion annually).

(b) Martin F. Shapiro et al., "Effects of cost-sharing on seeking care for serious and minor symptoms," *Annals of Internal Medicine* 1986;104:246-51.

(c) Robert Pear, "Few seek to treat mental disorders, a U.S. study says: Half of nation affected," *New York Times*, December 13, 1999, A1.

(d) Steven M. Asch et al., "Measuring underuse of necessary care among elderly Medicare beneficiaries using inpatient and outpatient claims," *Journal of the American Medical Association* 2000;284:2325-2333.

(e) David J. Hyman and Valory N. Pavlik, "Characteristics of patients with uncontrolled hypertension in the United States," *New England Journal of Medicine* 2001;345:479-486.

(f) Marianne Laouri et al., "Underuse of coronary angiography: Application of a clinical method," *International Journal For Quality In Health Care* 1997;9:15-22 (Schuster et al. included this study in their review); Pushkal P. Garg et al., "Understanding individual and small area variation in the underuse of coronary angiography following acute myocardial infarction," *Medical Care* 2002;40:614-626.

(g) Ronald Kessler et al., "The epidemiology of major depressive disorder: Results from the National Comorbidity Survey Replication," *Journal of the American Medical Association* 2003;290:3095-4105.

(h) Alison A. Galbraith et al., "Newborn early discharge revisited: Are California newborns receiving recommended postnatal services?" *Pediatrics* 2003;111:364-371. The authors defined early discharge as "a post-delivery stay of less than 48 hours for vaginal deliveries and 96 hours for Caesarean sections" (364). This standard was endorsed in 1992 by the American Academy of Pediatrics (AAP) and the American College of Obstetricians and Gynecologists. By 2001, 43 states had passed legislation requiring third-party payers to meet these postnatal stay recommendations. The AAP amended its guideline in 1995 to add recommendations on how quickly in-office or home follow-up should occur.

(i) Report by Oral Health America, described in "'Silent epidemic' continues: Poor oral health," Minneapolis *Star Tribune*, January 29, 2002, A3.

(j) American Diabetes Association, http://www.diabetes.org/info/diabetesinfo. jsp, accessed December 8, 2003.

(k) Lucian L. Leape et al., "Underuse of cardiac procedures: Do women, ethnic minorities, and the uninsured fail to receive needed revascularization?" *Annals of Internal Medicine* 1999;130:231-233. The study by Leape et al. examined revascularization underuse rates for both insured and uninsured patients, and reported that insurance status had no bearing on underuse rates; 26 percent of both the insured and uninsured patients failed to get revascularization surgery. Laouri et al. also conducted a study of the revascularization underuse rate and reported a 25 percent

(Table 4-3 continued)

underuse rate among a group of both insured and uninsured, but the underuse rate for the uninsured was worse than for the insured (Marianne Laouri et al., "Underuse of coronary revascularization procedures: Application of a clinical method," *Journal of the American College of Cardiology* 1997;29:891-897).

(l) Jae Kennedy and Christopher Erb, "Prescription noncompliance due to cost among adults with disabilities in the United States," *American Journal of Public Health* 2002;92:1120-1124.

(m) Bradley C. Strunk and Peter J. Cunningham, *Treading Water: Americans' Access to Needed Medical Care, 1997-2001*, Center for Studying Health System Change, http://www.hschange.com/CONTENT/421/? topic=topic02, accessed December 17, 2002.

---

exercising; bleeding other than nose bleeds or periods not caused by accidents; loss of consciousness ... ; shortness of breath with light exercise or light work; [and] weight loss of more than ten pounds ... (unless you were dieting)."[40] For patients who had insurance *with* co-payments, the underuse was only slightly worse; just 18 percent of the cost-sharing patients sought care for serious symptoms. One might think that the authors' finding of an 80-percent rate of underuse among patients with serious symptoms warranted considerable discussion and follow-up research. But, remember, these were the early days of the managed-care juggernaut and researchers were far more interested in documenting overuse than underuse. The authors offered only this single, understated comment: "Finally, regardless of [cost-sharing], most persons reporting serious ... symptoms did not report seeing a physician."[41]

The rest of the studies listed in Table 4-3 were published in 1997 or later. I want to discuss several of these in some detail, partly to strengthen my argument that underuse is much worse than overuse, and partly to give you some idea of how much more difficult it is to measure underuse than it is to measure overuse. I begin with three studies of heart patients – the one that found that nearly half of insured patients who should have had an angiogram didn't get one, and two that reported that a fourth of patients who were told by their doctors they needed some form of heart surgery – coronary artery bypass graft (CABG) or angioplasty – didn't have it done.

These three studies, done in the late 1990s, contradicted appropriateness studies done in the late 1980s and early 1990s which found small amounts of overuse of these services. A study by Marianne Laouri et al. followed up on 352 patients who tested positive on a stress test for an angiogram.* They found 44 percent underuse: 44 percent of the patients who should have had an angiogram still hadn't gotten one within a year after their stress test.[42] Laouri et al. then followed up on the patients who had angiograms that indicated they should have had either bypass surgery or angioplasty (the two procedures are known collectively as "revascularization procedures").† They found that 25 percent of these patients who should have had bypass surgery or angioplasty got neither. The authors concluded, "Underuse of coronary revascularization procedures ... occurs to a significant degree even among insured patients attending private hospitals."[43] Similar findings were reported by Leape et al. in a study of New York cardiac patients; they found a revascularization underuse rate of 26 percent.[44]

Table 4-4 compares the *overuse* rates for CABG, angioplasty and angiography shown in Table 4-1 with the *underuse* rates for these procedures I have just reviewed. The underuse rates are much higher than the overuse rates. The difference between the overuse and underuse studies is that the overuse studies examined only those patients who received a service (a CABG, for example), while the underuse studies examined all patients who were *eligible* for the service.

But note that even these studies of underuse by heart patients were limited to patients who had contact with the medical system. We can state with certainty that many people, especially many uninsured people, who should be examined for heart disease do not visit a doctor – on a timely basis or at all. That means that the 44-percent rate of underuse for angiography and the 25- and 26-percent rates of underuse for revascularization shown in Table 4-4 do not reflect the real rates of underuse. The real rates are even higher. How much higher we can't

---

* In stress tests patients walk on a treadmill with sensors glued at various places on their torso to measure heart function. If the test suggests the patient's heart is not functioning normally, an angiogram may be ordered. An angiogram is a moving picture of the heart. The angiogram reveals narrowed (or "occluded") arteries.

† Angioplasty is a procedure in which a tube with a balloon on the end of it is inserted into an artery in the leg or arm and threaded into the blocked coronary artery. When the balloon reaches the area where the artery has become dangerously narrow, the balloon is opened up to flatten the artery walls and thereby expand the diameter of the artery.

## Table 4-4: Underuse of invasive cardiac procedures among insured patients is much worse than overuse

| Type of service | Extent of overuse (year of study) | Extent of underuse (year of study) |
|---|---|---|
| Angiography* | 17% (1987)<br>4% (1993) | 44% (1997) |
| CABG* | 14% (1988)<br>2% (1993)<br>2% (1995) | |
| Angioplasty* | 4% (1993) | |
| Revascularization* | | 25% (1997)<br>26% (1999) |

* An angiogram is a moving x-ray of the coronary arteries. CABG stands for coronary artery bypass graft. Angioplasty is a procedure in which a balloon is inserted into a coronary artery and expanded to open the artery. Revascularization refers collectively to CABG and angioplasty.

Sources: Overuse studies are cited in Mark A. Schuster et al., "How good is the quality of health care in the United States?" *Milbank Quarterly* 1998;76:517-563. The three underuse studies are: Marianne Laouri et al., "Underuse of coronary angiography: Application of a clinical method," *International Journal of Quality Health Care* 1997;9:15-22; M. Laouri et al., "Underuse of coronary revascularization procedures: Application of a clinical method," *Journal of the American College of Cardiology* 1997;29:891-897; and Lucian L. Leape et al., "Underuse of cardiac procedures: Do women, ethnic minorities, and the uninsured fail to receive needed revascularization?" *Annals of Internal Medicine* 1999;130:231-233.

say. The same cannot be said of the overuse studies listed in Tables 4-1 and 4-4; there is no unseen, unmeasured group of *over*users out there analogous to the unseen and unmeasured *under*users of cardiac services.

Unlike the studies of cardiac services, several of the underuse studies listed in Table 4-3 did examine underuse of both types – underuse by people who had contact with the medical system, and underuse by people who did not. The study on underuse of treatment for hypertension (high blood pressure) is an example. The authors of this study, which appeared in 2001 in the *New England Journal of Medicine*, did not merely examine records of people who had visited doctors. Instead they conducted a national survey of adults to determine the prevalence of hypertension (which means they actually had to take people's blood pressure) and whether people with hypertension were getting treatment. The authors reported an enormous amount of hypertension (42 million adults during the 1992-1994 period of the survey), and a very high rate of underuse among these hypertensives: 31 percent were unaware they had high blood pressure, and another 17 percent were aware of their hypertension but were not being treated for it. These two numbers yield a total underuse rate of 48 percent.[45*] The authors of this paper did not attempt to determine the reasons for this gross underuse (such as the high price of anti-hypertension drugs). They noted that the underusers saw a physician at least three times in the previous year, and that health insurance status (having health insurance or not having it) was not correlated with underuse. Rampant underuse of hypertension treatment is a serious problem; uncontrolled high blood pressure can lead to stroke and heart disease.

The studies on underuse of dental services, diabetes treatment, and mental health care in Table 4-3 were also based on surveys, which means their results reflect underuse of both types. One-third of Americans don't see a dentist even once a year, according to a 2002 report.[46] Five million of the nation's 16 million diabetics don't know they have diabetes.[47] In 1999 the U.S. Surgeon General released a report that concluded that "22 percent of the population has a diagnosable mental disorder" and that "nearly two-thirds of all people with diagnosable mental disorders do not seek treatment." The *New York Times* reported, "The report is significant because it meticulously analyzes huge amounts of data and puts the imprimatur of the government on the finding, just as the surgeon general's report on smoking and health did in 1964."[48] The Surgeon General attributed the failure to seek treatment to lack of

---

* Another 29 percent were being treated for hypertension, but their blood pressure was still high (above 140/90). Only 23 percent of Americans with high blood pressure were being treated for it and had their blood pressure within normal limits.

health insurance, gaps in health insurance, and to the stigma associated with mental illness.

With one exception, I did not include in Table 4-3 any studies on underuse of medical services caused by the current nurse shortage, a shortage that materialized around 1990 and promises to become disastrous by 2020. Numerous studies on the effects of the shortage exist, but the results generally can't be expressed in the easy-to-understand percentage terms shown in Table 4-3. These studies do tell us the nurse shortage is already harming patients in nursing homes and hospitals.

Reports issued by the Department of Health and Human Services in 2000 and in 2002 documented enormous gaps between the work force levels needed in the nation's nursing homes and the actual work force levels.[49] According to the 2002 report, "In 2000, over 91 percent of nursing homes had nurse aide staffing levels that fell below the thresholds identified as minimally necessary to provide the needed care" (this is the first study cited in Table 4-3). Problems created by staff shortages in nursing homes include severe bedsores, malnutrition, infections, and congestive heart failure. The 2002 report estimated that adequate staffing of nursing homes would require an 8 percent increase in total spending (or $7.6 billion annually).

Research has established a clear connection between quality of care in hospitals and the nurse-to-patient ratio. The strongest study appeared in the *Journal of the American Medical Association* in 2002. It found that mortality rates among surgical patients were 31 percent higher in hospitals where each registered nurse had to take care of eight or more patients than in hospitals where each RN cared for four or fewer patients. Linda Aiken et al. estimated that 20,000 patients die every year because they check into a hospital with overworked nurses.[50] Patients in wards inadequately staffed by nurses can suffer underuse in a variety of forms, including failure to get medications on time or at all, and failure to get timely care for serious symptoms.

The undersupply of emergency rooms and ER staff creates another form of underuse that is hard to measure precisely. The crisis in America's emergency rooms, which has been building for the last quarter-century, is intimately related to the nurse shortage, but the nurse shortage is not the only cause of the ER crisis. Over the last decade, a mountain of anecdotal evidence and a small body of scientific evidence has accumulated indicating that the supply of emergency care services is woefully insufficient to meet demand, in both urban and rural areas.[51] According to a survey released by the American College of Emergency Physicians and the American Hospital Association in 2002, six of ten hospitals report that their ERs are so near capacity that they cannot easily handle more patients.[52]

Evidence also indicates an enormous amount of underuse of home-care services. Families USA reported that 66 percent of the elderly who received long-term care services at home in 1993 received only unpaid services, and another 24 percent received both paid and unpaid services. Of the unpaid caregivers, 32 percent defined their own health as "fair or poor," yet these caregivers provided a total of 39 hours of care a week. It is sometimes difficult to distinguish the care one would expect family members to give one another from care that ought to be provided by health-care professionals.[53] Nevertheless, these statistics suggest that a substantial portion of unpaid home care is a source of emotional and physical distress to the caregivers and should, therefore, be provided by the health-care system. But it isn't.

If we had no other research to go on other than that which I have reported so far in this section, we would be justified in concluding that underuse is much worse than overuse. But we have one more very important study to review, and that study provides the most convincing evidence to date that the overuse problem pales in comparison to the underuse problem. In 2003, Rand Corporation analysts published in the *New England Journal of Medicine* the most comprehensive study to date on the issue of over- and underuse. It was the most comprehensive for three reasons. First, it examined both underuse and overuse (the vast majority of appropriateness studies examined only one or the other). Second, it examined both types of underuse – underuse by people who visited a doctor and by those who did not. Third, it examined an unusually large sample of people (13,000 adults in 12 cities) and an unusually large number of medical services (preventive care services plus hundreds of other services appropriate for 30 types of illness or conditions). The authors' findings came as a shock only to those who had been listening too closely to the health insurance industry's propaganda. The authors found that the rate of underuse was more than four times the rate of overuse. "[W]e found greater problems with underuse (46.3 percent of participants did not receive recommended care ...) than with overuse (11.3 percent of participants received care that was not recommended and was potentially harmful)," they wrote.[45]

It is ironic that the Rand Corporation, which did so much to nourish the overuse myth with its appropriateness studies of the late 1980s and early 1990s, was the source of this latest study, a study which drove an enormous stake deep into the heart of the overuse myth. The myth that the average American overuses health care, however, does not survive on truth. It owes its existence, rather, to incessant repetition by the health insurance industry and its allies. These people will not cease to peddle the overuse myth merely because the evidence against the myth is now very strong. The livelihood of the insurance industry depends on the perpetuation of the myth. And so, as seriously wounded as it is, the myth will continue to stagger about the theater of American politics for years to come, demanding with great irritation that the spotlight be trained exclusively on it.

## Comparisons of American utilization rates with those of other countries

Comparisons of American medical use rates with those of other countries reinforce the conclusion that underuse is a serious problem in the U.S. and that overuse cannot explain the high cost of U.S. medical care. If excessive use of services (whether caused by doctors or patients) were the primary driver of total spending in the U.S., one would expect to find that citizens of other countries utilize medical care less often than Americans do. With the exception of several surgical procedures such as bypass surgery and C-sections, the evidence indicates Americans get fewer, not more, medical services.

Table 4-5 indicates that Americans are more likely than Canadians and Germans to experience denial of medical services or to have to postpone necessary medical care for financial reasons. One-and-a-half to twice as many Americans said they were not able to get, or had to postpone, needed medical care in 1995. Notice the enormous differences in out-of-pocket expenses. Americans paid an average of $993 out of their own pockets in 1995, three times what the average Canadian or German paid that year.

---

## Table 4-5: Americans are underinsured compared to Canadians and Germans: Out-of-pocket expenditures, and percent of Americans, Canadians, and Germans unable to get needed care, 1995

| | United States (n = 1,214) | Canada (n = 1,472) | Germany (n = 1,210) |
|---|---|---|---|
| Out-of-pocket expenditures last year | $993 | $302 | $328 |
| Not able to get needed medical care | 12% | 8%* | 6%* |
| Postponed needed medical care | 30% | 16%* | 13%* |
| Serious problem having enough money to pay doctor or hospital bills | 20% | 6%* | 3%* |
| Discouraged from medical treatment | 19% | 12%* | 6%* |

\* Statistically significant at .05 level.

Source: Karen Donelan et al., "All payer, single payer, managed care, no payer: Patients' perspectives in three nations," *Health Affairs* 1996;15(2):254-265.

---

Tables 4-6 and 4-7 also contradict the argument that "excessive" use of services explains high U.S. health-care costs. Table 4-6 compares the number of acute care hospital beds and hospital use rates of the countries with the ten most expensive health-care systems. You can see that the U.S. has far fewer beds available per capita than do the other countries, and, not surprisingly, that Americans have the lowest hospital use rates. In only two countries (Canada and the Netherlands) are patients less likely to be admitted to a hospital (the table uses discharge rates, which correspond closely with admission rates), and in only two countries (Iceland and France) are patients kicked out faster than Americans are. But only in America are *both* the admission rate and the average length of stay low. The result is that the total number of days in the hospital per 100 citizens (see the fourth column) is lowest in the U.S.

Table 4-7 examines data for doctors and nurses for the same ten nations listed in Table 4-6. It indicates America has a very low doctor-to-population ratio, Americans see their doctors infrequently, and America has a very low nurse-to-population ratio relative to other nations with expensive health systems. Canada, which spends just a little

---

**Table 4-6: Americans use fewer hospital services: Hospital capacity and use rates in the ten most expensive health-care systems as of 2001**

| Country | Hospital beds per 1,000 population[a] | Discharges per 100 population | Average length of stay (days) | Discharges x ALOS |
|---|---|---|---|---|
| US | 2.9 | 9.8 | 5.8 | 57 |
| Switzerland | 4.0 | na[b] | 9.2 | na[b] |
| Norway | 3.1 | 16.0 | 5.8 | 93 |
| Germany | na[b] | 20.1 | 11.6 | 233 |
| Canada | 4.7[c] | 9.1 | 7.3 | 66 |
| Luxembourg | 5.9 | 17.9 | 7.6 | 136 |
| Iceland | 3.7[c] | 15.6[d] | 5.7[d] | 89 |
| Netherlands | 3.3 | 9.1 | 8.6 | 78 |
| France | 4.0 | 25.2 | 5.7 | 144 |
| Australia | 3.7 | 15.7 | 6.1 | 96 |

(a) Some nations use a substantial portion of their hospital beds for long-term care patients. The numbers in this column are for acute care beds only.

(b) Na means "not available" from the source cited below.

(c) 1995 data.

(d) 1998 data.

Source: Organization for Economic Cooperation and Development, *OECD Health Data 2004*, *3rd ed.*, http://www.oecd.org, accessed June 6, 2005.

---

over half of what the U.S. spends on health care per capita, has many more nurses per person than we do, and Canadians see their doctors more often than we do.

Table 4-8 presents the findings of an article published in *Lancet*, the highly regarded British medical journal. This study found that Japanese doctors (doctors who practice in Japan) are nearly *twice* as likely to order three different types of treatment for terminally ill gastric cancer patients than are Japanese-American doctors (doctors of Japanese descent practicing in America). Specifically, Japanese doctors were much more likely to order blood transfusions for patients losing blood through their intestines; parenteral nutrition (getting food into the body by injection

## 4-7: Americans have fewer doctors and nurses: Physician- and nurse-to-population ratios, and physician visits per person, in the countries with the ten most expensive systems as of 2001

| Country | Practicing physicians per 1,000 population, 2003 | Visits to physicians per person | Practicing nurses per 1,000 population, 2003 |
|---------|---------|---------|---------|
| US | 2.4 | 5.6[a] | 7.9 |
| Switzerland | 3.5 | 10.7 | |
| Norway | 3.0 | 10.4 | |
| Germany | 3.3 | 7.3[b] | 9.9 |
| Canada | 2.1 | 6.2[a] | 9.4 |
| Luxembourg | 2.5 | 10.6 | |
| Iceland | 3.0 | 13.7 | |
| Netherlands | 3.3 | 5.6[c] | 12.8 |
| France | 3.3 | 6.9[a] | 7.3 |
| Australia | 2.5 | 6.2[d] | 10.2 |

(a) 2001 data.
(b) 2000 data.
(c) Year not listed in the source.
(d) 2002 data.
Sources: Physician-to-population ratios are from Organization for Economic Cooperation and Development, *OECD Health Data 2004, 3rd ed.*, http://www.oecd.org, accessed June 6, 2005. Physician visits are from Gerard F. Anderson and Peter S. Hussey, *Multinational Comparisons of Health Systems Data, 2004*, Commonwealth Fund, http://www.cmwf.org., accessed June 7, 2005. Nurse-to-population ratios are from *OECD Health Data 2005*, http://www.oecd.org/document/16/0,2340,fr_2649_34631_2085200_1_1_1_1,00.html, accessed July 20, 2005.

into muscles or veins) for patients whose cancer is causing them to be malnourished; and drugs called "vasopressors" that raise blood pressure (by causing blood vessels to constrict) in patients who, because of blood loss, have low blood pressure. The study did not seek to identify the causes of these differences. The spread of HMOs in the U.S. during the 1980s and 1990s, which increased pressure on doctors not to order services, no doubt played an important role. Japan, like all other industrialized nations, puts much more emphasis on controlling the *price* of health-care services than it does on the *volume* of services.

There is some evidence that America's shorter hospital stays are actually *adding* to total health-care spending because patients ejected from the hospital too early wind up needing additional services when their conditions worsen. A study published in the *Journal of Thoracic and Cardiovascular Surgery*, for example, found that this is the case for patients who undergo bypass surgery. The average length-of-stay for bypass patients in U.S. hospitals fell from nine days to 5.4 days between 1990 and 1998, but during that time readmissions to hospitals and use of extended care facilities rose. In 1990, almost all bypass patients went home after leaving the hospital and only 0.5 percent had to be readmitted. But by 1998, 43 percent left the hospital and stayed for more than

---

## Table 4-8: Doctors in Japan order more services for cancer patients than Japanese-American doctors do: Percent of Japanese and Japanese-American doctors who would recommend life-sustaining treatment for terminally ill patients with gastric cancer

|  | Japanese doctors | Japanese-American doctors |
|---|---|---|
| Blood transfusions for gastrointestinal bleeding | 74% | 42% |
| Total parenteral nutrition for malnutrition | 67% | 33% |
| Vasopressors for life-threatening hypotension | 61% | 34% |

Source: A. Asai et al., "Attitudes of Japanese and Japanese-American physicians towards life-sustaining treatment," *Lancet* 1995;346:356-59.

ten days at an extended care facility and only 57 percent went home, while 5 percent had to be readmitted.[55]

As I noted earlier, a few studies indicate that Americans get more of certain types of treatments, particularly surgery, than do citizens of other countries. On the other hand, a few studies indicate Americans get an average amount of other types of expensive services. Table 4-9 shows that the American consumption of bone marrow transplants for leukemia occurs at a rate midway between France's (the high rate) and Germany's (the low rate). Bone marrow transplantation is a very expensive procedure (it cost $140,000 in the U.S. in 1994).

## Closing thoughts on the excessive volume excuse

To sum up, the preponderance of the evidence indicates (a) underuse of the U.S. health-care system is much more extensive than overuse, and (b) the average American may receive more of a few expensive services than do citizens in other industrialized countries, but Americans get fewer hospital and physician services (the core of every nation's health system) and they complain more often about not getting needed medical care. The excessive-use-of-services excuse, it turns out, is not true of the average American – the average American underuses health services – and, in any case, overuse cannot explain why the U.S. system is twice as expensive as the systems of the rest of the industrialized world.

Advocates of managed competition and large deductibles have a common interest in persuading the public that excessive volume, not excessive price, is the problem. They differ, however, in who they think is to blame for excessive volume. Managed-competition advocates blame doctors primarily, while large-deductible advocates blame patients. But the fundamental premise both camps share – that volume is excessive – is wrong. Rather than prattle on about excessive use of services, both camps should acknowledge that America suffers some overuse and a lot of underuse. This they will be reluctant to do, however, because it makes their solutions look silly. How can you argue that the fee-for-service system is the great engine of inflation, and that managed-care tools are needed to combat fee-for-service incentives, if underuse is worse than overuse? How can you argue that patients should be exposed to deductibles of thousands of dollars when millions of Americans, many of them insured with small deductibles, are already underusing the system?

## Table 4-9: Americans get an average number of bone marrow transplants: Annual rate of allogeneic bone marrow transplants per 100,000 population in ten nations, 1989 through 1991

| | |
|---|---|
| France | 1.34 |
| Sweden | 0.90 |
| Canada | 0.89 |
| Australia | 0.88 |
| United Kingdom | 0.82 |
| United States | 0.81 |
| Denmark | 0.78 |
| Netherlands | 0.78 |
| New Zealand | 0.74 |
| Germany | 0.56 |

Source: George Silberman et al., "Availability and appropriateness of allogeneic bone marrow transplantations for chronic myeloid leukemia in ten countries," *New England Journal of Medicine* 1994:331:1063-1067.

Managed care and large deductibles may reduce unnecessary care, but they will also reduce *necessary* care. The solution to overuse is more research on what works, and more education of doctors and patients about that research. The solution to underuse is more education of patients and doctors, little or no out-of-pocket costs (at least for low-income people), and universal health insurance. For the true believers in managed care and large deductibles, these solutions don't glitter like the city on the hill they dream of. Research and education are, by comparison to these grand schemes, rather prosaic. They do not require a PhD in economics to comprehend. But they do have one important advantage: They will work much more effectively.

# Endnotes

[1] Steven Foldes and Andy Czajkowski (then president and CEO of Blue Cross and Blue Shield of Minnesota), "Managed care holds down costs, doesn't hurt quality," Minneapolis *Star Tribune*, January 3, 1998.

[2] Bill Brubaker, "Aetna's unmet claims," *Washington Post*, February 25, 2001, F1.

[3] Ceci Connolly, "Health care's soaring cost takes a toll: Squeeze hits workers, firms and government," *Washington Post*, July 9, 2002, A1, http://www.washingtonpost.com/ac2/wp-dyn?pagename=article&node=&contentId=A41642-2002Jul8&notFound=true, accessed October 12, 2002.

[4] Michael Tanner, "Chapter 2: What's wrong with the present system," in Grace-Marie Arnett, ed., *Empowering Health Care Consumers Through Tax Reform*, University of Michigan Press, Ann Arbor, September 1999, http://www.galen.org./book.asp, accessed December 31, 2003.

[5] Julie Appleby, "Finger pointers can't settle on who's to blame for health costs," *USA Today*, August 20, 2002, http://www.usatoday.com/money/industries/health/2002-08-20-blame-game_x.htm, accessed September 23, 2003.

[6] CBS Evening News, "Health insurance keeps hiking," reported by CBS News Correspondent Wyatt Andrews, August 14, 2002.

[7] John Wennberg and Alan Gittelsohn, "Small area variations in health care delivery," *Science* 1973;182:1102-1108.

[8] J. E. Wennberg, "Dealing with medical practice variations: A proposal for action," *Health Affairs* 1984; 4(2):6-32.

[9] J. E. Wennberg, "Population illness rates do not explain population hospitalization rates," *Medical Care* 1987;25:354-359.

[10] K. McPherson et al., "Small-area variations in the use of common surgical procedures: An international comparison of New England, England, and Norway," *New England Journal of Medicine* 1982;307:1310-1314.

[11] Mark Chassin et al., "Variations in the use of medical and surgical services by the Medicare population," *New England Journal of Medicine* 1986;314:285-290, 285.

[12] Francis C. Notzon et al., "Comparison of national cesarean-section rates," *New England Journal of Medicine* 1987;316:386-389. The average for the countries other than the U.S. and Canada was derived by the author from Table 1 of this paper.

[13] Organization for Economic Cooperation and Development, *OECD Health Data 2004, 3rd ed.*, http://www.oecd.org, accessed June 6, 2005.

[14] Dan Vergano, "Operations often depend on where you live," *USA Today*, September 19, 2000, http://www.usatoday.com/life/health/surgery/lhsur019.htm, accessed November 19, 2001.

[15] Chassin et al., op cit., 289.

[16] Bradford H. Gray, "The legislative battle over health services research," *Health Affairs* 1992;11(4):38-66, 62.

[17] The Pepper Commission: U.S. Bipartisan Commission on Comprehensive Health Care, *A Call For Action: Final Report*, U.S. Government Printing Office, Washington DC, 1990, 40.

[18] Robin Marantz Henig, "The unkindest cut of all: Unnecessary operations raise costs, risks to patients," *AARP Bulletin*, September 1992, 4.

[19] Mark R. Chassin et al., "Does inappropriate use explain geographic variations in the use of health care services? A study of three procedures," *Journal of the American Medical Association* 1987;258:2533-2537.

[20] Ibid., 2535-2536.

[21] Judith Wilson Ross, "Practice guidelines: Texts in search of authority," in *Getting Doctors to Listen: Ethics and Outcomes Data in Context*, Philip J. Boyle ed., Georgetown University Press, Washington, DC, 1998, 41-70, 41.

[22] Mark A. Schuster et al., "How good is the quality of health care in the United States?" *Milbank Quarterly* 1998;76:517-563, 521.

[23] Wayne Guglielmo, "The new Medicare law," *Medical Economics*, January 9, 2004, 37, 39.

[24] U.S. General Accounting Office, *Health Care Reform: "Report Cards" Are Useful but Significant Issues Need to be Addressed*, September 1994, 36.

[25] Lawrence C. Kleinman et al., "The medical appropriateness of tympanostomy tubes proposed for children younger than 16 years in the United States," *Journal of the American Medical Association* 1994;271:1250-1255.

[26] Gert Jan van Der Wilt and Peter F. de Vries Robbe, "The quest for the trial to end all trials," in *Getting Doctors to Listen: Ethics and Outcomes Data in Context*, Philip J. Boyle, et al., Georgetown University Press, Washington, DC, 1998, 86-99, 89.

[27] Ibid.

[28] Kleinman et al., op cit., 1251.

[29] Robert Lowes, "Straightforward UR – or a 'machine of denial'?" *Medical Economics*, May 8, 2000, 180-206.

[30] Ross, op cit., 62.

[31] Julie Kosterlitz, "Cookbook medicine," *National Journal*, March 9, 1991, 574-577, 575.

[32] Robert Brook, "Practice guidelines and practicing medicine: Are they compatible?" *Journal of the American Medical Association* 1989;262:3027-3030, quoted in Charles E. Phelps, "The methodological foundations of studies of the appropriateness of medical care," *New England Journal of Medicine* 1993;329:1241-1245, 1241.

[33] Lauren Chambliss and Sharon Reier, "How doctors have ruined health care," *Financial World*, January 9, 1990, 46-52, 47.

[34] Henig, op cit., 2.

[35] "Wasted health care dollars," *Consumer Reports*, July 1992, 435-448, 435.

[36] Judith Yates Borger, "Is the sky the limit?" *Corporate Report Minnesota*, February 1990, 62, 66.

[37] R. L. Kravitz and M. Laouri, "Measuring and averting underuse of necessary cardiac procedures: A summary of results and future directions," *Joint Commission Journal on Quality Improvement* 1997;23:268-76.

[38] Mark R. Chassin, "Quality of care: Time to act," *Journal of the American Medical Association* 1991;266:3472-3473, 3472.

[39] Schuster et al., op cit.

[40] Martin F. Shapiro et al., "Effects of cost sharing on seeking care for serious and minor symptoms: Results of a randomized controlled trial," *Annals of Internal Medicine* 1986;104:246-251, Table 1.

[41] Ibid., 250.

[42] Marianne Laouri et al., "Underuse of coronary angiography: Application of a clinical method," *International Journal For Quality In Health Care* 1997;9:15-22.

[43] Marianne Laouri et al., "Underuse of coronary revascularization procedures: Application of a clinical method," *Journal of the American College of Cardiology* 1997;29:891-897.

[44] Lucian L. Leape et al., "Underuse of cardiac procedures: Do women, ethnic minorities, and the uninsured fail to receive needed revascularization?" *Annals of Internal Medicine* 1999;130:231-233.

[45] David J. Hyman and Valory N. Pavlik, "Characteristics of patients with uncontrolled hypertension in the United States," *New England Journal of Medicine* 2001;345:479-486.

[46] Report by Oral Health America, described in "'Silent epidemic' continues: Poor oral health," Minneapolis *Star Tribune*, January 29, 2002, A3.

[47] American Diabetes Association, http://www.diabetes.org/main/application/commercewf?origin=*jsp&event=link(B1), accessed March 6, 2002.

[48] Robert Pear, "Few seek to treat mental disorders, a U.S. study says: Half of nation affected," *New York Times*, December 13, 1999, A1.

[49] Robert Pear, "U.S. recommending strict new rules at nursing homes," *New York Times*, July 23, 2000, A1; and Robert Pear, "9 of 10 nursing homes lack adequate staff, study finds," *New York Times*, February 18, 2002, http://www.healthcoalition.ca/nyt.html, accessed April 11, 2003.

[50] Linda H. Aiken et al., "Hospital nurse staffing and patient mortality, nurse burnout, and job dissatisfaction," *Journal of the American Medical Association* 2002;288:1987-1993.

[51] Scott Brown et al., "Do you want to die?" *Time*, May 28, 1990, 58; Carey Goldberg, "Emergency crews worry as hospitals say, 'No vacancy,'" *New York Times*, December 17, 2000, Section 1, 27.

[52] "ED overcrowding is pervasive," *American Medical News*, April 22/29, 2002, 5.

[53] Families USA Foundation, *Doing Without: The Sacrifices Families Make to Provide Home Care*, Washington, DC, July 1994.

[54] Elizabeth A. McGlynn et al., "The quality of health care delivered to adults in the United States," *New England Journal of Medicine* 2003;348:2635-2645, 2641.

[55] "Shorter stays create added costs," *American Medical News*, June 4, 2001, 22.

# 5

# Other Excuses for the High Cost of American Health Care

## Introduction

In the last chapter, we saw that excessive use of health care cannot explain the high cost of the U.S. system. In this chapter, I discuss the remaining five excuses for the high cost of American health care listed in Table 3-8. They are:

(1) Americans are getting older;
(2) Americans have bad lifestyles;
(3) Americans sue for malpractice too often;
(4) Americans are violent; and
(5) U.S. quality is superior.

These excuses are made either by way of explaining why U.S. costs are high relative to those of other countries, or why U.S. health-care inflation has accelerated. But these factors – overuse, aging, lifestyles, litigation, violence, and quality – can explain neither high U.S. costs nor spurts in health-care inflation.

## Excuse number 2: Americans are older

When health-care inflation got worse between 1987 and 1992 and again after 1996, some apologists for the U.S. health insurance industry blamed the aging of the population. Here is an example from a 1992 edition of *Mayo Today*, the newsletter for Mayo Clinic doctors: "The relation of an aging population to the rising cost of care is obvious," said the newsletter. "Spending on health care is directly related to age. As individuals grow older, they generally become sicker and need more care. This is one of the biggest factors contributing to increases in health-care expenditures."[1] Here's another typical example from a 2001 article in the *New York Times* reporting that health insurance companies were raising their premiums by 15 percent, the highest rate since 1991: "[T]he average age of the American population is increasing, and that means more medical bills."[2]

The aging of the American population cannot explain changes in the health-care inflation rate over short periods of time. If the Mayo Clinic and the *New York Times* had set out to explain why U.S. health-care costs were very high in 2000 compared with some time decades earlier, say 1940, then a discussion of the change in average age that occurred over those 60 years would be appropriate. But it is ludicrous to suggest that an outbreak of aging played a role in the sudden increase in premium inflation that occurred across the U.S. after 1996, for example. The average age of America's population changes at a glacial pace compared to the speed with which health-care costs grow. But that is the implication of the explanations like those offered in the Mayo Clinic newsletter and the *New York Times*. By their odd logic, average age must have stopped growing between 1992 and 1996 when America enjoyed a health-care inflation lull. Of course, that didn't happen either. There was no cessation of aging in 1992, and no outbreak of aging in 1996.

The age excuse not only fails to explain the ups and downs of medical inflation, it also fails to explain differences between the health-care costs of the U.S. and other nations. If high American health-care costs were due to America's average age, one would expect to find that Americans are older than citizens of other industrialized nations. But as Table 5-1 indicates, the opposite is true. Column one in Table 5-1 lists the same ten countries we examined in Chapter 4 – the countries with the ten most expensive health systems. Column two lists the percent of these countries' populations over 64. The U.S., relative to the other nine countries, is a young country. Only Iceland's population is younger than ours. Yet our costs are double those of the rest of the industrialized world.

## Excuse number 3: Americans have worse lifestyles

Americans unquestionably do things, or fail to do things, which result in worse health and, often, higher health-care costs. Obesity, drug abuse, smoking, failure to practice safe sex, and failure to wear

---

**Table 5-1: Americans are not older than people of other countries, and tend to smoke and drink less: Percent over 64, percent who smoke, and alcohol consumption in ten nations with the most expensive health systems**

| Country | % over 64 (2002) | % smokers (2001) | Alcohol consumption, liters per capita (2001)[a] |
|---|---|---|---|
| US | 12.3 | 18.5 | 8.3[b] |
| Switzerland | 15.5 | 25.3[c] | 11.0 |
| Norway | 14.9 | 30.0 | 5.5 |
| Germany | 17.3 | 24.3[d] | 10.4 |
| Canada | 12.7 | 18.0 | 7.8 |
| Luxembourg | 13.9 | 30.0 | 15.3 |
| Iceland | 11.8 | 23.6 | 6.3 |
| Netherlands | 13.7 | 34.0 | 10.0 |
| France | 16.3 | 27.0 | 10.5[b] |
| Australia | 12.7 | 19.8 | 9.9[e] |

(a) The denominator used for this column is people over age 14.
(b) 2000 data.
(c) 2002 data.
(d) 2003 data.
(e) 1999 data.
Source: Organization for Economic Cooperation and Development, *OECD Health Data 2004*, 3$^{rd}$ *ed.*, http://www.oecd.org, accessed June 6, 2005.

---

seat belts are examples of behaviors that damage health and, thereby, add to health-care costs. Politicians and experts often state or imply that this fact warrants the conclusion that dumb lifestyle choices are the primary cause of America's high health expenditures. Minnesota's former Governor Jesse Ventura is an example. Speaking at a Minneapolis hospital about his "big plan" for health-care reform, Ventura said, "We can control costs if people are taking responsibility for their own health. This is not about them being triathletes or marathon runners, but they could just go for a walk after dinner."[3] Here is another example of the "lifestyles are to blame" argument, this one from a paper by Michael Tanner of the Cato Institute: "There are many reasons that Americans spend so much on health care. They include … [l]ifestyle. The United States has much higher rates of such social problems as AIDS, drug abuse, [and] teen pregnancy, … all of which lead to increased health-care costs. Costs also are affected by such lifestyle decisions as smoking, diet, and exercise."[4] Tanner offered not a single footnote for these claims.

It is true that America could reduce its health costs substantially if enough Americans began to exercise, quit smoking, kick drug habits, and changed their diets. For both health and financial reasons, public policies designed to promote healthier living should be part of any health-care system. But an exclusive focus on this truth obscures a more fundamental problem with the lifestyle excuse: It can't account for the huge difference between America's per capita health-care expenditures and those of the rest of the developed world.

What little literature I've seen comparing American lifestyles to those of people in other industrialized countries shows little difference in behaviors – certainly not enough to account for a two-fold difference in health costs. People all over the world drink, smoke, and suffer from sexually transmitted diseases. The obesity epidemic we hear so much about in the U.S. is not limited to the U.S.; obesity is spreading rapidly in other countries, including Third World countries.[5]

Table 5-1 also presents data on smoking and drinking in the ten nations with the most expensive health systems. You can see that the percent of Americans who smoke is quite low, and the amount of alcohol we consume per person is somewhat low, compared with the other nine countries. Moreover, if smoking and drinking are in fact contributing more to U.S. health-care costs than they are to the costs of other nations, it is not obvious from the data on hospital use and doctor visits shown in Tables 4-6 and 4-7.

A 1999 survey of tenth-grade students in Europe and the U.S. reported that European students were more likely to smoke cigarettes and drink alcohol but less likely to use illicit drugs such as marijuana and Ecstasy. Thirty-seven percent of European students, but only 26 percent of U.S. students, had smoked at least one cigarette in the previous 30 days, and 61 percent of European tenth-graders, but only 40 percent of U.S. students, had drunk alcohol in the last 30 days. On the other hand, one in four American students used illicit drugs compared with, at most, one in ten in European countries.[6] In view of the substantial amount of research implicating tobacco and alcohol in human disease, it is difficult to conclude from this survey that drug-consumption habits of American teens are adding more to U.S. health-care costs than the habits of European teens are adding to European costs. It may well be that the smoking and drinking habits of European teens are putting a heavier strain on European health systems.

## Excuse number 4: Americans sue too often

Malpractice lawsuits have been filed in noticeable numbers in America since the 1930s. But the myth that malpractice suits are excessive and play a major role in health-care inflation did not begin to take hold until the 1970s when the first of three "malpractice crises" occurred. In the early 1970s, again in the mid-1980s, and in several states in the early 2000s, the premiums doctors and hospitals paid for malpractice liability insurance soared. Interestingly, the premium inflation of the 1980s was accompanied by inflation in premiums for other types of liability insurance, including insurance for day care centers, schools, and truckers. It is interesting, obviously, because it suggests that something besides the behavior of patients and the size of malpractice awards from juries caused the inflation in malpractice premiums in the 1980s.

The American Medical Association, which today represents a third of the nation's physicians, responded to each of these bursts of inflation with a national campaign to convince politicians and the public that malpractice premiums were rising because Americans sued doctors too often.* The AMA, with help from the insurance industry and the Chamber of Commerce, has been very successful. All 50 states have passed legislation enacting some version of what the AMA considers to be malpractice reform, and in the early 1990s the AMA persuaded the Republican leadership in Congress and the White House to support even more "reform" at the federal level. During the 1992 presidential debate, former President George Bush asserted that "the malpractice trial lawyers' lawsuits ... are running the costs of medical care up $25 to $50 billion."[7] George W. Bush has made the same claim repeatedly. In his January 28, 2003 State of the Union address, for example, Bush claimed malpractice litigation was "one of the prime causes" of health-care inflation.

Table 5-2 indicates most Americans had bought the AMA line by the early 1990s. You see that "malpractice lawsuits" was the most frequently cited factor in a poll conducted in 1993. Fifty-nine percent of Americans said "malpractice lawsuits" contributed "a great deal ... to high health-care costs," and 44 percent said the same about "defensive medicine" (the ordering of unnecessary medical goods and services by doctors to minimize the likelihood of malpractice lawsuits by patients and their families). (Make sure to glance at the last two items in Table 5-2; they indicate the public doesn't buy the overuse and age excuses.) Other polls confirmed this finding. The *Wall Street Journal* reported that 60 percent of Americans think malpractice litigation is "one of the biggest causes of spiraling U.S. health-care costs,"[8] and the Robert Wood Johnson Foundation (a prolific funder of health-policy research) reported that 64 percent of Americans think malpractice suits are "to blame" for health-care inflation.[9]

But the AMA's claims about malpractice suits are wrong or, at best, grossly misleading. First, only a small fraction of patients harmed by malpractice sue. Second, malpractice suits cannot possibly be "one of

---

* For example, *American Medical News*, a newspaper published every two weeks by the AMA, reported, "The AMA and the National Medical Association, the nation's largest African-American physicians' group, ... held a joint news conference to repeat the argument that the current liability system raises health care costs" (Diane M. Gianelli and Brian McCormick, "Pushing tort reform before the Senate," May 8, 1995, 1).

---

## Table 5-2: The public thinks malpractice suits cause health-care inflation: Results of a poll, 1993

| Factor | Percent saying the factor contributes a great deal |
|---|---|
| Malpractice lawsuits | 59 |
| Waste and abuse | 58 |
| Fraudulent claims | 50 |
| Doctors practicing defensive medicine to avoid suits | 44 |
| AIDS | 44 |
| New expensive drugs | 43 |
| New technology | 39 |
| Urban problems, like crime and drugs | 34 |
| An aging population | 29 |
| Expectations of the public for the best possible treatment for any condition | 25 |

Source: Robert J. Blendon et al., "Bridging the gap between expert and public views on health care reform," *Journal of the American Medical Association* 1993;269(19):2573-78.

---

the prime causes" of health-care inflation because malpractice costs amount to 2 or 3 percent of total health-care spending. Third, the real cause of the "malpractice crisis" is an unacceptable level of errors that result in injury to patients. If you look again at Table 5-2, you will notice that the scholars who conducted this poll didn't give their respondents an opportunity to comment on "malpractice by doctors." That tells you something about how completely bamboozled the American public has been by the AMA propaganda. Even experts think there's no point in including a question about malpractice itself in a survey about causes of health-care inflation.

Let me walk you through the evidence supporting the statements I just made, beginning with the statement that malpractice costs are no more than 2 or 3 percent of health expenditures. According to a 2004

---

## Table 5-3: Malpractice costs amount to 2 percent of total health-care costs when defensive medicine is included: Costs of malpractice insurance and defensive medicine, 1994, $s

| | |
|---|---|
| Malpractice premiums for all US doctors and hospitals | 9 billion |
| Defensive medicine | 12 billion |
| Total | 21 billion |
| | |
| US health-care expenditures | 949 billion |

$21 billion = 2% of $949 billion

Savings from AMA-recommended malpractice reform in 1994:
    In dollars                           4.3 billion
        As percent of total health-care spending     0.5*

* Total health-care spending in 1994 was $949 billion. $4.3 billion is 0.5 percent of $949 billion.

Sources: The estimates of the cost of malpractice premiums, defensive medicine, and savings from malpractice reform are those of the National Medical Liability Reform Coalition, which included the American Medical Association, the American Hospital Association, the National Association of Manufacturers, and MMI Companies (a hospital liability insurer). The coalition contracted with a consulting firm then known as Lewin/VHI to prepare its estimates. The Lewin/VHI estimate of $4.3 billion in savings is reported in Brian McCormick, "Study: Defensive medicine costs nearly $10 billion," *American Medical News*, February 15, 1993, 4. The 1994 Lewin/VHI estimates of premiums and defensive medicine costs are cited in Spencer Rich, "Malpractice curbs won't work, Nader says," *Washington Post*, Health, June 15, 1993, 5. The 1994 spending total is from Katharine R. Levit et al., "Health care spending in 1994: Slowest in decades," *Health Affairs* 1996;15(2):130-144.

---

report by the Congressional Budget Office, total premiums paid for malpractice insurance by doctors and hospitals came to $24 billion in 2002, or "less than 2 percent of overall health-care spending." The U.S. spent $1.559 trillion on health care in 2002, which means the exact proportion of our health-care bill attributable to malpractice costs was 1.5 percent. The AMA argues that "defensive medicine" must be added to the cost of liability insurance. The CBO, however, refused to attribute a cost to defensive medicine on the ground that the evidence for its existence is weak and the savings from reducing it, if any, would be "very small."[10]

But even if we take AMA estimates of the cost of defensive medicine at face value, the conclusion remains the same – total malpractice costs are just too tiny compared to total health-care spending to contribute a "great deal" to health-care inflation. Table 5-3 presents an estimate of the cost of our malpractice system as of 1994, broken into two components: premiums paid for malpractice insurance by doctors and hospitals, and the cost of defensive medicine. Total premiums paid to liability insurance companies came to $9 billion in 1994. According to a coalition of organizations that included the AMA, defensive medicine cost $12 billion that year. When you add $9 billion in premiums to $12 billion for defensive medicine, you get $21 billion, which turns out to be just 2 percent of total health spending in 1994.*

Gerard Anderson et al. conducted the only study I'm aware of that compared malpractice costs in the U.S. with those of another country. They calculated the "cost of defending U.S. malpractice claims" against physicians only (hospitals were excluded from this study) in 2001 with the cost in Canada. The authors concluded that these costs absorbed 0.46 percent of total health-care spending in the U.S. versus 0.27 percent of Canada's total health-care spending.[11] Obviously the difference – two-tenths of a percent – explains almost none of the huge difference in U.S. and Canadian per capita spending on health.

No one, not even the AMA, is proposing to abolish the court system and deny all victims of malpractice the right to sue. That means the savings from malpractice "reform" will be an even tinier portion of total health-care spending than 2 percent. According to the AMA, the "reform" measures it supported during the first half of the 1990s would

---

* Other proponents of the malpractice excuse said total malpractice costs were even lower than $21 billion in 1994. When former Representative Rod Grams (R-MN) introduced a malpractice "reform" bill in 1994 at the request of the AMA, he announced, "Defensive medicine and frivolous lawsuits cost Americans over $15 billion each year. How can the president and Democratic leadership ignore this part of the health-care debate?" (Tom Hamburger, "Grams offers legislation seeking major reform on medical malpractice," Minneapolis *Star Tribune*, July 21, 1994, 15A).

have saved a grand total of $4 billion in 1994, which amounts to just 0.5 percent of the $949 billion the U.S. spent on health care that year.

Given the great hue and cry about malpractice costs over the last three decades, you might think American scholars would have published numerous studies on how many Americans are hurt by malpractice and what percent of these sue. You would be flat wrong. Very few studies on this question exist.* Two of the best studies focused on hospitals, which is where 80 percent of malpractice occurs (that's because more risky forms of treatment occur in hospitals). One study, based on 21,000 patient records from 23 California hospitals, concluded that only 4 percent of malpractice victims were compensated for their injuries.[12] The second study, based on 30,000 records of patients treated in 51 New York hospitals, reported that just 2 percent of malpractice victims sued. (These studies didn't indicate what percent of those who sued received compensation but, obviously, not all of them won their suits.) Interestingly, the latter study was conducted by scholars at the schools of medicine, public health, law, and government at Harvard University. The study was published as a series of articles in the *New England Journal of Medicine*.[13] The authors concluded, "[T]here is no basis for the charge that the amount of malpractice litigation is excessive. On the contrary, there seems to be a major 'deficit' of litigation."[14] The implication of the California and Harvard studies is that enormous obstacles stand between malpractice victims and the courts. The stories of three people I knew personally, presented in Appendix A, illustrate some of these obstacles.

If only a tiny fraction of malpractice victims are suing and winning compensation for their injuries, true malpractice reform – reform which eliminated all unnecessary lawsuits and compensated all legitimate malpractice victims – would probably *raise* the total cost of malpractice, not lower it. This should remind you of the one-sided debate about overuse

---

* The authors of one of these studies took note of the contrast between the attention paid to malpractice premiums and the attention paid to the number of people hurt by malpractice. "Curiously, ... the problem of medical injury has received comparatively little attention...." they wrote (Lucian L. Leape, et al., "The nature of adverse events in hospitalized patients: Results of the Harvard Medical Practice Study II," *New England Journal of Medicine*, 1991;324:377-338, 377).

and underuse we discussed in Chapter 4. Just as the AMA would have you believe that frivolous lawsuits are rampant and uncompensated victims of malpractice don't exist, so the insurance industry would have you believe that overuse is rampant and underuse does not exist. But once we get a balanced picture of these problems, it becomes apparent that solving them might well raise, not lower, total health-care costs.

Until recently, the debate about malpractice costs minimized the role that malpractice itself played in the "crisis." But that changed dramatically in 2000 when the Institute of Medicine (IOM) published a report on medical errors entitled *To Err is Human*. The IOM estimated that preventable errors in U.S. hospitals caused somewhere between 44,000 and 98,000 deaths.[15] The IOM did not say that all of these deaths were caused by malpractice; rather, the IOM called them "preventable errors." Nevertheless, it is errors, whether they are tantamount to malpractice or not, that trigger lawsuits, and it is lawsuits that drive up malpractice liability insurance premiums. The IOM documented a lot of dying in hospitals due to error. If we add *injuries* in hospitals due to preventable errors, and preventable deaths and injuries *outside* of hospitals, we are looking at medical death-and-injury rates in the hundreds of thousands every year.

In criticizing those who claim America's health-care inflation can be blamed on malpractice suits, I don't mean to imply that the malpractice litigation system is beyond reproach. There is much that is wrong with the current system, including its inaccuracy. Too many victims of malpractice do not sue, and too many patients who are not malpractice victims do sue. I support any reform that makes the malpractice system fairer and more efficient.* But to say the malpractice system needs reform is quite different from saying it is a cause of America's very high health-care costs.

---

* One of those reforms, not so incidentally, would be universal coverage. One important reason victims of serious medical injury sue is to ensure that they have enough money to pay for their future medical needs. If we had a universal health insurance system in place, patients who were injured, including those whose injuries were not caused by negligence, would have much less incentive to sue. The presence of a universal health insurance system in Canada unquestionably contributes to Canada's lower expenditures on malpractice litigation.

## Excuse number 5: Americans are more violent

This is an excuse I rarely hear anywhere, and I never see it in the professional journals – the health-policy and medical journals. On the rare occasions when I have encountered this argument, it was not supported with citations to anything, much less professional journals. The president of the AMA, for example, told the House Ways and Means Committee in 1992, apparently without any citations to evidence, "When you compare our country to Canada, we have a very different demography. We have more violence."[16] The Cato Institute's Michael Tanner alleges, "The United States has much higher rates of ... violent crime, which lead[s] to increased health-care costs."[17] As was the case with Tanner's claim that "lifestyle" explains America's high health-care costs, this claim was not documented.

We can dismiss the violence excuse for the same reason we can dismiss the malpractice excuse – the total cost is just too tiny to have much influence on total health-care spending. The few people who claim that violence is a driving force behind U.S. health-care inflation apparently have gun violence in mind. Those who have studied the al-

## Table 5-4: Gun violence accounts for a tiny portion of total U.S. health-care costs: Cost of injuries caused by guns, U.S., 1990 and 1994

|  | Cost of treating gunshot injuries ($, billions) | Total US health care expenditures ($, billions) | Gunshot costs as percent of total expenditures |
|---|---|---|---|
| 1990 | 1.4 | 699.4 | 0.2 |
| 1994 | 2.3 | 947.7 | 0.2 |

Sources: The estimate of the cost of gun injuries for 1990 is from Wendy Max and Dorothy P. Rice, "Shooting in the dark: Estimating the cost of firearm injuries," *Health Affairs* 1993;12(4):171-185; the estimate of the cost of gun injuries for 1994 is from Philip J. Cook et al., "The medical costs of gunshot injuries in the United States," *Journal of the American Medical Association* 1999;282:447-454; total spending figures are from Katharine R. Levit et al., "Health spending in 1998: Signals of change," *Health Affairs* 2000;19(1):124-132, Exhibit 1.

leged violence-cost connection focused on gun violence. The reasons are obvious: Violence with fists or weapons other than guns causes much less damage to human beings; and gun violence is more common in the U.S.[18] I have seen two studies that examined the cost of medical care required for gun victims, and both concluded that the total cost came to 0.2 percent of health-care spending (see Table 5-4). The two studies cited in the table appear to be the most thorough ever done on the subject of gun-violence costs.

Both studies included in their definition of gunshot costs the costs of ambulance services, hospitalization, physicians, drugs, physical therapy, and home health care. The earlier of the two studies, done by Max and Rice, also included the cost of home modification, vocational rehabilitation, health insurance, and "other" expenses. Max and Rice did not distinguish gun injuries inflicted intentionally from those inflicted unintentionally or which were self-inflicted. Cook et al., the authors of the second study, did make that distinction; they found that 74 percent of gunshot injuries were caused by assaults. So if we restrict the definition of medical costs caused by "violence" to gunshot wounds *inflicted intentionally by others* (which is what U.S. apologists apparently have in mind when they offer "violence" as an excuse for our high health-care costs), the total cost was even less than two-tenths of a percent of total spending.

I have never seen a study comparing the cost of gunshot wounds in the U.S. to the cost in other countries. But in view of how small the costs of gunshot wounds are compared to total costs, we may predict with certainty that such a study would throw no light on the question of why U.S. health costs are so much higher than those of other countries.

## Excuse number 6: Quality of care in the U.S. is superior

We have now examined five justifications for the high cost of American health care: overuse, age, lifestyle, malpractice suits, and violence. We have seen that they explain little or nothing about why U.S. costs are so high relative to other countries, or why health-care inflation rises faster at some times rather than others. We have one last explanation to consider: that quality of care is superior in the U.S. With the exception of the overuse excuse, this may be the most common of the six excuses for high U.S. costs.

"The United States now has the best health-care system in the world." Thus spake Senator Phil Gramm, the former Republican senator from Texas, back in the early 1990s when one could still hear occasional discussions about the health systems of other countries.[19] But Senator Gramm is wrong. It *is* accurate to say the U.S. has some of the world's finest health-care professionals and medical centers. But that's not equivalent to the claim that our system is the best.

Comparing the quality of the U.S. health-care system to the quality of other systems is difficult because health-care systems are complex. We're talking about huge systems in which hundreds of thousands of health-care professionals deliver thousands of different types of treatments to millions of patients. In the U.S., we have 720,000 practicing physicians,[20] 2.2 million registered nurses,[21] 20,000 home health-care providers,[22] tens of thousands of other professional healers such as pharmacists, acupuncturists and chiropractors, 5,800 hospitals,[23] 16,500 nursing homes,[24] 6,800 home health agencies,[25] and tens of thousands of pharmacies, chemical dependency treatment agencies, and manufacturers of drugs, pacemakers, wheel chairs, and many other goods that American patients need. For physicians alone (never mind chiropractors, acupuncturists and other types of healers), the number of services they bill for is on the order of 8,000. That's the number of codes listed in *Current Procedural Terminology*, the book that tells physicians what code to enter on insurance claim forms to describe the type of treatment given.

In part because of the lack of interest within the U.S. health-policy community in other nation's health systems, and in part because health systems are so complex, studies comparing one nation's system to another's are scarce. The few studies that exist (at least in the English language) tend to compare only the U.S. and Canada. And much of that research was done in the 1980s and early 1990s when there was a glimmer of hope that a single-payer system would get an honest debate in Congress. Research on other systems, especially research on public opinion about those systems, became scarcer after 1993 when the White House and numerous federal and state politicians endorsed managed competition as the solution to the health-care crisis.

The complexity of health-care systems means that any comparison of systems must rely on a variety of measures. The types of measures used fall into three categories: polling data, "vital statistics" (such as infant mortality rates and average lifespans), and studies that compare the quality of particular treatments, such as heart surgery. Each category has its strengths and weaknesses. The advantage of polls and vital statistics is that they are *global* measures – they tell you something about the entire system, not just one part of it, say, emergency services or treatment of back pain. Conversely, the advantage of studies that focus on the quality of care given to particular types of patients is that they can tell you something about small pieces of the system. I examine each of these three types of evidence – polling data, vital statistics, and studies of particular treatments – next.

## The quality excuse: Evidence from surveys

We begin with the surveys. There aren't many of them. The most comprehensive survey was done by Robert Blendon and his colleagues at Harvard and two other institutions. It was done 15 years ago, but because it was so comprehensive, and because subsequent polls dealing with fewer countries have not altered the basic findings of this survey, I describe it here. Blendon and colleagues asked a thousand citizens in each of ten countries whether they thought their "health-care system" needed "only minor changes," needed "fundamental changes," or must be "completely rebuil[t]." The ten countries, ranked in order of score, are listed in Table 5-5. The U.S. ranked tenth out of ten (ours was the least popular of all ten systems studied), while Canada ranked number one. Only 10 percent of Americans were willing to say their system needed just minor change, while 60 percent wanted fundamental change, and 29 percent wanted the revolution. Meanwhile, 56 percent of Canadians said their system needed only minor change.

The column on the right side of Table 5-5 presents per capita expenditures on health for each nation in 1987. You see an interesting pattern. You see a general correlation between spending on health care and the popularity of the health system. In other words, as spending declined, the popularity of the system declined. You will notice, however, one flaming exception to this trend – America. We vastly outspent the other

### Table 5-5: Americans are unhappier with our system than citizens in nine other countries are with theirs: The public's view of their health system in ten nations, 1990; per capita health expenditures, 1987

| | Minor changes needed[a] | Fundamental changes needed[b] | Completely rebuild system[c] | Per capita health exps ($) |
|---|---|---|---|---|
| Canada | 56% | 38% | 5% | 1,483 |
| Netherlands | 47% | 46% | 5% | 1,041 |
| W. Germany | 41% | 41% | 13% | 1,093 |
| France | 41% | 42% | 10% | 1,105 |
| Australia | 34% | 43% | 17% | 939 |
| Sweden | 32% | 58% | 6% | 1,233 |
| Japan | 29% | 47% | 6% | 915 |
| UK | 27% | 52% | 17% | 758 |
| Italy | 12% | 46% | 40% | 841 |
| US | 10% | 60% | 29% | 2,051 |

(a) The survey question was worded as follows: "On the whole, the health-care system works pretty well, and only minor changes are necessary to make it work better."

(b) The question was, "There are some good things in our health-care system, but fundamental changes are needed to make it work better."

(c) The question was, "Our health-care system has so much wrong with it that we need to completely rebuild it."

Source: Robert J. Blendon et al., "Satisfaction with health systems in ten nations," *Health Affairs* 1990;9(2);185-192.

nine nations, and yet there we sat, at the bottom of the heap in terms of citizen satisfaction.

The survey presented in Table 5-5 has not been repeated. The Commonwealth Fund has, however, conducted surveys in five English-speaking countries annually since the late 1990s. These surveys have

## Table 5-6: Americans are more dissatisfied than are citizens of four other countries: The public's view of their health-care system in five nations, 1990 and 2004

| | Rebuild completely | | Minor changes needed | |
| --- | --- | --- | --- | --- |
| | 1990 | 2004 | 1990 | 2004 |
| United States | 29% | 33% | 10% | 16% |
| Australia | 17% | 23% | 34% | 21% |
| New Zealand | | 19% | | 19% |
| Canada | 5% | 14% | 56% | 21% |
| United Kingdom | 17% | 13% | 27% | 26% |

Sources: 1990 data are from Robert J. Blendon et al., "Satisfaction with health systems in ten nations," *Health Affairs* 1990;9(2);185-192; 2004 data are from Cathy Schoen et al., "Primary care and health system performance: Adults' experiences in five countries," *Health Affairs*, Web Exclusives, July-December 2004, W4 487-503.

asked the same questions (whether the system needs minor change or complete rebuilding) that Blendon et al. asked in their 1990 survey. Results of the 2004 survey using these questions are shown in Table 5-6 along with the 1990 data for four of these countries. These results indicate that Americans were considerably unhappier with their health-care system than were the citizens of the other four countries.

Another way to assess the quality of a country's health-care system is to ask its doctors what they think. In 1991, Blendon et al. asked doctors in the U.S., Canada, and Germany the same questions they asked in the previously mentioned surveys. The researchers reported that "both West German and Canadian physicians were more satisfied with their systems than were U.S. physicians."[26] The differences were large, especially between the German and U.S. doctors (see Table 5-7). Nearly half the German doctors were willing to say their system works well while less than a quarter of U.S. doctors were willing to say that.

However, none of these international surveys – the ten-nation survey, the survey of five English-speaking nations, and the survey of doctors in three countries – can be treated as measures of quality only. That's

**Table 5-7: German and Canadian doctors like their system better than American doctors like ours: Percent of U.S., Canadian and German doctors who say their system works "pretty well and only minor changes are needed," 1991**

| | |
|---|---|
| Germany | 48% |
| Canada | 33 |
| US | 23 |

Source: Robert J. Blendon et al., "Physicians' perspectives on caring for patients in the United States, Canada, and West Germany," *New England Journal of Medicine* 1993;328:1011-1016.

**Table 5-8: Americans are slightly less satisfied with care: Proportion of citizens of five nations who rated their physician and hospital care as excellent or very good, and per capita spending on health care, 2001**

| | Aus | Can | NZ | UK | US |
|---|---|---|---|---|---|
| Care received from doctor in last year | 63% | 54% | 67% | 53% | 57% |
| Care received from hospital in last two years | 55% | 54% | 67% | 53% | 57% |
| Per capita spending 2001 | $2,513 | $2,792 | $1,710 | $1,992 | $4,887 |

Sources: Survey data from Robert J. Blendon et al., "Inequities in health care: A five-country survey," *Health Affairs* 2002, 21(3)182-191; cost data from Uwe Reinhardt et al., "U.S. health care spending in an international context," *Health Affairs* 2004;23(3):10-25.

because the questions the pollsters used were not limited to quality. The pollsters asked people to comment on their "health-care system," which means people were asked to think about both the *quality* of their system *and* its cost. It's possible that the greater dissatisfaction expressed by Americans reflects more anger about the high cost of health care here than about quality of care. But we can say this: At minimum, these surveys lend not one iota of support to those who claim our health-care system is expensive because quality is superior.

The Commonwealth Fund surveyors also asked their respondents to rate the quality of care they get from their doctor and hospital. Obviously, these questions focused just on quality. Americans satisfaction levels were about equal to those of the Brits and Canadians, and were lower than those of the New Zealanders and Australians (see Table 5-8). Table 5-8 provides no evidence for the claim that America's health-care system is twice as expensive because it's twice as good.

## The quality excuse: vital statistics

Now let's shift from surveys to the second category of data comparing national health systems – vital statistics. The quality of a nation's health-care system is not the only factor affecting infant mortality rates and longevity, but it is certainly an important factor; in the case of infant mortality (which is the percent of babies born alive who die in their first year), it may be the most important factor. For decades the U.S. has ranked low among industrialized nations on these measures. In 2001, the U.S. ranked 24th in infant mortality among 26 industrialized nations and 22nd in life expectancy for both males and females among 28 industrialized countries.* The few countries that performed worse than the U.S. tended to be Eastern European countries like Poland and the Czech Republic. For example, the U.S. infant mortality rate of 6.8 per 1,000 was higher for every one of the 26 nations for which data were available in 2001 except Poland and Hungary. Even poorer countries like Portugal and the Slovak Republic had lower infant mortality rates than we did.[27]

---

\* These are data from the Organization for Economic Cooperation and Development. Thirty countries were members by 2001. Because two of these – Mexico and Turkey – are not usually counted among developed nations, and because their vital statistics are considerably worse than the other 28 OECD countries, I excluded them from my calculations.

In 2004, the *Journal of Epidemiology and Community Health* reported on the perceptions Americans, Canadians and Europeans have of their own health. I could have classified this study with the polling data we just reviewed, but because self-reported health status has been shown to be correlated with mortality, I report it in this section on vital statistics. The study found that the percent of adults who define their own health as poor was about the same in the U.S., Canada and 15 European countries for adults age 20 to 24, but as the respondents got older Americans were much more likely to say they were in poor health than were respondents in Canada and Europe. In the over-59 age brackets, the percent of Americans who said they were in poor health was roughly ten points above the percent of Europeans who said they were in poor health, and roughly five points above the Canadian rate. For example, among adults age 60 to 64, about 13 percent of Europeans, 17 percent of Canadians, and 23 percent of Americans said they were in poor health.[28]

## The quality excuse: studies of particular types of treatment

Now we move from the survey and vital statistics data – the data that give us a bird's-eye view – to studies of the quality of particular types of health care. Unlike surveys and vital statistics, these studies tend to focus on just two countries at a time, and most of these compared the U.S. and Canada. I will discuss the U.S.-Canadian studies in a little more detail in Chapter 11 (see Table 11-6). Here I describe two studies, one which examined the primary care sectors of the health-care systems of ten countries, and another which examined the quality of ten types of surgery in the U.S. and Canada.

Primary care is defined as the care people get when they first contact their medical system, that is, before they are referred to more specialized health-care professionals. Family doctors, internists, pediatricians, and obstetrician-gynecologists are usually described as primary care doctors. A 1991 study of the quality of primary care in ten countries concluded that primary care in the U.S. was inferior to that of most of the other countries studied.[29] Here is how the Minneapolis *Star Tribune* summarized the study:

A study of the primary health care offered to citizens of ten industrialized nations has found the United States at the bottom. Dr. Barbara Starfield of the Johns Hopkins School of Hygiene and Public Health compared Australia, Belgium, Canada, Denmark, Finland, West Germany, the Netherlands, Sweden, United Kingdom, and the United States on three levels.... The United States ranked near the bottom in all three categories. The Netherlands, Canada and Sweden fared well across the board.[30]

In a 1998 article, Dr. Starfield repeated her conclusion that the U.S. system is inferior to those of other countries, primarily because of its relatively poor primary care.[31]

The study described in Table 5-9 is one of the best of the three dozen studies comparing the U.S. and Canada. It was done by researchers affiliated with Dartmouth, the University of Manitoba, and the Manitoba Center for Health Policy and Evaluation. It compared three-year mortality rates of Canadians (Manitobans) and Americans (New Englanders) over 64 who underwent one of ten types of surgery. The study found that Canadian mortality rates were lower for eight of the ten procedures, higher for open prostatectomy, and almost identical for hip fracture repair.[*]

## The quality excuse: recapitulation

The evidence we've just reviewed – surveys, vital statistics, and studies comparing the quality of certain types of care in the U.S. and other countries – indicates that quality of care in the U.S. is not better

---

[*] The authors noted that the Canadian surgeons may have outperformed the American surgeons even on open prostatectomy and hip fracture repair. They stated that the New England men who underwent open prostatectomy may have been healthier than the Canadian men, which would have given the American patients a survival edge that had nothing to do with the quality of American surgery. The authors also noted that differences in "geographic distribution of patients and hospitals" in the two regions may have biased the hip surgery results against Manitoba. Because New England is compact and densely populated while Manitoba is more rural, the average New Englander who breaks a hip is

than, and may actually be somewhat inferior to, that of other countries. By no stretch of the imagination does this evidence support the claim (a claim usually made implicitly) that quality of care in the U.S. is so superior to that of other countries that it warrants paying twice as much

---

**Table 5-9: Canadians are more likely to survive surgery than Americans: Manitoban versus New England mortality rates for ten types of surgery among elderly patients, 1980s***

| | Three-year mortality rate (%) | |
|---|---|---|
| Procedure | Manitoba | New England |
| Total hip replacement | 8.35% | 10.56% |
| Simple cholecystectomy | 10.37 | 16.53 |
| Open prostatectomy | 15.64 | 12.23 |
| Carotid endarterectomy | 15.02 | 21.73 |
| Transurethral prostatectomy | 20.45 | 22.15 |
| Cholecystectomy with exploration of common bile duct | 19.65 | 23.19 |
| Coronary artery bypass surgery | 12.43 | 15.99 |
| Heart valve replacement | 19.81 | 24.94 |
| Repair of hip fracture | 42.13 | 41.83 |
| Concurrent valve replacement/bypass surgery | 27.72 | 29.43 |

* The Manitoba results were for surgery done between 1980 and 1986; the New England results were for surgery done in 1984 and 1985.

Source: Leslie L. Roos et al., "Health and surgical outcomes in Canada and the US," *Health Affairs* 1992;11(2):56-72.

---

much closer to a hospital than the average Manitoban. The authors reported that Manitobans were in fact more likely to experience a delay in surgery than New Englanders were. In sum, this study said Canada's doctors outperformed America's doctors in eight out of eight contests in which the playing field was level.

## Table 5-10: America publishes an average number of medical articles: Medical articles published per million population, 1990

| | |
|---|---|
| Israel | 819 |
| Sweden | 781 |
| UK | 594 |
| US | 526 |
| Canada | 520 |
| Germany | 354 |
| Japan | 250 |

Source: David U. Himmelstein and Steffie Woolhandler, *The National Health Program Book*, Common Courage Press, Monroe, ME, 1994, 109.

## Table 5-11: America spends an average amount on research: Total health research and development expenditures per capita, 1994

| Country | Dollars per capita |
|---|---|
| Switzerland | 164 |
| UK | 78 |
| Denmark | 71 |
| France | 63 |
| US | 59 |
| Japan | 35 |
| Canada | 22 |

Source: OECD, presented in Steffie Woolhandler and David U. Himmelstein, *For Our Patients, Not for Profits: A Call to Action*, The Center for National Health Program Studies, 1998, 114.

for it. As the *Philadelpia Inquirer* put it at the beginning of a series of articles about the U.S., Canadian, and German health-care systems, "Americans pay more than people in other advanced countries, but aren't healthier. Canada and Germany get good care for less."[32]

## The quality excuse: The U.S. does more research

A relatively rare variation on the quality excuse is that America does more research than other countries. This claim is not supported by the evidence. Whether research effort is measured in terms of results (medical articles published; see Table 5-10) or expenditures (see Table 5-11), the U.S. effort appears to be about average. An unpublished paper presented to the Federation of European Cancer Societies in 2001 confirms this conclusion. The study, conducted by Dr. Francesco Grossi of the National Institute for Research on Cancer in Genoa, Italy, examined the number and "impact" of papers on cancer treatment published in the U.S. and 11 other industrialized nations. Dr. Grossi found that U.S. scientists placed fifth in "impact" behind Canada (in first place), Holland, Britain and Australia. Seven other countries "closely followed" the U.S., according to the newspaper article about this study.[33]

---

## Endnotes

[1] "The rising cost of healthcare – why?" *Mayo Today*, February 1992, 6.

[2] Milt Freudenheim, "High cost of being well: Benefits at a premium," *New York Times*, October 16, 2001, C1, C16.

[3] Glenn Howatt, "Ventura talks up his health care proposal," Minneapolis *Star Tribune*, February 2, 2001, B5.

[4] Michael Tanner, "Chapter 2: What's wrong with the present system," in Grace-Marie Arnett, ed., *Empowering Health Care Consumers Through Tax Reform*, University of Michigan Press, Ann Arbor, September 1999, available at http://www.galen.org./book.asp, accessed December 31, 2003.

[5] Clifford Krauss, "Do doughnuts make Canada too well rounded?" *New York Times*, August 5, 2002, A4; Norimitsu Onishi, "On U.S. fast food, Okinawans are super-sized," *New York Times*, March 30, 2004, A1.

[6] Kate Zernike, "Study finds teenage drug use higher in the U.S. than in Europe," *New York Times*, February 21, 2001, A10.

[7] David Klingman et al., "Measuring defensive medicine using clinical scenario surveys," *Journal of Health Politics, Policy and Law* 1996;21:185-217, 186.

[8] "Doctors are spurring effort to remedy the nation's ailing malpractice system," *Wall Street Journal*, March 1, 1993, B1.

[9] American Political Network, *American HealthLine*, May 17, 1993.

[10] Congressional Budget Office, *Limiting Tort Liability for Medical Malpractice*, January 8, 2004, http://www.cbo.gov/showdoc.cfm?index=4968&sequence=0, accessed June 10, 2005.

[11] Gerard F. Anderson et al., "Health spending in the United States and the rest of the industrialized world," *Health Affairs* 2005;24:903-914.

[12] Described in Physician Payment Review Commission, *Annual Report to Congress*, 1991, Washington, DC, 369.

[13] Troyen A. Brennan et al., "Incidence of adverse events and negligence in hospitalized patients: Results of Harvard Medical Practice Study I," *New England Journal of Medicine* 1991;324:370-376; and Lucian L. Leape et al., "The nature of adverse events in hospitalized patients: Results of the Harvard Medical Practice Study II," *New England Journal of Medicine* 1991;324:377-384.

[14] Paul C. Weiler et al., "Proposal for medical liability reform," *Journal of the American Medical Association* 1992; 267:2355-2358, 2358.

[15] Linda T. Kohn et al., eds., *To Err Is Human: Building a Safer Health System*, National Academy Press, Washington, DC, 2000.

[16] Colin Gordon, *Dead on Arrival: The Politics of Health Care in Twentieth-Century America*, Princeton University Press, Princeton, NJ, 2003, 209.

[17] Tanner, op cit.

[18] Donald G. McNeil, Jr., "Not only in America: Gun killings shake the Europeans," *New York Times*, May 11, 2002, A3.

[19] Tom Hamburger et al., "What the death of health reform teaches us about the press," *Washington Monthly*, November 1994, 35-41, 37.

[20] National Center for Health Statistics, U.S. Department of Health and Human Services, *Health, United States, 2004*, http://www.cdc.gov/nchs/data/hus/hus04trend.pdf, accessed June 10, 2005.

[21] Ibid.

[22] Jill Burcum, "House calls," Minneapolis *Star Tribune*, April 2, 2002, E1.

[23] National Center for Health Statistics, op cit.

[24] Ibid.

[25] Ibid.

[26] Robert J. Blendon et al., "Physicians' perspectives on caring for patients in the United States, Canada, and West Germany," *New England Journal of Medicine* 1993;328:1011-1016, 1012.

[27] Organization for Economic Cooperation and Development, *OECD Health Data 2004, 3rd ed.*, http://www.oecd.org, accessed June 6, 2005.

[28] M.S. Kaplan et al., "Spending more, feeling worse: Medical care expenditures and self-rated health," *Journal of Epidemiology and Community Health*, letter, 2004;58:529-530.

[29] Barbara Starfield, "Primary care and health. A cross-national comparison," *Journal of the American Medical Association* 1991;266:2268-2271.

[30] "Study ranks primary health care in US lowest in group," Minneapolis *Star Tribune*, October 23, 1991, 11A.

[31] Barbara Starfield, "Is U.S. health really the best in the world?" *Journal of the American Medical Association* 1998;284, http://jama.ama-assn.org/issues/v284n4/ffull/jco00061.html, accessed October 15, 2002.

[32] Susan FitzGerald et al., "Healing in three nations: Care at what cost? A reprint of a series published in The Philadelphia Inquirer from April 25 to April 29, 1993," *Philadelphia Inquirer*, 1.

[33] Associated Press, "Health roundup," Minneapolis *Star Tribune*, October 24, 2001, A7.

# 6

# Waste in the System: Administrative Waste and Excess Capacity

## A mental map of the waste

If you accept my arguments that the six excuses reviewed in Chapters 4 and 5 cannot explain the high cost of American health care, then your mind should be wide open to accepting the argument I make in this chapter and the next: The cause of America's high cost is wastefulness in the health-care industry. Or, to frame it in the volume-versus-price terms I was using back in Chapter 3, your mind should be open to the argument that excessive prices, driven by wasteful practices, is the main problem, not excessive use of health care.

When I speak of the health-care industry, I mean the health-care *provider* sector and the health *insurance* sector. When I say the industry is wasteful, I mean two things. First, I mean that the industry spends a lot more money than is necessary to produce the medical goods and services we buy. Second, I mean that some players within the industry set their prices higher than is necessary, even taking into account their wasteful practices, which permits them to make enormous profits. Let me offer two examples to illustrate both types of waste.

The hospital industry is wasteful primarily in the first sense – its prices are high because it spends a lot of money on things it doesn't need to serve patients, such as advertising, empty beds, idle diagnostic machinery, clerks whose sole function is to deal with numerous insurance companies seeking to avoid paying bills, and enormous salaries for top management. But the hospital industry is not wasteful in the second sense I mentioned, that is, it doesn't set its prices so high above its costs that it makes huge profits. Profits in the hospital sector as a whole have never been unusually high (median hospital profits have hovered around 3 to 6 percent over the last decade), and for some rural and inner-city hospitals profit is so low they are in danger of going bankrupt.*

Thus, when we read a study indicating that U.S. hospitals charge much more for a good or service than independent suppliers do, or Canadian hospitals do, we should not conclude that American hospitals are making enormous profits. We should conclude, rather, that they are inefficient. For example, one study reported that American hospitals charged 20 times more than Canadian hospitals for syringes, needles, and swabs and three times more for blood cell counts.[1] In view of the relatively reasonable profits of most U.S. hospitals, it is unlikely that these high prices were due to excessive profit-taking by U.S. hospitals. For the average U.S. hospital, it is far more likely that inefficient hospital practices explain high charges.

The drug industry, however, is an example of a sector within the health-care industry that is wasteful in both senses – it spends enormous sums of money on activities it shouldn't spend money on, and it sets its prices at such sky-high levels that it enjoys obscene profits despite its inefficiency. Examples of wasteful expenditures include the huge sums the drug companies spend on lobbying, advertising, cajoling doctors to prescribe their drugs, and researching "me too" drugs. The evidence that the drug industry often corrupts the research it funds is accumulating so fast that it may soon be fair to state that a large portion of the drug industry's expenditures on research are worse than a waste of money; they

---

* Because the great majority of hospitals in the U.S. are nonprofit, it is more accurate to speak of the hospital industry's "margins" rather than its "profits." "Surplus" is what accountants call the excess of revenue over costs of *non*profits, and "profit" is used to describe the excess of revenue over costs of *for*-profits. "Margins" refers to both profits and surpluses. I use "profit" in the text because it's a term most readers are familiar with, and even nonprofit hospital staff sometimes refer to their "profit."

are expenditures that actually increase risks to patients. The evidence that the drug industry is guilty of price-gouging is the huge profits they make despite their wasteful expenditures. The drug industry makes profits three to four times those of the average Fortune 500 company, year in and year out. I will amplify these arguments in Chapter 7.

The waste in our health-care system can be divided into four categories: Administrative waste, excess capacity, excessively high fees and prices, and fraud. I have listed these in Table 6-1. After you've read the descriptions of the four categories of waste listed in Table 6-1, I believe you'll agree that any type of waste in the health-care industry you can think of can be assigned to one of these categories.

"Administrative waste" refers to *excessive* administrative expenditures. Every human enterprise, be it a business or a high school choir,

---

## Table 6-1: Waste in the American system can be divided into administrative waste, excess capacity, excessively high fees and prices, and fraud

Administrative waste*
        Insurance company overhead
        Provider (doctor and hospital) overhead
Excess capacity
High fees and prices
        High fees
        High drug prices
Fraud

* Ideally, other types of administrative waste should be listed here, not just excessive insurance company and provider overhead. The drug industry is unquestionably another source of excessive administrative costs. But the few studies that estimated administrative waste did not attempt to estimate excessive administrative expenditures by the drug industry. (Getting reliable data on drug industry administrative costs is probably impossible for anyone without subpoena power and millions of dollars to spend on auditors). Nor did those studies measure the variety of administrative costs employers and consumers incur in shopping for insurance and doing battle with insurance companies that refuse to reimburse doctors or authorize services.

---

has to spend some money on administration. The issue is not whether we should be able to reduce administrative spending to zero, but whether the amount of money the U.S. health-care industry spends on administrative functions (clerical services, advertising, and other services that do not constitute medical care) is excessive. The answer is clearly yes. "Excess capacity," the second category of waste, refers to too many buildings and too much equipment. This is primarily a problem within the hospital industry. "High fees and prices" needs no further explanation. Fraud is estimated to siphon off as much as 10 percent of U.S. spending on health care. I will discuss administrative waste and excess capacity in this chapter, and excessive fees and prices and fraud in Chapter 7.

## Waste category number one: Administrative waste

In 1993, the year that Bill and Hillary Clinton led the nation's policy makers and pundits in mass genuflection to the theory of "managed competition," the *Washington Monthly* published a fascinating article entitled, "Dead on arrival: Why Washington's power elite won't consider single payer health reform."[2] The authors – Tom Hamburger, then the Washington bureau chief for the Minneapolis *Star Tribune*, and Ted Marmor, a health policy expert at Yale – blamed the self-reinforcing behavior of Washington's "three established tribes: the politicians, the press, and the experts." Hamburger and Marmor reported that politicians refused to discuss the single-payer proposal because they were "terrified" of the health insurance industry; reporters generally failed to inform their readers of the details of single-payer and other health policy proposals because they were "too focused on politics, not on substance"; and experts didn't write articles and speak about single-payer because foundations generally refused to fund research on single-payer and because experts were fearful of "being dismissed as cranks or out-of-touch with *realpolitik*."

To this analysis I would add one other factor: The health insurance industry pours money into the nation's colleges, universities, and think tanks to fund professors and projects to the industry's liking. For example, the American Association of Health Plans, the former trade group for HMOs (which has since merged with the Health Insurance Association of America, the trade group for the non-HMO wing of the industry), gave money to two professors at the University of California San Francisco to write an article which claimed that scientific research demonstrates that HMO care is not inferior to the care offered by doctors outside HMOs.[3] (I wrote a rebuttal to this article for the *American Journal of Public Health*).[4] Blue Cross and Blue Shield of Minnesota has funded a position at the University of Minnesota called the "Blue Cross Professor of Health Insurance," now occupied by Roger Feldman, an economist who claims managed care saves money and who advocates market solutions to the health-care crisis.[5] Stephen Shortell is the Blue Cross of California Distinguished Professor of Health Policy and Management at UC Berkeley.[6] Glenn Melnick is the Blue Cross of California Professor of Health Care at the University of Southern California.[7] Aetna, the nation's largest private-sector insurer at the time, "gave a grant to the University of Pennsylvania for reworking the medical school curriculum to cover managed care issues," reported *American Medical News.*[8]*

We have already seen that health policy researchers paid much more attention to overuse than underuse of medical services. But nothing illustrates the bias of the nation's health policy experts better than their disinterest in the administrative costs of the U.S. system. With the exception of a few scholars associated with Physicians for a National Health Program (PNHP), a group representing 13,000 physicians who support a single-payer system, the health policy experts in this country have published no research on the total cost of administering the U.S. system. Most of what little research has been published on this subject

---

* The practice of buying influence at universities is not peculiar to the health insurance industry. American students may now sit at the feet of professors who occupy the Yahoo! chair of information systems technology (Stanford), the Coca Cola distinguished professor of marketing (University of Arizona), the Taco Bell distinguished professor of hotel and restaurant administration (Washington State University) (Paul Starr, "Your name here," *The American Prospect*, September-October 1998, 96), the Kmart professor of marketing (University of West Virginia), and the Freeport McMoRan (a mining company accused of despoiling the environment) chair in environmental studies (Tulane) (Eyal Press and Jennifer Washburn, "The kept university," *Atlantic Monthly*, March 2001, http://srd.yahoo.com/goo/%22The+kept+university%22/4/T=1010929679/ F=dbd95fd3bfc0858f38faf12a4fb7da7c/*http://www.newamerica.net/articles/ article.cfm?pubID=134&T2=Article, accessed January 13, 2002).

appeared between 1991 and 1993, largely in response to two papers published in 1991, one by Steffie Woolhandler and David Himmelstein, leaders of PNHP who teach at Harvard Medical School, and the other by the U.S. General Accounting Office, a research arm of Congress.* The Woolhandler-Himmelstein paper, published on May 2, 1991 in the *New England Journal of Medicine*, measured total administrative spending in the U.S.[9] The GAO report, which had been requested by Representative John Conyers (D-MI), a single-payer supporter, addressed a slightly different question: How much money would the U.S. save in administrative expenses if it adopted Ontario's single-payer system (Ontario is Canada's largest province)?[10]

---

* The Woolhandler-Himmelstein paper and the GAO report provoked a conference on the subject of administrative costs. The conference, funded by the Robert Wood Johnson Foundation and conducted by the Alpha Center (an arm of the Robert Wood Johnson Foundation), was held in February 1992. Not surprisingly, this conference produced a number of papers sympathetic to the managed-care plan industry, including: Anne K. Gauthier et al., "Administrative costs in the U.S. health care system: The problem or the solution," *Inquiry* 1992;29:308-320; and Kenneth E. Thorpe, "Inside the black box of administrative costs," *Health Affairs* 1992;11(2):41-55. The paper by Gauthier et al. asserted, for example, "New administrative structures are needed for the more difficult management tasks facing our society, such as ... controlling costs, managing care, improving patient outcomes, producing useful data, and changing provider behavior" (317). The unabashed and undocumented claim that (a) all these things need doing and (b) must be done by health insurance companies should have embarrassed these authors.

*Health Affairs* published several articles on the issues raised by Woolhandler-Himmelstein and the GAO in its spring and summer 1992 editions, and *Health Care Financing Review* published an article on administrative costs of several nations. These and a half dozen other papers constitute the entire body of peer-reviewed literature on the cost of administering the U.S. system.

The media's interest in administrative costs has been as lukewarm as the experts'. In the early 1990s, newspapers published several articles about the overhead costs generated by managed care. (See, for example, Mariann Caprino, "Sick of paper," Minneapolis *Star Tribune*, January 15, 1993, 1; and Thomas M. Burton, "Firms that promise lower medical bills may increase them," *Wall Street Journal*, July 28, 1992, A1). With the exception of a few articles generated by government investigations of managed-care plans, the media has ignored the subject of administrative costs.

The widespread apathy among experts toward administrative spend-ing stands in stark contrast to the enormous size of administrative costs. In their 1991 paper, Woolhandler and Himmelstein estimated that ad-ministering our system absorbed 22 percent of our health-care dollar in 1983, and 24 percent in 1987. In a subsequent paper, they estimated the total cost had risen to 31 percent in 1999.[11] To put it another way, only two-thirds of our health-care dollar actually goes to doctors, nurses, pharmacists, home care workers etc. to take care of patients.

To repeat, it's not possible for any group or business to devote all of its revenue to its "mission" or "program" and zero money to overhead. The issue is not whether all administrative expenditures our health sys-tem incur are wasted. The issue is whether *some portion* of it is wasted. The small body of research available on this subject indicates that about half of the 31 percent of our health-care dollar spent on administration is necessary and the other half is wasted.

The wasted half is due to two features of our health insurance sys-tem: (1) The system is dominated by managed-care plans (MCPs); (2) the system is dominated by hundreds of private sector plans which are less efficient than government insurers like Medicare. The problem of unnecessary administrative costs is aggravated by the absence of true competition in the insurance industry. I'll talk about the impact of managed care and multiple payers in this chapter. I'll talk about the absence of competition in the industry in Chapter 9 where I discuss the defects of managed competition.

## Waste generated by managed care

It appears that no one has published an analysis of the change in administrative expenditures for the entire health-care system during the period that managed care spread. However, we do have some data and a few studies that permit us to examine changes in administrative costs for portions of the system. Let's look first at the insurance sector.

Table 6-2 presents data for the HMO industry in Minnesota. This table reports what happened to the administrative expenses of Minnesota's HMOs compared with their health-care expenses (that is, their expenditures on patients) between 1980 and 1991, a period during which HMO enrollment in Minnesota more than doubled. You see that HMO administrative expenses rose 403 percent compared with a 255 percent increase in their health-care expenditures. Given that HMO enrollment more than doubled, the rapid increase in administrative expenditures is astonishing. In most industries, a doubling of production would *reduce* overhead (another term for administrative costs) per unit produced. The fact that overhead per insured patient rose so dramatically during the 1980s in Minnesota was probably due to "competition" among HMOs to tighten their grip on doctors and cut the volume of medical services, which in turn required the HMOs to hire a lot more people to police the doctors. As was the case around the country, the huge increase in enrollment in Minnesota HMOs during the 1980s came at the expense of traditional insurers like Blue Cross. The Blues and other traditional insurers responded by adopting managed-care tactics, which drove up their administrative costs.

A handful of data reveal the same pattern at the national level. During the period 1981 to 1991, when managed-care enrollment accelerated, administrative costs for all private-sector insurers rose 265 percent while claims paid increased only 171 percent. During this same time period, Medicare's administrative costs fell from 2.9 cents to 2.1 cents per dollar of claims paid.[12] During the period 1987 to 1993, the period in which MCPs completed their takeover of the U.S. health-care system, the growth rate of private-sector health insurance administrative expenditures soared compared to the growth rate of health insurance premiums. Administrative expenditures by health insurers, per person covered, rose by 236 percent while premiums rose only 70 percent for non-HMO plans and 71 percent for HMOs.[13]

The spread of managed-care tactics also drove up administrative costs for providers. The following excerpt from a report by the Public Advocate for the City of New York on how MCPs in New York delay and deny medical care illustrates some of the problems managed care creates for doctors:

> Rita Paciullo ... handles administration for a Bronx medical practice which includes prominent physicians at Montefiore Medical Center. She said it is "difficult to get through" to many MCOs [managed-care organizations] to obtain a pre-authorization and she cited Aetna ... in particular. To begin with, she explained,

"the phone number on the card" that the physician is supposed to call "is not necessarily the right office at the HMO for that [patient] ID number or that group number. So often you are 20 minutes on hold and then you find out you're supposed to call a different number." She continued, "You have to listen to maybe four recorded messages, hope you punched in the right number, and when you finally get to talk to an employee in the right place you may have to fax them notes of what you want them to approve. And then you have to keep calling them back to see if they got the fax – they never call you. So we've had to increase staff. We have people doing nothing but getting on phone [*sic*] with insurance companies."[14]

---

## Table 6-2: HMO administrative costs shot up as HMOs spread: Minnesota HMO expenditures, 1980 and 1991 (per HMO member per month)

| Expense category | 1980 | 1991 | Percent change[a] |
|---|---|---|---|
| Health care | $30.11 | $106.73 | 255% |
| Administrative | $3.14[b] | $15.78[b] | 403% |
| Total | $33.44 | $122.43 | 266% |
| | | | |
| Total HMO enrollment | 451,105 | 1,193,800 | |

(a) Percent changes calculated by the author. The figures for this column reported in the original source were wrong.

(b) These figures understate the HMOs' administrative costs. If you divide the $15.78 of overhead in 1991 by $122.43, you get 13 percent. Other data indicate the percentage is higher, possibly two to three times as high (see discussion in Appendix B). The Minnesota Department of Health, the source for these data, requires HMOs to file annual reports on their expenditures. The Department permits HMOs to allocate some administrative services to the medical services category.

Source: Bert McKasy, Minnesota Commissioner of Commerce, and Marlene E. Marschall, Commissioner of Health, *Study of Health Care Management Companies*, St. Paul, MN, March 1993.

## Table 6-3: Administrative personnel have grown much faster than medical staff: Full-time-equivalent medical personnel (thousands) in the U.S., 1968 and 1993

|                               | 1968  | 1993   | Percent change |
|-------------------------------|-------|--------|----------------|
| All medical personnel         | 3,976 | 10,308 | 159%           |
| All administrative personnel  | 719   | 2,792  | 288            |
| Physicians                    | 430   | 761    | 77             |
| Registered nurses             | 544   | 1,434  | 164            |
| Licensed practical nurses     | 250   | 537    | 115            |

Source: David U. Himmelstein and Steffie Woolhandler, "Who administers? Who cares? Medical administrative and clinical employment in the United States and Canada," *American Journal of Public Health* 1996;86:172-178.

## Table 6-4: Hospital administrative expenditures shot up as managed care spread: Percentage change in full-time-equivalent hospital personnel* per 1,000 adjusted patient days, adjusted for changes in patient health, 1981-1993

| Total              | 11.3%  |
|--------------------|--------|
| Nursing            | -7.3%  |
| Technicians        | 16.2%  |
| Nonprofessional    | 19.5%  |
| Administration     | 46.5%  |
| Other professional | 50.0%  |

\* "Nursing" personnel included registered nurses, licensed practical nurses, and aides; "technicians" included clinical technical personnel, such as pharmacy technicians; "nonprofessional" included nonclinical support personnel; "administration" included nonclinical administrative staff; and "other professional" included clinical professional staff such as dietitians, physical therapists, and social workers.
Source: Linda H. Aiken et al., "Downsizing the hospital nursing workforce," *Health Affairs* 1996;15(4): 88-92.

Table 6-3 reports the results of a study that examined job growth in the provider sector between 1968 and 1993. You can see that growth in administrative jobs that support medical personnel – the people who deliver health care directly to patients – greatly exceeded growth in medical jobs. Between 1968 and 1993, the number of *medical* personnel working in the U.S. grew 159 percent, way below the 288 percent by which *administrative* personnel grew. Table 6-4 shows administrative costs ballooned in the *hospital* industry between 1981 and 1993. You see that total hospital employment rose by 11 percent during that period, but administrative personnel rose by 47 percent and, perversely enough, nurses were cut by 7 percent. Other research indicates that 95 percent of physicians believe the spread of managed care increased their paper-work,[15] and that "managed care imposes requirements on substance abuse treatment facilities that significantly increase their administrative burden."[16] According to *U.S. News and World Report*, Riverside Methodist Hospitals, a 1,063-bed medical complex in Columbus, Ohio, needed 66 employees in its billing department as of 1992, twice the number it needed ten years earlier.[17]

This evidence that the spread of managed care drove up administrative costs explains why the MCP industry was unable to reduce health-care inflation. Many pundits are mystified by the apparent contradiction between the established fact that MCPs reduce the use of medical services and the MCP industry's inability to reduce health-care inflation. But there is no mystery. The increase in administrative costs offset the savings realized through reduced services to patients. The net effect on health-care inflation may have been zero or, worse, to aggravate inflation.

## Administrative waste generated by multiple payers: insurance sector

Now let's turn to the question of how America's private-sector, multiple-payer system contributes to excessive administrative costs for insurers (we will look at the problem for providers in the next section). "Multiple-payer" means that America's doctors, hospitals and other health-care professionals are paid by many different insurance companies and government insurance programs. It is difficult to find solid data on the number of health insurers operating in America today.

That's probably due to the fact that the fifty states regulate the insurance industry, which means there is no single government agency in America with a list of all health insurance companies currently licensed to do business in the country. Estimates of the total number of private-sector insurers operating in the U.S. run from 1,500 to 2,000.*

In Minnesota, the state I'm most familiar with, over 200 health insurance companies are licensed to serve the state's 5 million residents. Like many other states, Minnesotans are also served by several federally funded agencies, such as Medicare, Medicaid (which operates as fifty different programs, one for each state), the Veterans Health Administration and other programs for military personnel, plus several state-funded programs that expand coverage beyond the poor people covered by Medicaid.

The private-sector, multiple-payer system (with or without dominance by MCPs) creates high administrative costs for both the insurance and the provider sectors. It creates high administrative costs for

---

* Here is how three papers from the health-policy literature put it:

Last year [1994], health-care providers submitted more than 4.8 billion claims to over 2,000 different commercial health insurance firms, health maintenance organizations, preferred provider organizations, Medicaid, and Medicare processors. ["Processors" refers to the private-sector insurance companies that process claims for Medicare.] (Stephen C. Gleason, "Health system deregulation: Some aspects of health care system reform need not be held hostage," *Journal of the American Medical Association* 1995; 274:1483-1486, 1484.)

The current [1992] insurance market consists of approximately 1,500 third-party payers offering an infinite variety of payment, incentive, and benefit.... (Anne K. Gauthier et al., "Administrative costs in the U.S. health care system: The problem or the solution?" *Inquiry* 1992;29:308-320, 309.)

Nation-wide, hospitals currently deal with over 1,500 separate insurers.... (John F. Sheils and Randall A. Haught, *The Health Care For All Californians Act: Cost and Economic Impacts Analysis*, The Lewin Group, January 2005, A-16).

America's Health Insurance Companies, the insurance industry's trade group, claims to have 1,300 members (http://www.ahip.org, accessed June 11, 2005).

the insurance sector because private-sector insurers spend money on things public insurers spend little or nothing on, namely, marketing, underwriting (a strange word that means the insurer spends money to discover a patient's health history and to adjust premiums accordingly), lobbying, high salaries and lavish perks for executives, and, in the case of for-profit insurers, dividends for stockholders. (As I just noted, those payers that use managed-care tactics incur additional administrative costs, primarily in the form of salaries for people who supervise and second-guess doctors.) The multiple-payer system generates high costs for providers because it forces providers to deal with dozens, hundreds, or thousands of different insurers, all operating with different rules and forms. Below I offer evidence that administrative costs for both insurers and providers are higher in multiple-payer systems. But before we turn to that evidence, let me first describe in a little more detail how existing single-payer systems work.

Canada's system is administered at the provincial and territorial level (Canada has ten provinces and three territories). The Canadian federal government provides the majority of the funding and sets minimum standards each provincial and territorial program must meet. The provincial health ministry is the single-payer, which means it is the sole source of funding for providers. Moreover, the health ministry has the authority to set limits on physician fees and to negotiate budgets with hospitals. Even though Canada's national health insurance program provides spotty coverage for prescription drugs (the poor and the elderly are usually the only populations covered), Canada imposes price controls on drugs at the national level, and the provinces cut their drug costs even further by buying drugs in large volumes from drug manufacturers, which gives them the clout to negotiate prices even below the national price ceilings. As you can see, the phrase "single payer" is really shorthand for two features: One payer reimburses doctors and hospitals, and that one payer has the authority to set limits on what doctors, hospitals, and drug companies can charge. The one-payer feature, and the fact that this one payer doesn't attempt to supervise doctors as America's insurers do, accounts for Canada's very low overhead of 1 percent of revenues.

Traditional Medicare (the non-HMO portion of Medicare which enrolls 87 percent of all Medicare beneficiaries) resembles a true single-payer but is by no means an ideal single-payer. Medicare resembles a single-payer primarily because it is the sole payer of clinics and hospitals which treat Medicare beneficiaries for services insured by Medicare. Moreover, traditional Medicare pays these providers directly, that is, it does not funnel payments through insurance companies so that the insurance company can scrape 15 to 35 percent off the top before passing the rest on to providers. (For a discussion of the evidence underlying this estimate, see Appendix B.) Finally, Medicare sets limits on the fees doctors can charge. But (and here's where Medicare departs from a true single-payer), Medicare does not negotiate budgets for American hospitals. Instead, Medicare pays hospitals for each patient treated, and sets limits on what it will pay. Note I have said nothing about whether Medicare controls prices for drugs. Why? Because between 1966, when Medicare began, and 2006, when limited outpatient drug coverage will be added to Medicare, Medicare didn't cover outpatient drugs; Medicare only covered drugs administered in a hospital, such as intravenous antibiotics. Medicare's inability to control drug prices will not change in January 2006 when the program begins to offer meager drug coverage. Republicans saw to it that the law creating the drug coverage prohibited Medicare from negotiating with drug manufacturers to reduce drug prices.

With this explanation of Canada's system and of traditional Medicare, you're equipped to make sense of Table 6-5 which compares the overheads of the Canadian system and the U.S. Medicare program (the entire program, not just traditional Medicare) with those of private U.S. insurers. As you can see, the overhead costs of the Canadian system (1 percent of total revenues) and of Medicare (2 percent) are small compared with the 15-to-35-percent overhead of U.S. insurance companies. If these differences shock you, I urge you to consult the source materials I cite in Table 6-5. Better yet, use your common sense. Ask yourself, What administrative activities do private-sector insurers engage in that Canada's national insurance program and traditional Medicare pay very little for or do not engage in at all? Answer: marketing, underwriting (doing research on applicants to see how sick they are and setting premiums accordingly), policing doctors (in the case of MCPs but not traditional insurers), lobbying, paying spectacular sala-

## Table 6-5: Single-payers have lower overhead: Administrative costs for Canada's system, Medicare, and private health insurance companies as a percent of total revenues or expenditures*

Canada: 1%

Medicare: 2%

Average, all private-sector health insurance companies: 15-35%

* The paper from which Canada's overhead is derived expressed Canada's percent as a percent of *expenditures*. I had the option of expressing Medicare's overhead as a percent of *revenues* but chose to use expenditures instead because Medicare's revenues, by design, consistently exceed their expenditures in order to build up a reserve for future generations of beneficiaries. The 15-35-percent estimate of overhead for health insurance companies is based on research which expressed the percent in terms of both revenues and expenditures. As is the case with virtually all companies that are financially viable over long periods of time, insurance company expenditures and revenues are approximately equal.

Sources: For Canada, Steffie Woolhandler et al., "Costs of health care administration in the United States and Canada," *New England Journal of Medicine* 2003;349:768-775; for Medicare, author's calculations based on data reported in 2002 through 2005 editions of *Annual Report of the Boards of Trustees of the Federal Hospital Insurance Trust and Federal Supplementary Medical Insurance Trust Funds*, http://www.cms.hhs.gov/publications/trusteesreport, accessed July 29, 2005; for health-insurance-company figures, see Appendix B.

ries to management, and paying dividends to stockholders (in the case of for-profit insurers but not nonprofits).

*Modern Healthcare*, a trade journal for the health-care industry, reported my favorite example of private-sector administrative waste. In the early 1990s, the U.S. Senate investigated Blue Cross Blue Shield plans in the District of Columbia and several eastern states. The Senate report found numerous unexplained trips to exotic places by executives of the District of Columbia Blue Cross Blue Shield. *Modern Healthcare* offered this tidbit: "Also on the travel bill: a trip by the plan's president, Joseph Gamble, that took him to London, Paris and finally Zimbabwe at a cost of nearly $8,000. The reason for the trip? Mr. Gamble had to give a speech in Zimbabwe on fraud in the insurance industry."[18]

A 2001 audit of the books of Allina, a mammoth Minnesota non-profit HMO, by Attorney General Mike Hatch turned up numerous examples of clearly wasteful administrative expenditures. Allina, which did business only in Minnesota, Wisconsin and the Dakotas, paid for more than 1,000 trips to California and Florida, more than 30 trips to Hawaii, and trips to Aruba, London, France, Italy, Amsterdam, Athens, Mexico and Puerto Rico between 1998 and 2000. One of the California trips was taken by eight Allina executives to the beautiful city of Monterey to take a seminar on how Allina could find its "moral center." One dinner for these ethically challenged executives was served in a restaurant overlooking the 18th hole of the Pebble Beach Golf Course. Cost: $1,500.[19]

Lobbying legislators and the public is another administrative expense private-sector insurers incur that Canada's system and traditional Medicare do not incur. The single best known example of such lobbying is the series of "Harry and Louise" ads prepared for the Health Insurance Association of America (which recently merged with the American Association of Health Plans to become the obnoxiously entitled America's Health Insurance Plans). These ads attacked Bill Clinton's 1993 Health Security Act. Other examples of lobbying by the insurance industry include expensive media campaigns against single-payer ballot initiatives in California in 1996 (Proposition 186) and in Oregon in 2002 (Measure 23). The insurance industry outspent the proponents of Proposition 186 by three to one, and the proponents of Measure 23 by ten to one.

I have no idea how much the insurance industry spent to defeat the Patient Protection Act, a bill introduced by Senator Paul Wellstone in 1994, but it was no doubt a lot of money. The industry's campaign to defeat this bill included helping Republicans fundraise,[20] and, at least in Minnesota, pressuring insurance company employees to call members of Congress. On July 20, 1994, the Minneapolis *Star Tribune* reported that Blue Cross and Blue Shield of Minnesota's (BCBSM) had been caught urging its employees to lobby against the Patient Protection Act that Senator Wellstone had just introduced with support from the American Medical Association. Worse, the employees had been told to hide their connection to BCBSM. The memo asking BCBSM employees to do this came from BCBSM's "legislative director," Tom Lehman. The letter had gone to all BCBSM employees in Minnesota's Third Congressional District, which was represented by Representative Jim Ramstad (R), who was considering sponsoring the Wellstone bill in the House of Representatives. According to a spokesman for Ramstad, Ramstad had gotten only 20 calls, all positive, regarding the Patient Protection Act prior to the mailing of the Lehman memo. After Lehman's memo went out, Ramstad's office got 58 calls, all opposing the Patient Protection Act.[21] Polling data suggest that the vast majority of Americans consider the money spent on lobbying like this to be a waste of premium dollars.

If Canada's single-payer, and the traditional Medicare program in the U.S., do not pay for expensive advertisements and sales forces, do not underwrite, do not pay their managers millions of dollars and send them on junkets to exotic places, do not lobby politicians and take out ads to defeat federal legislation and initiatives on state ballots, do not tell doctors how to practice medicine, and do not have to make a profit for stockholders, is it any wonder that these public insurers are vastly more efficient than private-sector insurers?

## Administrative waste generated by multiple payers: provider sector

In the previous section, we examined the effect that multiple payers have on administrative expenditures by insurers. In this section, we examine the effect of multiple payers on the administrative expenditures of doctors and hospitals.

The administrative waste generated by multiple payers is probably higher, measured in total dollars systemwide, for the provider sector than it is for the insurance sector. Whereas the insurance sector in a multiple-payer system wastes money on marketing, underwriting, policing doctors, lavish executive salaries and perks, lobbying, and profit, the provider sector wastes money (a) dealing with multiple insurers, and (b), in the case of hospitals, keeping track of every service and item in order to document it in a bill to an insurer. I have seen no research describing the average number of payers clinics and hospitals deal with nor the average number of employees per clinic or hospital it takes to deal with these payers. However, I can pass on anecdotes, such as these:

In my urban practice I participate in 29 different managed-care plans, each with its own panel of physicians, consultants, hospitals, and diagnostic facilities.... It ... is a time-consuming burden to locate the consultants for each plan.... The snarled referral process depletes the physician's energy and drives up administrative costs. It can take hours to accomplish what used to be achieved with a simple note or telephone call to a trusted colleague. I have added one full-time administrative person whose time is almost entirely devoted to arranging managed-care referrals. The myriad plans, with complexities of primary and secondary billing, have also made my billing extraordinarily expensive and complex. What was once handled by one person now requires two-and-a-half employees, an expensive computer system, and expensive maintenance contracts for hardware and software. (Letter from a physician to the *New England Journal of Medicine*)[22]

In my office [with a dozen physicians], we take all health insurance. We have 350 individual contracts for different health plans, and we are supposed to remember 350 different types of options that insurance companies or plans may cover – which is impossible. (Statement of a Minnesota physician)[23]

Some urban teaching hospitals must deal with as many as 100 different so-called utilization review firms, "all of whom have different criteria," says Adrienne Levatino, vice president at the Illinois Hospital Association.[24]

Large American hospitals (those with more than 400 or 500 beds) cope with payers totaling in the hundreds, and occasionally thousands, and they need 50 to 70 employees in their billing departments versus ten to 15 people in large Canadian hospitals (which deal with one payer primarily) and German hospitals (which deal with many payers, but these payers have to follow similar billing procedures).* One of the best pieces published by the U.S. media about the health-care reform debate was a 1993 series of articles in the *Philadelphia Inquirer* that examined the U.S., Canadian, and German systems by focusing on a single hospital in each country: Lankenau Hospital (475 beds) in Wynnewood, Pennsylvania; North York General Hospital (473 beds) in Toronto, Canada; and Schwabing Hospital (1,372 beds) in Munich, Germany. These articles described the experiences of patients treated at these three hospitals. I thought the following description of the billing departments of these three hospitals was priceless:

> [T]he billing office [at Lankenau in Pennsylvania] was a blur of activity. There, dozens of hospital staffers were chasing after hundreds of pending hospital bills. Sitting in cubicles with computer terminals and reams of files, these employees tracked bills both old and new, some stretching back two years. In all, 53 people would spend this day at Lankenau making sure the hospital got the money it needs to operate. This was no easy task, considering how many ways there are in the U.S. to pay medical bills.... It's such a complicated, time-consuming business that Lankenau's finance section is larger than its departments of pediatrics or obstetrics or radiol-

---

* Because Canada's national health insurance system does not cover everything for sale in the Canadian health system, two-thirds of Canadians have supplemental insurance. The insurance covers items like drugs and private rooms in hospitals. For some patients hospitalized in Canada, the hospital may have to bill more than one insurer, but the calculations required are far simpler than those required of U.S. hospitals. Unlike Canada, Germany has a multiple-payer system, but the multiple insurers (called "sickness funds") are heavily regulated. Among the regulations they must abide by are regulations that make coverage uniform. These regulations minimize overhead costs for *providers*, but they do not appear to reduce the overhead costs of the German *insurers*. According to OECD data, *insurer* overhead as a percent of health expenditures in 1990 was higher in Germany than it was in the U.S., and much higher than it was in Canada (David U. Himmelstein and Steffie Woolhandler, *The National Health Program Book: A Source Guide for Advocates*, Common Courage Press, Monroe, ME, 1994, 123).

ogy…. Every plan [that Lankenau deals with] offered a different type of coverage. One had a $1,500 deductible, another had a $300 deductible plus a $150 deductible for every hospital admission, and another had a $125 deductible and 80 percent coverage until the patient spent another $400, after which full coverage kicked in. North York General in Toronto doesn't have to spend its time or money badgering insurance companies. Because its budget is almost totally funded by the government at the start of every year, it can make do with a dozen people in its billing office…. The German billing system is equally hassle-free, and Schwabing [in Munich] – with three times as many beds as Lankenau – needs only 18 people to do the job.[25]

First prize for the highest number of payers a hospital or clinic has to suffer goes to the Mayo Clinic in Rochester, Minnesota. According to the *New York Times*, "The billing office at Mayo deals with more than 2,400 insurers, each with its own standards. To ease the crunch, the 70 employees in the office have subspecialized, for example, with one in psychiatry and another in rehabilitation medicine. Together they make an average of almost 500 phone calls a day to insurers…."[26] (If Mayo is dealing with 2,400 payers, it must be dealing not only with the 1,500 to 2,000 U.S. insurers, but several hundred foreign payers as well.)

In addition to the myriad differences in coverage among payers, doctors must cope with bewildering diversity in obligations imposed upon doctors by their various payers. Ironically, an Aetna attorney relied on this fact in arguing to a federal judge that the judge should not consolidate several lawsuits involving 600,000 physicians against several MCPs, including Aetna, alleging the MCPs cheated them out of more than $1 billion. According to the Aetna lawyer, the lawsuits should not be consolidated into a single class-action lawsuit because each MCP is unique in the rules it uses to control and reimburse doctors. Aetna, he said, uses 22,000 different physician fees and more than 1,500 different physician contracts.[27]

It is occasionally alleged that Medicare's true overhead costs are higher than the 2 percent that Medicare's trustees report because

**Table 6-6: Medicare gives doctors less "hassle": Results of a survey of Ohio physicians\* (4-point scale with 4 representing the ideal)**

| | |
|---|---|
| Medicare | 2.20 |
| Aetna | 2.04 |
| Nationwide Health Plans | 2.03 |
| Medical Mutual of Ohio | 1.94 |
| United HealthCare | 1.94 |
| Anthem | 1.89 |
| CIGNA | 1.89 |
| Ohio State University Managed Care | 1.86 |
| Ohio Health Group's Health Reach | 1.82 |
| Medicaid | 1.70 |

\* The survey was prepared by MaternOhio Management Services, which "handles business tasks for ob-gyn practices in the Columbus area," according to *American Medical News*. The survey asked doctors to score the insurers on the quality of their billing, collections, patient identification cards, pre-certification for treatments, and other responsibilities. Only 36 of 180 clinics responded, which is generally regarded as a low response rate.

Source: Mike Norbut, "Ohio physicians rate insurers in HMO report card twist," *American Medical News*, August 11, 2003, 17.

Medicare "offloads" administrative work onto doctors and hospitals at a greater rate than private-sector insurers do. It is true that Medicare's paperwork for doctors and hospitals can be a royal pain, but there is no evidence that Medicare's paperwork is more burdensome than the private sector's. Because of the experts' indifference to administrative costs, no studies on this question have been published in the professional literature. The only studies I'm aware of are two surveys of doctors, one by the American Medical Association (AMA) and another by an Ohio company that provides business services to clinics. The AMA asked doctors how much time it takes them to prepare a Blue Shield claim versus a Medicare claim. The doctors indicated it took their staff about one hour for each type of claim.[28] The Ohio survey asked doctors to rate the ease of dealing with Medicare and 11 other insurers on a one-to-four-point scale, with 4 representing the ideal. As Table 6-6 indicates, Medicare won by a large margin over its nearest rival, Aetna. (The low score by Medicaid is probably because Medicaid in Ohio, as in most states, had been largely privatized, that is, turned over to MCPs, by the time the poll was taken.)

## Are administrative expenditures wasteful?

We have now examined administrative costs for both sectors of the health-care industry – the insurance sector and the provider sector. We have seen that administrative costs are driven up by the near-universal use of managed care, the multiplicity of payers, and the dominance of the multiple-payer system by private-sector insurers which incur administrative expenses that public-sector insurers do not incur.

Defenders of our system argue that all the money we spend on administrative costs is wholly or partially justified by benefits Americans allegedly derive from managed care and multiple payers. They argue that managed care improves quality of care and reduces costs. They claim multiple payers provide consumers with "choice of insurance company," and this choice is valued by all or most consumers. Neither argument is valid. Let's take the apologies for managed care first.

Here is an example of an ostensibly neutral health policy expert justifying the high administrative costs associated with managed care. Glenn Melnick, the Blue Cross-sponsored economist at USC we met earlier, offered this argument to the *Washington Post*: "Let's say you have two hospitals, one that has a single administrator and one with a large administrative staff. If that staff is looking at the cost-effectiveness of health care and studying outcomes, its administrative costs will be higher, but its cost per patient will be lower."[29] Melnick is implying that the enormous increase in hospital administrative costs that occurred during the era of managed care can be attributed to a large increase in scientists on hospital staffs who are finding ways to reduce hospital costs while maintaining or improving "outcomes," health policy jargon for the effect of treatments given to patients.

There is no published evidence to support Melnick's assumption that the primary cause of rising administrative costs at either the hospital or system level is an increase in scientists measuring "effectiveness of health care" and "outcomes." There is little evidence to support

Melnick's claim that the alleged presence of these hospital scientists has improved quality of care for the average hospital patient. Finally, there is no published evidence to support Melnick's claim that the additional costs of hiring these scientists (as opposed to other types of hospital employees) has been more than offset by a decrease in hospital costs. I will discuss what evidence we have on the effect of managed care in more detail in Chapter 9. I'll summarize the scientific evidence here:

(1) The evidence that managed care has saved America money is inconclusive; the fairest conclusion is that managed care has not saved any money.
(2) The evidence indicates managed care has, on balance, damaged quality.

In short, there is no good evidence supporting the claim by proponents of managed care that the extra administrative costs generated by managed care are justified by comparable benefits, either in the form of lower costs or improved quality.

Now let's examine the claim that the existence of multiple insurance companies for consumers to choose from is a blessing. The claim that Americans get some benefit from having numerous insurance companies to choose from never comes from the average consumer. In my 20 years of talking to average Americans about our health-care system, I have never once heard this argument made. The argument is made only by experts, typically economists, talking to one another at conferences or in the pages of professional journals. "Argument" is actually too fancy a word for what they offer. They simply assert that Americans "value choice" of insurer; they offer no documentation and no elaboration. Here are two examples, the first from the U.S. General Accounting Office, and the second from Patricia Danzon, a conservative economist:

> In the United States, multiple entities – some federal, some state, and some private – have a role in financing, administering and reimbursing the health-care system. The lack of a single entity managing the system results in piecemeal measures to control costs. On the other hand,

the decentralized competitive system offers the possibility of greater consumer choice concerning the level and nature of health-care benefits for some Americans. It has also led to the development of innovative approaches to health-care delivery, like HMOs and managed care.[30]

[T]he diversity of insurance plans that emerges in competitive insurance markets reflects the diversity of patient preferences.... The flip side of higher overhead costs accompanying a health-care market that offers choices among plans is that diverse consumer preferences are better satisfied than if all consumers must accept a uniform public plan.[31]

The claims made here that "greater consumer choice" and "choices among plans" are benefits Americans value are examples of naked ideology at work. Evidence abounds that Americans value the right to choose their own *doctor*. But there is no scientific evidence, nor, to my knowledge, any anecdotal evidence, that Americans place any value, much less a high price, on the "right" to choose between, say, Blue Cross and Prudential. The traditional Medicare program is a "one-size-fits-all" insurance program, to quote the contemptuous phrase used by conservatives who seek to privatize Medicare, yet the elderly who enjoy Medicare coverage are not clamoring for "choice" of insurer. Medicare is a very popular program (see further discussion in Chapter 11).*

The claim that Americans value choice of insurer is undermined by the fact that roughly half of all nonelderly insured don't have the option

---

* In their campaign to privatize Medicare, Republicans have deliberately sought to confuse seniors about what they are up to. They religiously use the phrase "giving seniors more choice," but they don't say choice of what. For example, in his third debate with Al Gore on October 17, 2000, George W. Bush stated, "In the Medicare reform I talk about it says ... we're going to give you choices to choose if you want to do so...." (Commission on Presidential Debates, http://www.debates.org/pages/trans2000c.html, accessed July 30, 2005). Astonishingly, Newt Gingrich admitted to this strategy in an interview with Jeff Goldsmith in *Health Affairs*. Gingrich claimed "Congressional Republicans won the debate over Medicare in 1996," a dubious claim, and that this was accomplished

to choose among insurance companies. For these Americans, choice of health plan is non-existent because their employer tells them what plan will be available.* For those whose employer gives them a choice, their options are rarely more than two or three, and, for most employees, these options long ago ceased to include a traditional insurer. The only Americans with lots of choices in the primary insurance market (as opposed to insurance that supplements Medicare) are the 4 or 5 percent of us who have to buy health insurance on our own and who have the money to do so. It is illogical to argue that Americans attach much value to choice of insurer when so few of us have it.

The only conceivable argument in favor of the claim that "Americans value choice of insurance company" is the selfish assertion that the healthy should have the option to choose an insurance company that avoids the sick and thereby keeps its premiums below average. But this argument that "Americans" want choice so "we" can avoid having to subsidize the sick appeals only to a portion of the American populace. Judging from opinion surveys on related topics, this portion is a very small minority. Large majorities of Americans support traditional Medicare, which is a uniform public plan subsidized by all of us, and large majorities support national health insurance or the principles underlying national health insurance. Harris polls indicate, for example, that 91 percent of the nation in 1987, and 88 percent in 1994, felt that "everybody should have the right to get the best possible health care – as good as a millionaire gets."[32]

In fact, considerable anecdotal evidence exists that Americans view "choice among plans" as a liability. Unlike conservative economists who

---

because "[e]veryone of our members had been trained. We all knew the right language; we all had the right answers." Goldsmith asks, "And what was the message?" Gingrich replies, "The message was, 'We guarantee you will get to keep Medicare, but you should have the right to choose:' No bureaucrat or politician should limit your right to choose." Goldsmith asks, "Choose what?" "That was the message," Gingrich replies cryptically. "Oh, OK," says Goldsmith, and Gingrich scampers on to another topic (Jeff Goldsmith, "Politics, technology, and transformation: A conversation with Newt Gingrich," *Health Affairs*, Web Exclusives, July-December 2003, W3-511-520, 513).

* Estimates of the percent of workers who have a choice of two or more plans vary, from 45 percent (1993 figure) to 60 percent (2001 figure) (Thomas Rice et al., "Workers and their health plans: Free to choose?" *Health Affairs* 2002;21(1):182-187).

have nothing better to do with their time than shop on the Internet for health insurance, the average American is frustrated by the difficulty of shopping for health insurance in the chaotic American insurance bazaar. As we shall see in Chapter 8, the typical American would much prefer a national, universal health insurance system that provided uniform coverage.

We may conclude this section, then, by observing that we pay higher administrative costs for the privilege of funneling our health-care dollar through hundreds of insurance companies, managed or unmanaged, and we incur administrative costs as well for the privilege of having these insurance companies tell our doctors how to practice medicine. Neither of these features – the multiplicity of insurers, and the use of managed care by insurers – can be justified on the ground that consumers want them and are benefiting from them. We may conclude, therefore, that the administrative expenditures associated with these features are wasted dollars.

## Waste category number two: Excess capacity

Let me begin this section by giving you a concrete example of how excess capacity raises the cost of our health-care system. Researchers affiliated with two federal agencies, the National Institutes of Health and the Food and Drug Administration, published a study in 1990 demonstrating that 10,000 mammography machines were in use in the U.S. that year, but only 2,600 were needed. That meant that each mammogram facility was doing an average of six mammograms per machine per day at a cost of about $110 per mammogram. According to the authors, if fewer machines existed, and they each did 20 to 30 mammograms a day, the cost per mammogram would drop to $50. The reason for this dramatic difference in price is that mammography facilities have very high fixed costs (costs that do not vary with the utilization rate of the machines); as these fixed costs are spread out over more mammograms, the cost per mammogram falls.[33] Observing these statistics, historian and managed-care proponent Paul Starr said, "Only in America are poor women denied a mammogram because there is too much equipment."[34]

Like the problem of excessive administrative costs, the problem of excess capacity – too many idle machines and facilities – is a woefully understudied phenomenon. Like excessive administrative costs, excess capacity is a relatively unpopular subject with the experts and the health-care industry because it places blame on the supply side (particularly hospitals) rather than consumers. Moreover, the persistent problem of excess capacity reveals a serious defect in the theory that competition works in the health-care industry and can be counted on to make the system efficient and keep price inflation to a minimum.

The literature on this subject consists of news stories and a very small number of scientific studies, most of which were published prior to the mid-1990s when the MCP industry was completing its takeover of the health-care system. This literature demonstrates that between the 1960s (and possibly earlier) and the 1990s, hospitals "competed" with one another not by lowering prices but by purchasing every conceivable medical device, regardless of whether the community in which this "competition" was occurring was already saturated with more than enough devices to meet demand. This form of competition between hospitals was called "an arms race."[35] The literature on the "arms race" suggests that it continued after the mid-1990s, the only difference being that by then the combatants had changed from individual hospitals to hospital chains, MCPs that owned hospitals, and large physician groups.

To give you some idea of how the arms race works, consider this excerpt from an article that appeared in the *Wall Street Journal* in 1990:

> [Dateline] Kalamazoo, Mich. – When the two archrival hospitals here found out that both planned to launch helicopter ambulance services, they flew into action. Borgess Medical Center quickly found a copter, called photographers and was first to get pictures in the local paper. But Bronson Methodist Hospital struck back, getting its chopper into the air first and proudly proclaiming a nurse aboard every flight. Borgess retaliated three months later, boasting a doctor on every trip. Within a year, each hospital had upgraded to twin-engine choppers – making the announcement the same week. "There are only 90 helicopter ambulances in the whole country," an exasperated executive of Upjohn Co.,

the city's largest employer, said at the time, "and two of them are here. Not to mention two heart programs, two maternity wards, two state-of-the-art emergency rooms, and two radiology services.... In most businesses, competition cuts prices. But hospital bills in Kalamazoo ... are the second highest in Michigan and among the highest in the nation. In general, hospital costs in two-hospital towns like Kalamazoo are 30 percent higher than in one-hospital communities...."[36]

Or consider these excerpts from a *Wall Street Journal* article published in 1994:

The Gamma Knife is a medical device that costs $3 million. It emits gamma radiation to treat brain tumors and lesions. But it is used on only a few types of tumors, and most of the 16 Gamma Knives in the U.S. are idle for all but two days a week. By some estimates, just six of them could have treated all American patients last year.... For people worried by runaway costs, the Gamma Knife is a troubling case. "It all comes down to a race to see who can have the better toys," charges James Proffitt, health-benefits manager at McDonnel Douglas Corp. of St. Louis.... [I]n southern Florida, ... two nearby hospitals are battling to see which can make the most of the Gamma Knife. A midsize community hospital, Doctors Hospital in Coral Gables, acted first, installing one last October [1993]. On March 28 [1994], Miami's biggest teaching hospital, Jackson Memorial Medical Center, activated its Gamma Knife. Officials at both facilities concede it is ridiculous to have two such specialized machines only ten miles apart. Yet neither would dream of yielding to the other.[37]

According to other media reports, the "arms race" has also produced too many cardiac catheterization labs, cancer radiation facilities, rehabilitation services, magnetic resonance imagers, bone-marrow transplant facilities, neonatal intensive care units, and hospital beds.[38]

This anecdotal evidence suggests a perverse hypothesis: That hospitals that have competing hospitals nearby charge more than hospitals that do not have competitors in their neighborhoods. Several studies confirmed this hypothesis. I just quoted the *Wall Street Journal* finding that "hospital costs in two-hospital towns ... are 30 percent higher than in one-hospital communities."[39] A study involving the great majority of U.S. hospitals documented the existence of this goofy relationship between "competition" and price for the whole country during the 1970s and 1980s. The results of this study, shown in Table 6-7, indicate that hospital costs, whether measured as the cost of serving one patient for one day or as the cost per patient admitted, rose as the number of competitors within 24 kilometers (about 14 miles) rose. For example, hospitals that had 11 or more hospitals within 14 miles charged $373 per day (see second column) while hospitals with no competitors within 14 miles charged only $325 a day. This is, of course, Economics 101 turned upside down.

Because competition does not work in the hospital industry, many states passed laws limiting capital expenditures by hospitals in the 1970s, then, with the advent of MCPs, repealed them. A study by Cindy Bryce

---

## Table 6-7: Hospital fees rise as "competition" intensifies: Hospital costs in relation to number of competitors, 1982

| No. of neighboring hospitals within 24 km | Avg cost per patient day | Avg cost per patient admission |
| --- | --- | --- |
| 0 | $325 | $2,268 |
| 1 | $331 | $2,340 |
| 2-4 | $340 | $2,432 |
| 5-10 | $362 | $2,674 |
| 11+ | $373 | $2,859 |

Source: James C. Robinson and Harold S. Luft, "Competition and the cost of hospital care, 1972 to 1982," *Journal of the American Medical Association* 1987;257:3241-3245.

and Kathryn Cline of Pennsylvania's experience with lithotriptors (machines which pulverize kidney stones with sound waves) indicates that MCPs were no substitute for regulation. Prior to 1986, Pennsylvania had a regulation in place that limited the number of lithotripters in the state to five until such time as all five machines were performing at least 1,000 lithotripsy procedures annually. (Bryce and Cline reported that lithotripters can perform up to 2,000 procedures annually, and that Canada's lithotripters averaged more than 1,700 procedures in 1991.) But when this regulation was repealed in 1986, the number of machines in the state shot up and utilization rates per machine fell. Between 1988 and 1994, the number of machines rose from six to 13, but the total number of procedures performed rose only 40 percent, resulting in a decline in the average annual utilization rate from 773 to 489 procedures per machine. In 1988, *two* of the *six* machines were doing more than 1,000 procedures annually. By 1994, *none* of the *13* lithotripters was doing more than 1,000 annually. The authors estimated that if five of the 13 machines were eliminated, the average cost of a procedure would fall from $2,107 to $1,331.[40]

In the 1980s and early 1990s, the consensus of expert and industry opinion was that the arms race was driven primarily by hospitals' efforts to please doctors.* Doctors, of course, are the people who decide whether to admit patients to hospitals, and, with a few exceptions such as maternity and emergency patients, patients usually go to the hospital their doctor refers them to. In the days before MCPs took power away from physicians, physician control over hospitalization gave doctors great leverage over hospitals. "I get threats all the time from doctors who say if I don't give them what they want, they'll go across town to Ohio State or Mount Carmel," said Nancy Schlichting, CEO of Riverside Methodist Hospitals in Columbus, Ohio.[41] The *Wall Street Journal* offered the same explanation for the rapid spread of the Gamma

---

* For example, Carolyn W. Madden offered this explanation in an influential health policy journal: "Competition among hospitals actually encouraged overbuilding because competition was quality- and technology-based rather than cost- or price-based. Hospitals needed to have the full range of available equipment and facilities in order to attract and retain a medical staff...." ("Excess capacity: Markets, regulation, and values," *Health Services Research* 1999;33:1651-1682, 1653).

Knife. "Last fall, Mr. Proffitt of McDonnell Douglas [which merged with Boeing in 1997] ... tried to block a Gamma Knife purchase in Kansas City, arguing that the few patients who needed it could go to medical centers in Chicago or Denver. But when a top neurosurgeon hinted that he might leave Kansas City if he didn't get a Gamma Knife, opposition to the purchase collapsed."[42]

By the 1990s, research suggested that hospitals in many markets were beginning to exhibit pricing behavior more typical of truly competitive markets. That is, hospitals in areas with numerous nearby hospitals tended to charge *lower* prices than hospitals with monopolies or near-monopolies in their service areas.[43] Experts attributed this change to the rise of large MCPs that used their marketing clout to demand discounts from hospitals. In markets where MCPs had numerous hospitals to deal with, hospitals were more likely to lower their charges. But despite the new pressure from a more consolidated and powerful insurance industry for lower hospital charges, the arms race did not end. In fact, by the late 1990s it may even have gotten worse.[44]

There are two differences between today's arms race and the race as it was conducted in the 1970s and 1980s. First, today's "competing" hospitals are more likely to be members of large MCPs or hospital chains than to be independent hospitals. Second, physician groups are more likely to be direct participants in the arms race than they were in the 1980s. In the early days of the arms race, physicians contributed to the race primarily by putting pressure on hospitals to buy expensive equipment. Today physician groups contribute to the arms race by buying equipment themselves that used to appear only on the premises of hospitals, and by constructing their own imaging centers and same-day surgery facilities, commonly called "specialty hospitals" or "ambulatory care centers."

Excess numbers of MRI and CT (computed tomography) machines are commonly cited examples of excess capacity caused by increased purchases by physicians. Between 1998 and 2002, family practice medical groups increased their billings for radiology services by 75 percent, and cardiology groups doubled their radiology billings.[45] In 2001, the five counties surrounding Syracuse, New York, had 20 MRIs; by 2004 they had 27.[46] The addition of all this imaging capacity in the Syracuse area means one of three things: the MRIs are being used at

## Table 6-8: Compared with other countries, the U.S. supply of imaging devices is high: CT scanners and MRIs per million people in eight nations, 1996 and 2002[a]

| Country | CT scanners[b] 1996 | CT scanners[b] 2002 | MRIs[b] 1996 | MRIs[b] 2002 |
|---|---|---|---|---|
| Japan | 69.7 | 92.6 | 18.8 | 35.3 |
| US[c] | 26.9 | 12.8 | 16.0 | 8.2 |
| Australia | 18.4 | na[d] | 2.9 | 4.7 |
| Italy | 16.9 | 23.0 | 3.1 | 10.4 |
| Germany | 16.4 | 13.3 | 5.7 | 5.5 |
| France | 9.4 | 9.7 | 2.3 | 2.7 |
| Canada | 7.9 | 9.7 | 1.3 | 4.2 |
| UK | 6.3 | 5.8 | 3.4 | 4.0 |

(a) For some countries, the data are for years earlier than 1996 and 2002. Canada's data, for example, are for 1995 and 2001.

(b) CT means computed tomography, and MRI means magnetic resonance imaging.

(c) Anderson et al., the source for the 2002 data, warn that that U.S. figures "may be an underestimate since the numbers in locations with multiple scanners are undercounted."

(d) Na means not available.

Sources: Except for Italy, 1996 data are from *1998 Commonwealth Fund International Health Policy Survey*, Commonwealth Fund, (October 1998); 1996 figures for Italy are from Gerard Anderson, "In search of value: An international comparison of cost, access, and outcomes," *Health Affairs* 1997;16(6):163-171; all 2002 data are from Gerard F. Anderson et al., "Health spending in the United States and the rest of the industrialized world," *Health Affairs* 2005;24:903-914, Exhibit 2.

capacity on appropriate patients; the MRIs are being used at capacity but a substantial portion of the images taken are unnecessary; or the MRIs are being used at below-capacity levels. The first outcome seems unlikely given how rapidly MRI capacity grew. It seems far more likely that the addition of seven MRIs in three years added to waste in the system, either by inflating unnecessary use of MRIs or by increasing excess capacity.

Judging from the complaints of hospitals, the purchases of diagnostic machines, diagnostic imaging centers, and specialty hospitals by doctors is aggravating excess capacity in hospitals. Hospitals claim that the doctors setting up these facilities are typically those who work in money-making hospital departments such as cardiac care, cancer treatment, and radiology, not the doctors who work in money-*losing* hospital departments, such as emergency and mental health services. Construction of physician-owned specialty hospitals increased so rapidly during the latter half of the 1990s, and hospitals reacted with such hostility, that Congress asked the Government Accountability Office to prepare reports on specialty hospitals. In two reports issued in 2003, the GAO confirmed the hospitals' allegations. The GAO reported that specialty hospitals tend to be for-profit, to exist in states that don't require physicians to get permission from a state agency to construct new facilities, to focus on cardiology and surgery, not to have emergency departments, to treat fewer Medicaid patients, and to treat healthier patients. Congress responded by calling for more studies and inserting a provision in the 2003 Medicare Prescription Drug, Improvement and Modernization Act that suspended construction of specialty hospitals for a period of 18 months.[47] The day after that moratorium on construction ended in June 2005, the Centers for Medicare and Medicaid Services announced it would reduce payment rates to specialty hospitals and make it harder for them to qualify for participation in Medicare.[48]

No one has published an estimate of the cost of excess capacity for the whole country, much less for the U.S. and several other countries. So it is impossible to say with any confidence how much the excess-capacity problem contributes to the high cost of U.S. health care compared to other countries. But Table 6-8, which looks at just two types of equipment, suggests excess capacity accounts for at least some of the difference. Table 6-8 lists device-to-population ratios for CT and MRI scanners for eight countries for the years 1996 and 2002 (for a few countries, the data are for years one or two earlier than 1996 and 2002). You can see that the supply of CT scanners and MRIs in the U.S. in 1996 greatly exceeded that in the other nations with the exception of Japan. By 2002, the gap between the U.S. and other countries had closed somewhat (again with the exception of Japan). Japan's stellar showing in this table may reflect the power of the CT and MRI manufacturers in that country. It is impossible to tell from Table 6-8 what the appropriate number of these devices is. Judging from occasional stories of long waits for MRIs in Canada in the 1990s, Canada's 1.3 MRIs per million people shown for 1996 was too low.* The fact that Canada's MRI-to-population ratio tripled between 1995 and 2001 (Canada's data in this table had a one-year lag) suggests Canada's policy makers also thought a ratio of 1.3 per million was too low. On the other hand, the Bryce-Cline study of Pennsylvania's excess capacity reported that MRIs in that state operated at only 60 to 75 percent of the state's recommended volume level between 1987 and 1994. This suggests that the 16 MRIs per million people in the U.S., the national level as of 1996, was too high.

## Review and a quick quiz

We have now discussed the first two categories of supply-side waste (excess administrative costs and excess capacity) of the four listed in Table 6-1. I will present more evidence on the problem of administrative waste in Chapter 11 when I talk about why Medicare should be the centerpiece of a reformed health-care system. I'll take up the last two categories of waste – high fees and prices, and fraud – in the next chapter.

This is a good place to remind readers of the volume-versus-price distinction, and the demand-side versus supply-side distinction, I made earlier. In Chapters 4 and 5 we examined six conventional diagnoses of the health-care crisis – overuse, age, lifestyles, malpractice litigation, violence, and superior quality. We noted that the first five of these excuses characterized the public – the demand side of the health-care market – as the primary cause of the U.S. health-care crisis. We observed, conversely, that with the exception of the HMO industry's physician-blaming version of the overuse excuse, none of those six excuses cast any blame on the supply side. To put this another way,

---

* Some poor countries of the world don't have even one MRI or CT scanner. According to an Afghanistan pediatrician, "There is not a single CT scan [he must have meant "scanner"], MRI or dialysis machine in the whole country [of Afghanistan]" (Tim Weiner, "A bazaar is newly abuzz and the talk is of a new era: After the Taliban, What?" *New York Times*, November 29, 2001, B5).

these conventional excuses blame the public for demanding, directly or indirectly, too many services. But the data we reviewed in Chapters 4 and 5 indicated the six conventional diagnoses have little explanatory power. They tell us little about why U.S. health-care costs are very high relative to those of other countries, and they tell us nothing about why health-care inflation heats up over short periods of time (typically three to five years) and then cools off for another short period of time.

In this chapter, we have reviewed evidence that the supply-side – the insurers, hospitals, drug companies and, to some extent, physicians – don't want the public to dwell on. We have seen that administrative costs are very high, and that our multiple-payer, managed-care insurance system is the cause. We have also seen that the unregulated American version of "competition" creates excess capacity.

But diagnoses that implicate the supply side continue to be rare compared with diagnoses that blame the public. To test your ability to spot a conventional public-blaming diagnosis, and to separate useful analysis from ideology, I present several typical diagnoses from the mainstream media. What's wrong with these statements?

> The bottom line, economists say, is that the nation's health spending can be controlled only if the public eases up in its demand for the latest technology, regardless of the price (article in the *St. Paul Pioneer Press*).[49]

> Economists concede that they have pinned the blame on technology mainly by eliminating other factors that might account for spiraling costs. "It's just hard to imagine what [the driving force] is, if not technology," said Joseph P. Newhouse, professor of health policy and management at Harvard University (article in the *National Journal*).[50]

The author of the first statement (a reporter) obviously subscribes to the overuse, public-is-to-blame, school of thought. The American public, according to this author, is insisting on having tests and pills and surgeries that are not necessary, and this self-centered and ignorant behavior is the cause of health-care inflation. According to this reporter, the supply side is doing nothing wrong, or at least nothing so serious as to warrant discussion in an American newspaper.

The statement by Joseph Newhouse, the prominent health policy expert quoted in the second example, is a bit more sophisticated, but it conveys a similar message. By blaming "technology," Newhouse is presenting either the overuse excuse or the quality excuse. That is, he is either saying that patients are getting unnecessary high-tech tests and procedures, or he is saying the tests and procedures they get are medically necessary, in which case he is implying quality of care is improving and that's what accounts for health-care inflation. There is a kernel of truth to both interpretations, but both are very misleading. Yes, it is true, some patients overuse medical care some times, but underuse is more prevalent than overuse. Yes, it is true that technology has improved quality of care substantially, but technological change occurs slowly and affects the entire industrialized world, which means it cannot explain change in health-care inflation rates over periods of five to ten years (which is how the technology or quality excuse is often used in this country), and it cannot explain the huge differences in costs between industrialized countries. More importantly, Newhouse's diagnosis conveniently distracts attention away from waste in the health-care industry – excessive administrative costs, excess capacity, price-gouging, and fraud.

## Endnotes

[1] R. D. Hull et al., "Subcutaneous low-molecular-weight heparin versus warfarin for prophylaxis of deep vein thrombosis after hip or knee implantation. An economic perspective," *Archives of Internal Medicine*, 1997;157:298-303.

[2] Tom Hamburger and Ted Marmor, "Dead on arrival," *Washington Monthly*, September 1993, 27-32.

[3] Robert Miller and Harold Luft, "Does managed care lead to better or worse quality of care?" *Health Affairs* 1997;16(5):7-25.

[4] Kip Sullivan, "Managed care plan performance since 1980: Another look at two literature reviews," *American Journal of Public Health* 1999; 89:1003-1008.

[5] University of Minnesota site, http://www.econ.umn.edu/faculty/feldman, accessed November 25, 2002.

[6] Peter P. Budetti et al., "Physician and health system integration," *Health Affairs* 2002;21(1):203-210.

[7] USC School of Policy, Planning and Development site, http://www.usc.edu/schools/sppd/faculty/melnick.html, accessed November 25, 2002.

[8] Julie A. Jacob, "Aetna wants you to be glad it met ya," *American Medical News*, September 13, 1999, 1, 30.

[9] Steffie Woolhandler and David U. Himmelstein, "The deteriorating administrative efficiency of the U.S. health care system," *New England Journal of Medicine* 1991;324:1253-1258.

[10] U.S. General Accounting Office, *Canadian Health Insurance: Lessons for the United States*, Washington, DC, 1991.

[11] Steffie Woolhandler et al., "Costs of health care administration in the United States and Canada," *New England Journal of Medicine* 2003, 349:768-775.

[12] Citizens Fund, *Premiums Without Benefits*, October 1993, Washington D.C.

[13] Kip Sullivan, "On the 'efficiency' of managed care," *Health Affairs* 2000;19(4):139-148.

[14] Public Advocate for the City of New York, *Obstacle Course: How Managed Care Organizations Manage to Delay and Deny Health Care*, New York, NY, June 1999, 35-36.

[15] "Survey: Physicians dissatisfied with managed care," *Journal of the American Medical Association*, unnumbered page entitled "AMA Action," August 25, 1999.

[16] Jeffrey A. Alexander and Christy Harris Lemak, "The effects of managed care on administrative burden in outpatient substance abuse treatment facilities," *Medical Care* 1997;35:1060-1068, 1067.

[17] Jerry Buckley, "Why the prognosis for reform is so poor," *U.S. News and World Report*, November 23, 1992, 30.

[18] "Company tab," *Modern Healthcare*, February 8, 1993, 40.

[19] David Hanners, "Allina OK'd lavish travel," *St. Paul Pioneer Press*, September 7, 2001, A1; Josephine Marcotty and Jill Burcum, "Allina leader agrees perks were wrong," Minneapolis *Star Tribune*, September 7, 2001, A1; and Kip Sullivan, "Minnesota fat cats," *In These Times*, July 8, 2002, 18.

[20] Public Citizens, *Holding Patients Hostage: The Unhealthy Alliance Between HMOs and Senate Leaders*, 2000, http://www.citizen.org/pressroom/release.cfm?ID=865, accessed November 25, 2002.

[21] Gordon Slovut, "Blue Cross employees join to lobby by phone: Dialing orders: Hide link to Blues," Minneapolis *Star Tribune*, July 20, 1994, 1A.

[22] Michael K. Rees, letter to editor, *New England Journal of Medicine* 1993;328:390-391, 391.

[23] Statement by Dr. Timothy Komoto, family practice physician at the Bloomington Lake Clinic in Mendota Heights, Minnesota, "Minnesota health care roundtable: Allocating health care resources," *Minnesota Physician*, January 1999, 22, 25.

[24] Ron Winslow, *Wall Street Journal*, "Effort to curb health costs is hitting snags," August 8, 1991, B1.

[25] Susan FitzGerald et al., *Healing in Three Nations: Care at What Cost? A Reprint of a Series Published in The Philadelphia Inquirer from April 25 to April 29 1993*, 3.

[26] Elisabeth Rosenthal, "Insurers second-guess doctors, provoking debate over savings," *New York Times*, January 24, 1993, A1.

[27] Catherine Wilson, "Doctors press managed care lawsuit," http://dailynews.yahoo.com/h/ap/20010507/bs/managed_care_1.html, accessed May 8, 2001.

[28] American Medical Association, Center for Health Policy Research, "The administrative burden of health insurance on physicians," SMS Report 1989; 3(2):2-4), cited in Steffie Woolhandler and David U. Himmelstein, "The deteriorating efficiency of the US health care system," and in U.S. General Accounting Office, op cit., fn. 5, 66.

[29] David Segal, "Managed care generates a paperwork explosion," *Washington Post*, February 15, 1996, D9, D12.

[30] U.S. General Accounting Office, op cit., 27.

[31] Patricia Danzon, "Hidden overhead costs: Is Canada's system really less expensive?" *Health Affairs* 1992;11(1):21-43, 26, 38.

[32] Letter from Dolores Parker, Harris Interactive, November 16, 2001.

[33] Martin L. Brown et al., "Is the supply of mammography machines outstripping need and demand? An economic analysis," *Annals of Internal Medicine* 1990;113:547-552.

[34] "The problem," Minneapolis *Star Tribune*, October 25, 1993, 29H.

[35] Gordon Slovut, "'Arms race' at area hospitals could raise costs," Minneapolis *Star Tribune*, March 6, 1991, 1b; Andrew Pollack, "Medical technology 'arms race' adds billions to the nation's bills," *New York Times*, April 29, 1991, A1.

[36] Ron Winslow, "Competitive anomaly: Consumers pay more in 2-hospital towns," *Wall Street Journal*, June 6, 1990, A1.

[37] George Anders, "Hospitals rush to buy a $3 million device few patients can use," *Wall Street Journal*, April 20, 1994, A1.

[38] Buckley, op cit; Slovut, op cit.; "Wasted health care dollars," *Consumer Reports*, July 1992, 435-448; "194,000 hospital beds vacant every day – study," *Modern Healthcare*, May 21, 1990, 7; George Anders, "As outpatient care gains, communities need to trim their excess hospital beds," *Wall Street Journal*, February 22, 1993, B1.

[39] Winslow, op cit.

[40] Cindy L. Bryce and Kathryn Ellen Cline, "The supply and use of selected medical technologies," *Health Affairs* 1998;17(1):213-224.

[41] Buckley, op cit., 37.

[42] Anders, op cit., A1.

[43] Thomas L. Gift et al., "Is healthy competition health? New evidence of the impact of hospital competition," *Inquiry* 2002;39:45-55.

[44] Glenn Howatt, "An 'arms race' in health care worries state," Minneapolis *Star Tribune*, November 19, 2002, A1.

[45] Reed Abelson, "An MRI machine for every doctor? Someone has to pay," *New York Times*, March 13, 2004, A1.

[46] Ibid., B3.

[47] Markian Hawryiuk, "Specialty hospital growth put on hold," *American Medical News*, December 15, 2003, 5.

[48] Centers for Medicare and Medicaid Services, "CMS outlines next steps as moratorium on new specialty hospitals expires," press release, June 9, 2005, http://www.cms.hhs.gov/media/press/release.asp?Counter=1478, accessed July 30, 2005.

[49] R.A. Zaldivar, "Hi-tech medicine is big cause of higher costs," *St. Paul Pioneer Press*, August 1, 1993, 1A.

[50] Julie Kosterlitz, "Paying for miracles," *National Journal*, August 7, 1993, 1967-1971, 1969.

# 7

# Waste in the System: High Fees and Prices, and Fraud

## Introduction

In this chapter, we continue our examination of the waste in the U.S. health-care system. In Chapter 6, we reviewed the evidence indicating that America wastes a lot of money on administrative expenditures and excess capacity. In this chapter we review the third and fourth categories of waste listed in Table 6-1 – excessive fees and prices, and fraud.

## Waste category number 3: Excessive fees and prices, overview

When economists investigate whether the sellers in a given market have the power to set their prices so far above their costs that they can make unreasonably high profits, they begin by asking whether the market in question is competitive. There is general agreement among economists and health policy experts that competition does not work well in the health-care industry. This general agreement was clear even before managed-care plans (MCPs) took over the industry. Back then it was commonplace for experts to state that the entire health-care industry was inefficient because it was subject neither to the laws of competition nor to effective regulation. The Congressional Budget Office observed in 1992, for example, "[H]ealth care markets are not truly competitive and therefore do not work very well."[1] Former U.S. Surgeon General C. Everett Koop said, "We have a system that is distinguished by a virtual absence of self-regulation on the part of those who provide care ... but distinguished as well by the absence of such natural marketplace controls as competition in regard to price, quality, or service."[2] Alain Enthoven and Richard Kronick, authors of the 1989 article laying out the blueprint for managed competition, said, "[W]e have a system that is neither efficient nor fair."[3] As we shall see in Chapter 9, the spread of managed care, and the consolidation of the health-care industry that it triggered, weakened what little competition existed in the industry.

True competition, which means competition for customers on both price and quality (not "competition" in the form of promiscuous advertising or an "arms race") thrives only when both of the following conditions are met: (1) buyers and sellers are so numerous that no seller or buyer can influence price or quality; (2) buyers are well informed about both price and quality differences. These conditions rarely prevail in the health-care industry. The insurer, hospital, drug, and equipment markets are often so highly consolidated that one or a few sellers dominate. When a few large sellers confront numerous small buyers, sellers can dictate or at least influence their own prices, and they can get away with inferior quality. In rural areas, doctors and hospitals often have monopoly status (monopoly means one seller). But the second requirement (informed buyers) is equally important. If buyers can't distinguish the price or the quality of one seller from another, competition will be weak even where sellers are numerous. In most sectors of the health-care industry, buyers – the patients who buy medical care and the employers and individuals who pay insurance premiums – have little or no information about the quality of the goods and services they are buying. Making *price* comparisons of medical services and tests is very difficult in most sectors of the health-care industry as well.[*]

---

[*] For example, in all but three states, it is impossible for the public to find regularly published data on what hospitals charge for their services. What little data we have on hospital charges indicate they are all over the map. Thanks to a law that took effect in California in 2004, Californians now know, for example, that the price of a Tylenol tablet ranges from free to $9 among California hospitals, and the price of a CT scan ranges from $882 to $4,038 (Lucette Lagnado,

Because competition is weak throughout much of the health-care industry, it is possible that profiteering occurs throughout much of the industry. However, the physician and drug sectors are the only sectors for which extensive evidence indicates overcharging is a chronic problem, decade in and decade out. Therefore, I focus on these two sectors in this section on excessive prices.*

## Excessive physician fees

In 2000, the average U.S. physician took home $205,700 (after expenses, and before taxes).[4] According to a 2004 report, Allina, formerly an HMO and now a hospital-clinic chain operating primarily in Minnesota, annually pays its cardiologists $586,000 plus benefits worth at least $143,000 a year.[5] Are those income levels excessive? In other words, are they more than we need to pay to induce a sufficient number of qualified Americans to undergo the rigorous training necessary to become a doctor and to practice high-quality medicine? As was the case with two other forms of supply-side waste we have already examined

---

"California hospitals open books, showing huge price differences," *Wall Street Journal*, December 27, 2004, A1). One of the only other sources of hospital prices that I'm aware of – a 1983 report published by what was then called the Council of Community Hospitals, a trade group representing Twin Cities Hospitals – stated, "[V]ery few communities in the United States even have the data available to produce hospital price information" (*Twin Cities Hospital Prices*, 1983, Minneapolis, MN, 11). This report listed prices charged by 32 hospitals in the Twin Cities area for 25 procedures covering the period April 1982 through February 1983. Prices varied greatly. For example, the price of a cataract operation, with no complications, ranged from $1,068 at Lakeview Memorial Hospital to $2,436 at St. Paul-Ramsey Medical Center (now called Regions Hospital). The number of operations performed could not explain this price difference. During the study period, Lakeview Memorial did 47 uncomplicated cataract operations while St. Paul-Ramsey performed 51.

*Excessively high prices is not the only category of waste that owes its existence to the absence of strong competitive forces within the health-care industry. The first two types of waste listed in Table 6-1 – excessive administrative costs and excess capacity – also owe their existence to feeble competitive forces. In a truly competitive industry, suppliers couldn't pay unnecessarily high administrative and capacity costs; they'd be driven out of business. It is conceivable that a truly competitive industry would also do a better job of addressing fraud, the fourth category of waste listed in Table 6-1.

– excessive administrative costs and excess capacity – the research on this question is woefully thin. You can find numerous reports on how much physicians earn, and whether physician income is going up or down, but it is very difficult to find research in the medical and health policy literature that asks whether physician income is too high (or too low, for that matter).

A 1992 analysis of competition within the health-care industry by the Congressional Budget Office is one of the few studies that addressed the problem of overcharging by physicians. The CBO concluded that physicians in general are overpaid. The CBO didn't actually say "overpaid." They used the more formal language of economists; they said doctors were paid an amount "above the return needed to attract the appropriate supply" of physicians.[6] The CBO based this conclusion on three types of evidence: the large number of qualified applicants to medical school who are turned away; research indicating that investments in medical education produce larger returns than investments in training for "most other occupations"; and the difference between what U.S. doctors make and what doctors in other countries make. Because this last type of evidence is the most understandable to most people, I will examine it in some detail. Studies of physician incomes and the fees they charge indicate U.S. physicians make much more money than do physicians anywhere else in the world.

Table 7-1 presents one of the very few studies I know of that compares U.S. physician incomes (after expenses but before taxes) to incomes in several other countries (not just one other country), in this case, five other nations. Unfortunately, the data are old – they are for 1965 and 1991. You can see that U.S. doctors made 70 to 75 percent more than German and Canadian doctors, and three times what doctors in Australia, France, and the U.K. made in 1991. You can see that the gap between U.S. doctors and doctors in all other countries grew considerably worse during the 1965-1991 period. (Because growth in U.S. physician income slowed in the 1990s, this gap may have gotten smaller since 1991.) You can see also that the much larger income we paid to physicians did not create the highest doctor-to-population ratio. Our ratio of 2.5 doctors per 1,000 people was lower than the German and French ratios. As we saw in Table 4-7, the U.S. ratio was low in

## Table 7-1: U.S. physicians have long been the highest paid in the world: Average physician pre-tax income in six nations (dollars), 1965 and 1991

|  | 1965[a] | 1991 | Percent change | Physicians/ 1,000 people 1991 |
|---|---|---|---|---|
| United States | 125,218 | 171,000 | 37% | 2.5 |
| Germany | 85,006 | 101,640[b] | 20% | 3.1 |
| Canada | 82,243 | 96,512 | 17% | 2.1 |
| Australia | 65,160 | 59,340 | -9% | 2.3 |
| France | 50,943 | 56,524 | 11% | 2.7 |
| United Kingdom | na | 53,381 | na | 1.7 |

(a) Measured in 1991 dollars, after expenses. The actual incomes were much lower in 1965. For example, the actual average income of U.S. physicians in 1965 was $28,960.

(b) Figure is for 1992.

Sources: Income data from *1998 Commonwealth Fund International Health Policy Survey*, Commonwealth Fund (October 1998); physicians-per-10,000-residents figure from http://www.oecd.org/oecd/pages/home/displaygeneral/0,3380,EN-search-0-nodirectorate-4-5-no-0,FF.html, accessed October 23, 2001.

2003 compared with other countries with the most expensive health systems.

Two studies published in the early 1990s of fees paid to U.S. and Canadian physicians indicated Canadian doctors were paid less than half as much, on average, for the identical service as U.S. doctors. Table 7-2 presents the later of these two studies. This study, done by Welch et al., compared doctor fees paid by the four largest Canadian provinces (Ontario, Quebec, British Columbia, and Alberta)* in 1992 with the fees paid to U.S. doctors by Medicare. Welch et al. concluded that

---

* Welch et al. noted that the fees paid by the other Canadian provinces not included in this study were almost identical to those reported for the largest four provinces.

## Table 7-2: Canadian fees for medical services are barely more than half of U.S. Medicare fees: Canadian and Medicare fees for selected medical services, 1992 (dollars)

| Type of service | Canadian fee* | Medicare fee | Canadian-to-Medicare ratio |
|---|---|---|---|
| Office visit, established patient | $22.34 | $31.00 | 0.72 |
| Emergency room visit | 19.47 | 46.19 | 0.42 |
| Coronary artery bypass graft (three grafts) | 998.38 | 2,225.25 | 0.45 |
| Total knee replacement | 553.78 | 1,815.73 | 0.30 |
| Transurethral resection of prostate | 327.46 | 801.69 | 0.41 |
| Remove cataract, insert lens | 388.57 | 940.57 | 0.41 |
| Colonoscopy | 138.65 | 262.89 | 0.53 |
| Chest X-ray, two views | 5.40 | 10.54 | 0.51 |
| Left hand catheter, coronary angiography | 239.78 | 434.01 | 0.55 |

* Welch et al. made two adjustments to the Canadian fees. First, they converted the Canadian fees to equivalent U.S. dollars (the Canadian dollar has for decades been worth less than the U.S. dollar). Then they raised Canadian fees by 13.6 percent to reflect the higher overhead costs of American doctors. I saw no point in obscuring the true difference between Canadian and U.S. doctor fees just because the American multiple-payer, managed-care system imposes higher administrative costs on U.S. doctors. To undo this correction, I multiplied the Canadian fees presented by Welch et al. by 0.88.

Source: Medicare fee data are from W. Pete Welch et al., "Physician fee levels: Medicare versus Canada," *Health Care Financing Review* 1993;14(3):41-54, Table 1; Canadian fee figures and Canadian-to-Medicare ratio figures are my calculations based on data presented in Welch et al., Table 1.

Canadian fees were 59 percent of U.S. Medicare fees. Then they noted that U.S. private insurer fees were 150 percent of Medicare's fees. That means Canada's fees were 39 percent of U.S. private-sector fees in 1992. However, the disparity is even worse than Welch et al. reported. Welch et al. inflated the Canadian fees by 13.1 percent in order to reflect the advantage Canadian doctors have in lower overhead costs due to their single-payer system. Thus, if we want to separate out fee differences from the impact of Canadian-U.S. differences in administrative costs, we have to reverse the inflation in fees that Welch et al. built in to the fees they reported for Canada. If we do that, it turns out Canadian fees were 52 percent of U.S. Medicare fees and 35 percent of private-sector U.S. fees in 1992.*

The only other study that attempted to compare U.S. and Canadian fees compared the fees paid in Iowa by both private- and public-sector insurers with those paid in the Canadian province of Manitoba in 1985, and extrapolated those findings to all of Canada and the U.S. They concluded that Manitoba doctors were paid 46 percent of what Iowa doctors were paid and that the average Canadian doctor was paid 42 percent of what American doctors were paid.[7]

What could justify paying America's doctors two or three times as much as doctors in other countries? We have already discussed and rejected the argument that the quality of care in the U.S. is superior to – never mind twice as good as – the quality available in other countries. We saw there was no scientific evidence to support that claim, and even some evidence suggesting U.S. quality is slightly inferior. Go back and look at Table 5-9, the table that showed differences in survival rates of Manitobans and New Englanders following ten types of surgery. You see rates listed for transurethral prostatectomy and coronary artery by-pass surgery, procedures that also show up in Table 7-2.† Notice that the three-year death rate among New Englanders shown in Table 5-9 was worse for both of these types of surgery. Yet the study by Welch et al. indicates Canadian surgeons were paid less than half of what U.S. surgeons were paid for these procedures. Those data contradict the claim that the fees and incomes of U.S. physicians are double and triple

---

* This study was done, incidentally, for the Health Care Financing Administration (HCFA), the old name for the agency that runs Medicare and Medicaid. The study was done in the early 1990s and published early in 1993, just as the entire health policy establishment was rushing to embrace managed competition. HCFA, like most health policy experts and foundations that fund health policy research, has shown little interest since 1993 in studying price controls or single-payer systems.

† Tables 5-9 and 7-2 use different terms for the same procedure – "transurethral prostatectomy" and "transurethral resection of the prostate."

those of doctors in other countries because quality of care in the U.S. is double or triple that delivered in other countries.

Nor can it be argued that America's unusually high physician payments are necessary to induce a sufficient number of Americans to become doctors. We have seen that the supply of doctors on a per capita basis is relatively low in the U.S. even when we restrict our comparison to the world's most expensive health systems.

In a truly competitive market, the high incomes of doctors would attract an influx of new doctors, and this influx would drive physician fees and incomes down to the point where physician incomes were roughly equal to the incomes of other professions with similar training costs. According to the Congressional Budget Office, this has not happened, in part because the supply of new physicians is constrained by the admissions policies of the nation's medical schools, which are in turned influenced by the American Medical Association. "[T]he number of qualified applicants for medical school is far greater than the number of student slots available," said the CBO, "so the entry limits probably matter."[8] During the 1990s, applications to medical schools exceeded slots at medical schools by a factor of two or three to one. The peak occurred in 1996 when 46,968 students applied for 16,200 openings. Officials representing the nation's 125 medical schools confirm the CBO's statement that the people being rejected by medical schools are by and large qualified. "The application process is expensive, time-consuming and ego-bruising, so people don't apply to medical school unless they have a reasonable chance of acceptance," said Dr. Jordan J. Cohen, president of the Association of American Medical Colleges.[9]

I occasionally hear people argue that U.S. doctors should make as much money as they do because they graduate from medical school with large debts. There is no question that medical students graduate with huge debts; the average medical school graduate was $99,000 in debt in 2001.[10] But does a debt of $99,000 acquired at the beginning of a physician's career justify an income that is so high that the $99,000 debt is repaid dozens of times over by the time the physician retires? Of course not.[*]

We may conclude, then, that U.S. physicians are paid far more than physicians anywhere else in the world, and that this difference cannot be

---

[*] There are three ways to document my assertion that a typical medical school debt is paid many times over by the time a typical U.S. physician retires.

explained by greater quality of medical care in the U.S., by an unusually large supply of physicians in the U.S., nor by the debt that the average U.S. doctor bears upon graduation from medical school. Moreover, only a small portion of the difference in fees and gross incomes between doctors in the U.S. and elsewhere can be attributed to higher overhead for U.S. doctors. The evidence indicates, in short, that the average American doctor is overpaid.

Whether *all* U.S. doctors are overpaid is another matter. My own impression is that primary care doctors are not overpaid but specialists are. But that is an impression only. I have not seen international comparisons of physician income that report incomes separately for primary care doctors and specialists.

## Excessive drug prices

Americans pay much higher prices for prescription drugs than do citizens of other countries. Even the American drug manufacturers admit this. Whether we look at drug *expenditures*, which reflect both vol-

---

First, we can refer to two studies cited by the CBO in support of its statement that the return on investment in a medical degree is much higher than it is for other professions. Second, we can cite Welch et al. They said that even if Canadian medical school graduates had no debt at all (which is an incorrect assumption), differences in debt among U.S. and Canadian doctors would explain just 1.5 percent of the huge differences in physician fees in the two countries. Third, we can use some common sense and some fourth-grade arithmetic to demonstrate that the huge incomes physicians get more than compensate them for their medical school debt. Here's the arithmetic. A typical physician will practice for 35 years – from about age 30 to age 65. During those 35 years, the typical U.S. doctor will be paid roughly $120,000 to $170,000 more than doctors in other countries. If our sole concern is ensuring that U.S. physicians are paid enough to reimburse them for their $99,000 in debt, do we need to pay them $70,000 to $120,000 more per year every year for 35 years to accomplish that? No. If it is important to America that our physicians, unlike other professions, enter the work force debt-free, there are ways to accomplish that that don't rely on overpaying them throughout their entire career. We could, for example, subsidize medical education even more than we do today. Or we could, with Medicare-style limits on fees, reduce physician incomes to a level that would still suffice to attract the necessary number of physicians – let's say, using the 1991 figures shown in Table 7-1 – from $171,000 (the U.S. level) to the German level of about $100,000, and then add to that sum about $5,000 a year so that over 35 years physicians would be paid back their $99,000 debt plus the interest they paid.

ume and price, or just drug *prices*, we see the same picture – Americans are paying through the nose for prescription drugs.

The campaign to force the big drug companies to sell AIDS drugs at a price affordable to Third World countries has revealed some astonishing differences in the price at which drug companies sell drugs in different countries. Under pressure from AIDS activists, drug manufacturers recently agreed to sell a year's supply of the "AIDS cocktail" for one patient for $1,000. This was far below the $10,000 to $15,000 charged in the U.S. However, it was still higher than the $600 per year per patient that an Indian manufacturer said it could provide the drugs for. The Indian manufacturer – Cipla Ltd. of Bombay – made the offer to Doctors Without Borders, a group that had called on the drug multinationals to reduce the price of their AIDS medicines.[11]

Like defenders of excessive administrative costs, excess capacity, and excessive physician fees, defenders of excessive drug prices claim they are justified because they benefit Americans. The benefit, they say, is research – research by the drug industry on new drugs that cure disease. Any reduction in drug prices, say these advocates, will inevitably lead to less research on life-saving and life-improving drugs. The most aggressive proponent of this argument is, of course, the drug industry. The industry has been making this argument since at least 1959 when Senator Estes Kefauver (D-TN) opened his investigation into the high price of prescription drugs. The industry has promoted this argument even more vigorously since 1993 when President Bill Clinton called drug prices "shocking" and implied he might endorse drug price controls. In 1994, the industry even changed the name of its trade group from the Pharmaceutical Manufacturers Association to the grammatically tortured Pharmaceutical Research and Manufacturers of America (PhRMA).

PhRMA's Web site claims that the process of inventing new drugs and getting them approved for sale by the FDA exposes drug companies to "high risk" and that unless drug companies earn profits "commensurate with [that] high risk ... , investors will probably put their money elsewhere."[12] In May 2000, PhRMA's president, Alan F. Holmer, told the Senate Finance Committee, "Government price controls are unacceptable to the industry because they would inevitably harm our ability to bring new medicines to patients."[13] In his debate with Al Gore on October 17, 2000, presidential candidate George W. Bush responded as follows to a question from the audience about what he planned to do to reduce drug prices: "I'm against price controls. I think price controls would hurt our ability to continue important research and development. Drug therapies are replacing a lot of medicine as we know it. One of the most important things is to continue the research and development component."[14]

The argument that research on new drugs will be significantly reduced if drug prices are lowered is true only if all three of the following assumptions are true:

(1) Any effort to reduce drug prices will inevitably reduce drug industry revenues;
(2) Any reduction in revenues must inevitably come out of research and development (R and D) expenditures for "breakthrough" drugs, not other types of expenditures such as those on marketing, lobbying, profit, and "me too" drugs; and
(3) The drug industry finances all or most research.

None of these assumptions is true.

The first assumption (that any reduction in drug prices must lead to a reduction in industry revenues) may not be true if the drug-price reduction is limited to Americans without drug coverage. At least two studies have confirmed that if prices are reduced only for those Americans who have no health insurance or who have insurance that doesn't cover drugs, drug sales to this population will rise, and the result will be little or no net change in revenues. One of these studies was done by Alan Sager and Deborah Socolar at Boston University. In a report prepared for a coalition of eight Northeastern states, Sager and Socolar concluded that if the residents in those states with no drug coverage (they amounted to 23 percent of all residents in those states) were allowed to buy prescription drugs at a 42-percent discount, the increased sales that this price cut would trigger would cause the drug industry's total revenues to remain unchanged. Because the cost of producing the additional drugs would be inexpensive, profits would remain unchanged as well.[15]

But let's assume now that the first assumption *is* true – that drug industry revenues and profits *would* be substantially reduced by any price control proposal – and ask whether reduced revenues must inevitably lead to reduced research. For this to happen, the last two assumptions would have to be true – drug industry R and D expenditures would have to fall, and all or most R and D would have to be done by the drug industry.

It is extremely unlikely that drug manufacturers would reduce their budget for new-drug research in response to a decline in revenues. First, the portion of drug industry revenues that is devoted to research on breakthrough drugs (as opposed to drugs that are not significant improvements over existing drugs) is very small (it is on the order of 1 or 2 percent) which means there is plenty of room elsewhere in the industry's budget to cut back. Second, the industry's high profits depends on patents, and patents cannot be obtained without research.

Table 7-3 reports various estimates of how the drug industry spends its revenues. All of these estimates are based on industry data.* According to these estimates, the industry spends somewhere in the range of 11 to 17 percent of its revenues on R and D. Fifteen percent appears to be an average. Let's ignore for a moment the fact that the National Science Foundation says drug industry research amounts to only 10 percent of sales, and let's ignore as well the fact that not all of the 15 percent the drug industry claims it spends on R and D is for research on new drugs (some is for "me too" drugs, and some may be for marketing) and concentrate on the enormous portions spent on administration and profit. The data in Table 7-3 indicate the drug industry, by its own admission, spends 55 to 60 percent of its revenues on administration and profit.† That is a huge piece of the pie compared to the little 15-percent slice the drug industry claims is going to research. Why, we may ask, must any reduction in revenues come out of the 15 percent allocated to R and D when admin-

---

* PhRMA annually reports figures for industry-wide R and D spending based on its surveys of drug manufacturers; drug manufacturers report their expenditures, including expenditures on R and D, in documents filed with the Securities Exchange Commission. What the drug industry does not report is expenditures broken down by drug.

† In this discussion of drug industry expenditures, the definition of "administrative costs" differs slightly from the definition used in the discussion of insurer and provider administrative costs in Chapter 6. In Chapter 6, administrative costs referred to all non-medical expenditures, including profit. In this discussion of the drug industry, I am separating profit out from administrative costs in order to allow the reader to see how big drug industry profits are.

## Table 7-3: The drug industry spends more than half of its revenues on administration, marketing, and profit: Allocation of drug manufacturer costs, selected years

|                              | 1992[a] | 1997[b] | 1999 | 2002[c] |
| ---------------------------- | ------- | ------- | ---- | ------- |
| Materials and production     | 30%     | 34%     |      | 25%     |
| Administration               | 42%     | 36%     |      | 41%     |
| Research and development     | 15%     | 11%     | 17%  | 14%     |
| Profit                       | 13%     | 19%     |      | 21%     |
| Total                        | 100%    | 100%    |      | 100%    |

(a) The 1992 data were described by the Minnesota Department of Health as representative of the "U.S. drug manufacturer" (p. 87). This document distinguished marketing from administration; it indicated that marketing accounted for 20 percent of drug industry expenditures while other administrative costs accounted for 22 percent.

(b) The 1997 figures are averages for Merck and Pfizer.

(c) The 2002 figures are for "13 large ... pharmaceutical companies," according to the source.

Sources: 1992 data from *Prescription Drug Study: A Report to the Minnesota Legislature on the Prescription Drug Market*, Minnesota Department of Health (April 1994), 88; 1997 data from Rhoda H. Karpatkin, "Are prescription drugs too expensive?" *Consumer Reports*, October 1999, 7; 1999 figure for research is from PhRMA's Web site (the Web site didn't indicate what proportion was spent on the other categories, so only the 17-percent figure for research is shown); 2002 data are from Uwe E. Reinhardt, "An information infrastructure for the pharmaceutical market," *Health Affairs* 2004;23(1):107-112, Exhibit 1.

istration and profit are so large? "Administration" includes marketing and lobbying costs, to take two prominent examples. Why would these types of costs remain sacrosanct while R and D was cut? The industry's claim that any drop in its revenues must come out of the tiny slice allocated to research is not credible given the enormous slice allocated to administration and profit.*

---

* For the sake of simplicity, I will ignore here another option open to the drug industry in the event of a downturn in revenues – making its manufacturing operations and research more efficient.

To my eye, the 40 percent or so of revenues that the drug industry spends on administration is large compared with administrative
expenditures by other sectors of the economy. However, as is the case
with other forms of supply-side waste, the health policy community has
made no effort to determine whether drug-manufacturer administrative costs are high compared with other types of firms. Drug-industry
administrative costs are definitely high if we compare them to other
sectors of the health-care industry. U.S. hospitals spend 25 percent of
their revenues on administrative costs (including profit or, in the case
of nonprofit hospitals, surplus),[16] private-sector insurers spend 15 to 35
percent (this estimate also includes profit or surplus), and Medicare
spends 2 percent.

Data comparing the *profits* of the drug industry with the profits of
other industries are available, and they indicate drug-industry profits
are gargantuan. Since 1962, *Fortune* magazine has annually published
a report on the financial performance of the drug manufacturers large
enough to rank among the "Fortune 500" (the largest 500 U.S. for-
profit corporations) as well as for the entire Fortune 500.* During those
four-and-a-half decades, the median profit rate for the entire Fortune
500, measured as a percent of revenues, was nearly always in the range
of 3 to 5 percent. But since 1961, the drug industry has enjoyed profits
*double to quadruple* the Fortune 500 median, year in and year out.

The history of drug industry profits since 1961 falls into three
phases – 1961-1981, 1982-2002, and the years after 2002. Throughout
the entire 1961-81 period, the drug industry was either the first- or
second-most profitable industry – usually it was in second place. But
after 1981, the drug industry began to pull away from the rest of the
Fortune 500. You can see the numbers for the post-1980 era in Table
7-4. They indicate that from 1982 through 2002 the drug industry was

---

* *Fortune* published its first "directory" of the 500 largest U.S. corporations in
July 1956. In its June 1962 report (which contained data on the 1961 performance
of the Fortune 500), *Fortune* listed the drug industry as a separate industry for
the first time (it had been combined with "chemical companies" prior to that).
The *Fortune* reports provide data on the drug industry's profits, the profits of
two or three dozen other industries (the total number of industries grew as the
years went by), and the profits for the Fortune 500 as a whole for every year since
1961.

consistently *the* most profitable industry in America. In 2003 and 2004, the industry fell to number 3 as its sky-high profits dropped slightly, from the 17-to-19-percent range of the late 1990s and early 2000s to the 14-to-16-percent range of the mid-90s.* Any industry that racks up huge profits as consistently as the drug industry does cannot be described as "high risk."

So the drug industry's administrative expenditures *and* profits (55 to 60 percent of revenues in total) dwarf the industry's expenditures on R and D (15 percent according to the industry). Now let's examine the two questions we set aside moments ago: Does the drug industry really devote 15 percent of its revenues to R and D, and what portion of drug-industry R and D expenditures are devoted to *new* drugs? The evidence indicates drug manufacturers probably spend less than 15 percent on R and D, and that R and D spending on breakthrough drugs amounts to no more than 2 percent of revenues.

The National Science Foundation (NSF), an agency established by Congress in 1950 to provide Congress with "data on scientific and engineering resources" in America,[17] conducts surveys of American businesses in all sectors of the economy to determine how much R and D businesses are doing. In its 2003 report, the NSF reported that the pharmaceutical industry spent 10 percent of its revenues on R and D.[18] The NSF report did not explain why its figure was lower than the 15-percent figure touted by the drug industry. Interestingly, the NSF figure is based upon surveys that drug manufacturers fill out and return to NSF, which is the same methodology PhRMA claims to use for its estimates. Without further evidence to indicate whether the NSF or PhRMA methodology is better, it's impossible to state with confidence that NSF's 10-percent figure is the more reliable. Given

---

* For about half the years since 1961, *Fortune's* surveys also reported industry profits as a percent of industry *assets*. For most of those years, *Fortune* also reported profits as a percent of *stockholder equity* in the industry. The drug industry's profitability vis a vis other industries looks just as good if return on assets is used instead of return on revenues. If we use return on *stockholder equity* as the measure of profitability, the drug industry looks just as good in the post-1985 era, and not quite as good prior to 1985 (during the 1969-1984 period, the drug industry typically ranked number 3 on this measure). But because profit is defined as revenues minus costs, profit as a percent of revenues is the most appropriate measure of profit to use.

## Table 7-4: Drug industry profits are huge compared to those of other large corporations: Drug company profits as a percent of revenues compared to profits of Fortune 500 companies, 1981-2004

| Year | Profits as percent of revenues | Profitability rank[a] | Multiple of F500[b] |
|------|------|------|------|
| 1981 | 9.1% | #2 | 2.0 |
| 1982 | 9.9% | #1 | 2.8 |
| 1983 | 10.4% | #1 | 2.7 |
| 1984 | 10.0% | #1 | 2.2 |
| 1985 | 10.4% | #1 | 2.7 |
| 1986 | 13.1% | #1 | 3.2 |
| 1987 | 13.2% | #1 | 2.9 |
| 1988 | 13.5% | #1 | 2.9 |
| 1989 | 13.0% | #1 | 2.8 |
| 1990 | 13.6% | #1 | 3.3 |
| 1991 | 12.8% | #1 | 4.0 |
| 1992 | 11.5% | #1 | 4.3 |
| 1993 | 12.5% | #1 | 4.3 |
| 1994 | 16.1% | #1 | 3.5 |
| 1995 | 14.4% | #1 | 3.0 |
| 1996 | 17.1% | #1 | 3.4 |
| 1997 | 16.1% | #1 | 3.3 |
| 1998 | 18.5% | #1 | 4.2 |
| 1999 | 18.6% | #1 | 3.7 |
| 2000 | 18.6% | #1 | 4.1 |
| 2001 | 18.5% | #1 | 5.6 |
| 2002 | 17.0% | #1 | 5.5 |
| 2003 | 14.3% | #3 | 3.1 |
| 2004 | 15.8% | #3 | 3.0 |

(a) The number of industries ranked varied over the years. The numbers in this column indicate the drug manufacturing industry was the most profitable industry between 1982 and 2002.

(b) The numbers in this column are derived by dividing the drug industry's return on revenues by the median return on revenues for the entire Fortune 500. For example, the 2002 figure of 5.5 is derived by dividing the drug industry's return of

(Table 7-4 continued)

17.0 percent by the median return for the entire Fortune 500 of 3.1 percent.

Sources: Figures shown in columns 1 and 2 are from *Fortune*'s annual reports on the Fortune 500, 1982 to 2005. For example, the data for 2002 were reported in "How the industries stack up," *Fortune* April 14, 2003, F-26. Column 3 is based on calculations done by the author using the profits-as-a-percent-of-revenues figures in column 1 and median figures for all Fortune 500 industries reported in *Fortune*.

---

NSF's greater credibility on this issue, I'm inclined to accept NSF's figure over PhRMA's.

The next question is what portion of that 10-to-15 percent of revenues is spent on breakthrough drugs, that is, drugs that constitute cures for diseases previously considered incurable, or which constitute significant advances over existing treatments. This is the issue because the drug industry makes it the issue. The drug industry does not argue against price controls on the ground that high prices are needed to produce yet another heartburn or allergy pill, for example, that is no more effective than those already on the market. The drug industry argues, rather, that *breakthrough* medicines are at stake. Or, as George W. Bush put it, "drug therapies [that replace] medicine as we know it" are at stake.

Data from the U.S. Internal Revenue Service indicate research expenditures on new drugs account for no more than 10 percent of drug-industry revenues. (New drugs are those that require FDA approval before they can be sold, but which may or may not be a breakthrough drug. FDA approval may be required because a drug contains a "new molecular entity," that is, a chemical never before approved by the FDA, or because the drug contains a previously approved molecular entity but the makers of the drug propose that the drug be used for a disease or condition not previously approved by the FDA.) The IRS has information on new-drug expenditures because federal law grants drug companies tax credits for research on new drugs. The IRS annually reports (with considerable delay) data on drug company expenditures on new drug research that qualify for the tax credit, as well as sales revenues for these companies. These IRS data indicate that the drug industry spent 8 percent of sales revenue on research on new drugs in 1998, and 9 percent in 1999.[19]

Next question: What portion of the 8-to-9 percent spent on new drugs was for *breakthrough* drugs? Answer: 20 to 30 percent. This estimate is based on the percent of new drugs approved by the FDA that the FDA deems to be "significant" improvements over existing drugs. The FDA divides new drugs into those that are "a significant improvement" over existing drugs and those that are not. Those in the former category are given "priority review" status by the FDA, which means the approval process is speeded up; those in the latter category are given a "standard review" status.* The percentage of drugs given priority review status varies slightly depending on what time period one looks at. According to an analysis of FDA records by the National Institute for Health Care Management Foundation (a group funded heavily by health insurance companies), only 24 percent of the 1,035 drugs approved by the FDA between 1989 and 2000 got priority status.[20] If the cost of obtaining FDA approval is the same for priority and standard drugs, then we can say that only 2 to 3 percent (24 percent of 8 and 9 percent) of drug-industry revenues are spent on breakthrough-drug R and D.†

---

* The FDA gives a new drug priority review status if the drug "would be a significant improvement compared to marketed products ... in the treatment, diagnosis, or prevention of a disease" (James Love, *Evidence Regarding Research and Development Investments in Innovative and Non-Innovative Medicines*, Consumer Project on Technology, Washington, DC, Table RND 3.0-2, http://www.cptech.org/ip/health/rnd/evidenceregardingrnd.pdf, accessed June 19, 2005, 17). Clarinex is an example of a new drug that was not a significant improvement over existing drugs, in this case, Claritin. As the *Wall Street Journal* put it, "Schering-Plough Corp.'s new Clarinex is almost identical to its huge-selling allergy pill Claritin" (Laurie McGinley, "Drug study finds little innovation," May 29, 2002, A3). I am not arguing that copycat drugs are of no benefit and should be banned. The availability of several drugs for a given condition is often useful because some patients respond better to one drug than another. I am arguing only with the drug industry's claim that all or most of its research dollar is sunk in high-risk, new, breakthrough drugs. That just isn't true.

† Prior to the 1990s, the FDA used a typology different from the priority/standard-review typology it uses today to evaluate drugs. According to Lisa Bero and Drummond Rennie: "The proportion of all drugs approved by the U.S. FDA before 1990 that were rated A (important therapeutic gain over currently marketed drugs) was 13 percent, while 37 percent were rated B (moderate therapeutic gain), and 50 percent were rated C (little or no therapeutic gain)" ("Influences on the quality of published drug studies," *International Journal of Technology Assessment in Health Care*, 1996;12:209-237, 210).

According to James Love with the Consumer Project on Technology, the cost of bringing priority review drugs to market is a little over half that of the cost for standard review drugs. Love based this estimate on a study indicating that fewer patients are used in clinical trials testing the safety and efficacy of priority drugs than in trials testing standard drugs. When he adjusted the R and D costs for priority drugs downward to reflect this fact, he determined that the drug industry spends less than 2 percent of its sales revenues on R and D for priority-status drugs.[21] Finally, tax credits reduce this 2 percent even further. Donald Light and Joel Lexchin estimate tax credits reduce drug-industry expenditures on basic research by about half.[22] If this is accurate, it would mean the drug industry spends only about 1 percent of its own money on research into breakthrough drugs. Even if Love, Light and Lexchin are wrong, and R and D costs for priority-review drugs are higher, say two, three or four times higher, breakthrough drugs would still be only 2 to 4 percent of revenues. Two to 4 percent is still peanuts compared with the 55 to 60 percent the drug industry spends on administration and profit.

As if this weren't bad enough, it appears that the proportion of drug industry R and D devoted to basic research is dwindling. According to Gardiner Harris, reporting in the *Wall Street Journal*, the drug industry is doing less basic research in-house and is relying ever more heavily on research from small, independent companies that concentrate exclusively or primarily on research. "[T]he pharmaceutical industry is gradually shifting the core of its business away from the unpredictable and increasingly expensive task of creating drugs and toward the steadier business of marketing them," wrote Harris. "With more and more of the industry's research being conducted in biotech labs, its core competency increasingly is marketing, not discovery."[23]

But isn't it possible drug manufacturers would cut their relatively tiny R and D spending on breakthrough drugs rather than their administrative costs and their profits? After all, drug manufacturers are under pressure from their stockholders to maintain their high profits, and manufacturers clearly feel it is important to spend lavishly on marketing, lobbying and other expenses in the "administrative" category to maintain profits. Might they not cut research on breakthrough drugs just to bluff Congress and the public? This brings us to the second reason I listed above for rejecting the drug industry's claim that they will cut research if they suffer a decline in revenues.

The drug industry would be committing suicide if it stopped doing research. It is conceivable but unlikely it would cut back on research on "me too" drugs like Nexium and Clarinex, and *extremely* unlikely it would cut back on research on breakthrough drugs. The reason is simple: The drug industry's outlandish profits are possible only because they obtain patents on new drugs, and patents require research. Patents effectively confer upon drug companies monopoly status for the patented drug for a period up to 20 years. No one but the drug company that holds the patent on a drug may sell it. But you can't get a patent unless you do original research. To sum up: no research, no patent; no patent, no monopoly; no monopoly, no outlandish profits.

But let's assume, for the sake of argument, that reductions in drug prices lead to lower revenues for drug manufacturers, and that the manufacturers find they simply must make up for the losses by cutting the 1-to-2 percent they spend for research on breakthrough drugs rather than touch the 55 to 60 percent they spend on administration and profit. Would that mean new-drug research would come to a halt? Of course not. That's because the taxpayer has always been the primary financier of basic, path-breaking drug research.

The chief financier of breakthrough research, according to numerous studies and all observers including PhRMA, is the U.S. government. "Pharmaceutical companies conduct some of [the] basic research," said the drug industry in its newsletter *Patient Matters*, "but most is conducted by the federal government at the National Institutes of Health (NIH) or at universities."[24] A 1995 study at the Massachusetts Institute of Technology, for example, found that, of the 14 new drugs identified by drug industry officials as the most significant drugs introduced over the previous 25 years, 11 "had their roots in studies paid for by the government."[25] In other words, for these 11 drugs, the government did the basic research and incurred the risk that this research would produce no useful information. According to a paper published in *Health Affairs*, only 15 percent of scientific articles cited in drug patent applications were based on drug industry research.[26] According to an unpublished analysis by the National Institutes of Health completed in 2000, 85 percent of the scientific papers which led to the discovery and development of the five top-selling drugs in 1995 (Zantac, Zovirax, Capoten, Vasotec, and Prozac) were financed by American tax dollars or by foreign universities.[27]

It is difficult to understate the role the federal government, particularly the National Institutes of Health, has played in developing new drugs. Senator Bill Frist (R-TN), a physician-turned-conservative-politician, recently sang the praises of tax-financed research in the *Journal of the American Medical Association.* "Since World War II, government-funded research has sparked a stunning record of scientific and medical advances," Frist wrote. "The development of vaccines and their translation into the daily practice of medicine have helped reduce the incidence of, and in some cases eradicate, diseases such as smallpox, hepatitis B virus, measles, and polio. New treatments have been developed to treat cancer, heart disease, and mental illness."[28]

## Summing up

We have now examined all three of the assumptions that underlie the drug industry's claim that a reduction in drug prices will lead to a reduction or termination of breakthrough-drug research. These assumptions are: any reduction in drug prices must lead to a reduction in drug-industry revenues; a reduction in drug-industry revenues must come out of the 1-or-2-percent slice of revenues devoted to breakthrough-drug research as opposed to the huge 55-to-60 percent slice devoted to administration and profit; and the drug industry is the only, or the primary, financier of research into breakthrough drugs. We have seen that none of these assumptions is true.

The following are true statements:

- A reduction in industry prices may not reduce total industry revenues, especially if the price cuts are limited to a portion of the populace, because the increased volume of sales may offset reduced prices.
- If industry revenues are cut, the industry is extremely unlikely to stop what research on breakthrough drugs it is doing because (a) it spends only 1 to 2 percent of its revenues on such research and (b) it needs to have new patentable blockbuster drugs in the pipeline because its high profits depend on patents, and,

therefore, it is more likely to cut other types of expenditures, notably its enormous administrative costs.

- Even if the industry really had no choice but to cut back on the small slice of expenditures devoted to basic research, that would not mean the end of basic research in America because the U.S. government funds most basic research.

We may conclude that Americans are not receiving value commensurate with the high prices we pay for drugs. In fact, as we shall see in the next section, the billions we pay in the form of excessive prices is worse than wasted. Drug-industry-sponsored research is becoming increasingly corrupt. Industry research is actually harming some people.

## Biased drug research

The problem of corrupt industry-sponsored research has gotten worse over the last 15 years. The problem can be attributed primarily to these two developments: (1) a decline in the proportion of drug research funded by taxes and an increase in the proportion funded by pharmaceutical companies, and (2) the drug industry's effort to increase its influence over scientists who perform or evaluate its research. More tax-financed drug research may turn out to be very desirable regardless of whether the drug industry reduces its expenditures on research.

The creeping privatization of research is of relatively recent vintage. It was set off by the decline in government funding, primarily *federal* funding, of R and D that began midway through President Ronald Reagan's term in office. Reagan's large tax cuts and his increase in military spending led to a cut in domestic spending that was about equal to the increase in military spending. By 1988, Reagan's priorities had caused a reduction (measured in inflation-adjusted dollars) in federal spending on R and D of all types. In that same year, total spending on R and D by U.S. corporations, including drug companies, rose substantially and continued to rise until about 1992 when it leveled off.[29]

As the drug industry became the largest source of drug research dollars (but not the largest source of breakthrough research dollars), and as the industry became more consolidated through mergers, it used its new clout to increase its influence over the scientists who performed its research, as well as the scientists at the FDA who evaluated the research. Twenty years ago, drug manufacturers would contract with scientists, often physicians, at medical centers (clinics and hospitals) on university campuses to do their research for them, and these scientists would design the experiments and find the patients necessary for the experiments. But over the last decade manufacturers have shifted a large portion of their research to for-profit, private-sector firms, including advertising agencies, in order to enhance their control over researchers' final product.[30] This shift in turn put more pressure on academic medical centers to produce reports more to the liking of the drug manufacturers.[*] By the late 1990s, the drug industry's efforts to influence drug researchers had become so aggressive and widespread that a national debate about drug industry tactics erupted within medical journals and the media. In an article about a "government conference" convened in 2000 to discuss the problem, the *New York Times* reported, "The huge influx of money into biomedical research is creating unacceptable conflicts of interest for scientists and is eroding the public's trust in the data...."[31]

The corrupting effect of corporate money on research resembles the corrupting effect that MCP money has had on the U.S. health-care system, or that big money in general has had on democracy in America. It is pervasive, manifests itself in myriad ways, and is often hard to detect. The amount and variety of drug-company corruption of research is so extensive it would take a book or two to do the subject justice. Here I will merely offer a simple outline of the ways in which research is corrupted and offer a few examples.

We can divide the corrupt methods drug companies use into two broad categories: tactics which lead to the publication of erroneous, biased, or misleading studies; and tactics that conceal from doctors and the public studies and case reports that cast an unfavorable light on drugs. Subcategories of the first category of research corruption include:

---

[*] Another important cause of greater corporate control over drug research was federal legislation enacted in the 1980s that permitted universities to patent, and therefore profit from, their inventions, and legislation encouraging corporations to invest in academic research.

- The proposed new drug was not tested on patients who will use it (for example, it is tested on relatively healthy people when it will be prescribed for very sick people);
- the new drug was not compared with less expensive drugs or treatments such as exercise and changed diet, but rather only with equally or more expensive drugs;
- the new drug was compared with other drugs given at low doses known to minimize the effectiveness of the other drugs, or with other drugs given at high doses known to aggravate side effects;
- papers (either published articles or unpublished papers read at professional meetings or submitted to the FDA) summarize the research inaccurately (for example, the trial collected data from multiple hospitals or cities, but presented only data from sites with positive results);
- papers summarize the research accurately, but draw misleading conclusions;
- papers with the same data and the same conclusions are published in several different journals, leading doctors to think more favorable research has been done on a drug than has actually been done; and
- doctors are listed as the authors of a paper, but in fact the paper was ghost-written by drug company employees or contractors.[32]

A paper in *Archives of Internal Medicine* illustrated several of the corrupt methods listed above. The authors of the paper reviewed 52 articles published in journals describing a total of 56 experiments involving arthritis patients comparing one nonsteroidal anti-inflammatory drug (NSAID) with another (Advil, Aleve and Motrin are examples of NSAIDs). All these studies had one thing in common: One of the NSAIDs under examination was manufactured by the drug company that financed the study. The authors called this drug the "manufacturer-associated drug." The authors found that 48 percent of the experiments were rigged (the authors didn't use that word) by a very simple tactic: The authors used dosages of drugs that were not equivalent. Guess which drug was administered in a higher dosage? Yes, the manufacturer-associated drug. The authors also reported that papers reporting on 22 of the 56 experiments concluded that one NSAID was less toxic than the other, and of these alleged to be less toxic, 19 were the manufacturer-associated drug. Worse yet, "In almost half of these trials, this claim of less toxicity was not supported by a test of statistical significance,"[33] a test so fundamental to Western science that every introductory course in statistics teaches it.

Not surprisingly, these tactics affected the articles' conclusions. The authors reported that 29 percent of the experiments (or "trials," as scientists refer to them) found one drug superior to others, and in all of these cases the superior drug was the manufacturer-associated drug. In the other 71 percent of trials, the drugs were found to be comparable. In short, the manufacturer-associated drug was never inferior to other drugs, and often superior.

Examples of the second type of research corruption – concealing or delaying publication of adverse findings – are legion. I offer four examples here – the harassment of a university researcher, the editor of a medical journal, and two FDA employees.

Betty Dong, a clinical pharmacist at the University of California, San Francisco, is among the better known victims of drug-industry retribution because her story drew so much attention from the media, including *60 Minutes* and the *Wall Street Journal*. In the 1980s she did some preliminary research which indicated that Synthroid, a drug used to treat hypothyroidism, was more effective than its competitors. The manufacturer of Synthroid, then known as Boots Pharmaceutical, offered Dong $250,000 to conduct a more rigorous study. She accepted the money, did the research, and discovered that Synthroid was no more effective than three cheaper hypothyroidism drugs. The company, by now called Knoll Pharmaceutical, unleashed a vicious campaign against Dong. It refused to permit her to publish her results, it cleaned up her data and published its own study with more favorable findings, it attacked Dong's expertise, and it criticized her study when it was finally published in the *Journal of the American Medical Association* seven years after the research had been completed.[34]

Editors of medical journals have also been the victims of drug industry retribution. The *Annals of Internal Medicine* published a paper in 1992 that demonstrated that drug advertisements in medical journals are often misleading. Drug companies stopped advertising in the *Annals*, costing the journal $1 million to $1.5 million. According to the *New York Times*, the lost revenue was "a factor in" the resignation of the journal's co-editor, Dr. Suzanne Fletcher, now a professor at Harvard Medical School.[35]

The power of the drug industry to suppress research extends even into the cubicles of the FDA, the agency that is supposed to protect Americans from dangerous drugs. FDA officials have repeatedly harassed FDA staff who insisted on presenting evidence of harm caused by drugs to FDA advisory panels or, worse, to the American public. The two best known victims of FDA harassment today are Drs. Andrew Mosholder and David Graham.

In December 2003, Dr. Mosholder, an epidemiologist on the FDA staff, told his superiors that his review of studies of antidepressants indicated that children on antidepressants were twice as likely to show suicidal tendencies as children taking a placebo. Mosholder told his bosses he wanted to present his findings to an FDA advisory committee that was scheduled to meet in February 2004 and to urge the committee to recommend issuing a warning to doctors. But Mosholder's superiors refused to allow him to present his findings to the committee, and the committee decided only to call for more study of the issue. After the committee met, someone leaked Mosholder's findings to the press.[36] By the spring of 2004, two congressional investigations of the FDA's behavior were underway. In June, Senate Finance Committee Chairman Charles Grassley (R-IA) wrote a letter to the FDA, based on his staff's investigation of the incident, in which he concluded the FDA suppressed Dr. Mosholder's data. Senator Grassley demanded to know, "[I]n how many other instances has the [FDA] manipulated its advisory committee meetings to withhold from the public and misrepresent safety information about marketed drugs of critical importance to patient safety?"[37] In August 2004, someone leaked to the *Wall Street Journal* a draft of the study the advisory committee had asked for which concluded that Dr. Mosholder was right – that antidepressants do cause suicidal ideation in children.[38] The next month, Representative Joe Barton (R-TX), chairman of the House Energy and Commerce Committee, accused the FDA of withholding from his committee information on studies confirming Dr. Mosholder's findings. "The FDA's lack of cooperation with the committee … leaves me wondering whether this is sheer ineptitude or something far worse," Barton said.[39]

The best known victim of abuse by the FDA is Dr. David Graham, an FDA drug-safety officer and the man who blew the whistle on the arthritis drug Vioxx. In August 2004 Graham told his supervisor that his research, funded by the FDA, indicated Vioxx tripled the risk of heart attack and should be withdrawn from the market. Graham was told to keep his information to himself. FDA brass maligned Graham to the media (acting-director of the drug evaluation unit, Dr. Steven Galson, told reporters Graham's work amounted to "junk science"). The next month Merck, the maker of Vioxx, withdrew the drug from the market. In November 2004, Graham told the Senate Finance Committee that Vioxx had caused heart attacks in 88,000 to 139,000 people. "The FDA … is incapable of protecting America against another Vioxx," he added.[40] At about the same time, Graham and a professor at Stanford completed another study that reached similar conclusions about Pfizer's arthritis drugs Celebrex and Bextra. Graham was forbidden to present the study's findings to an advisory committee.[41] He has powerful allies in Congress, so it is unlikely he will be fired. But his job responsibilities have been changed, over his protests, and he has been ostracized by many of his colleagues.*

It is bad enough that the drug industry spends such a small portion of its revenues on basic research and then threatens to shut down its research if anyone tampers with its sky-high prices. But it is downright despicable for the industry to inject bias into what little research it does and to intimidate researchers who insist on reporting information

---

* The FDA's willingness to suppress information and harass whistle-blowers on its staff is an example of what some economists call "regulatory capture" – the development of undue influence over a regulatory agency by the industry the agency is supposed to regulate. Regulatory capture is only infrequently achieved with outright bribes. More commonly, it is achieved with intensive lobbying, promises of jobs after staff leave the agency, and consulting relationships between staff and the industry even while staff are still employed by the agency. The drug industry applies all these tools to the FDA and the FDA's advisory committees (Gardiner Harris and Alex Berenson, "Ten advisers voting on pain pills' sale have industry ties," *New York Times*, February 25, 2005, A1; *Pushing Prescriptions: How the Drug Industry Sells its Agenda at Your Expense*, Center for Public Integrity, http://www.publicintegrity.org/rx, accessed August 7, 2005).

antithetical to the industry's bottom line. If the drug industry were ever to follow through on its threat to cut research on "miracle drugs," Americans should reply, "Good riddance," and vote to use the savings from reduced prices to finance a higher level of tax-financed research. Paying independent scholars at universities and government agencies with tax dollars to do much more of the research necessary to bring a drug to market is one of the most important steps we could take to improve the integrity of drug research. The public thinks this is a good idea. A 2003 Harris poll, conducted for the *Wall Street Journal*, found that 42 percent of adults think universities should conduct most medical research while only 16 percent believe corporations should.[42]

## Waste category number four: Fraud

Health-care fraud that adds to the cost of health care falls into three categories:

- fooling a *patient* into undergoing, and an *insurer* into paying for, services or goods that were not needed;
- fooling an insurer or other payer into paying for services that were never rendered or goods that were never provided; and
- fooling a patient or payer into paying more for a service or good than they would have had they known what the item was worth.*

In my two decades of monitoring the U.S. health-care system, I've read some very strange stories. But none was stranger than this story told first by ABC's "Prime Time Live" in the summer of 1991, and later that year by *Newsweek* magazine. It's an example of the first type of

---

* Note that all three of these bulleted clauses begin with "fooling." The difference between fraud and the examples of excessive price and unnecessary services discussed earlier is that fraud requires intention on the part of the seller to deceive. A doctor who hospitalizes an asthma patient who other physicians think could have been treated in a less expensive, non-hospital setting, is not guilty of fraud if there is no deception. Similarly, a drug company that sells a drug at 20 times the cost of producing the drug is not guilty of fraud; the person paying the outrageous price was not fooled into thinking the price was lower or that the drug was something that it was not.

fraud (fooling patients into accepting services they don't need). Here is how the *Newsweek* article began:

> Sid Harrell, a retired Army medical technician in Live Oak, Texas, was chewing a pork chop in front of the television one evening last April when he looked out the front window and saw a pair of beefy private-security agents confronting his wife and his 14-year-old grandson, Jeremy. The men announced that the child would have to come with them. Mrs. Harrell asked why, but they weren't sure themselves. "You'll have to call Colonial Hills," one of them explained.
>
> Colonial Hills is a private psychiatric hospital in San Antonio [owned by National Medical Enterprises, now Tenet Healthcare, a huge multi-state hospital chain]. The Harrells had recently sent Jeremy's troubled 12-year-old brother to Colonial Hills for treatment (the Harrells are the boys' legal guardians). Jeremy himself was well adjusted and getting good grades in school. But Mrs. Harrell has testified that when she called Colonial Hills to clear up the apparent confusion, a counselor told her the hospital was seizing Jeremy under the state's involuntary-commitment law to evaluate and treat him for drug abuse. Mrs. Harrell become hysterical, but Jeremy assured her he would be fine, and Mr. Harrell reluctantly let the agents take him away.

The doctor who had ordered Jeremy detained had never met him. Yet, according to the Harrells, the hospital held Jeremy for five days, and released him only after a state senator secured a court order. The doctor subsequently resigned and was stripped of his Texas medical license.[43]

The story of Jeremy's kidnapping caused other people to accuse other National Medical Enterprises hospitals of kidnapping them or holding them after they indicated they wanted to leave. By the end of 1992, National Medical found itself the subject of several lawsuits filed by patients and ten insurance companies, and the object of investigations by 14 state and federal agencies.[44] These investigations revealed that National Medical's chief executive, Richard Eamer, who earned $20 million in 1991, had put enormous pressure on his hospital directors to turn a large profit. One of the allegations in the lawsuits was that Eamer's hospitals paid "bounty hunter" fees of up to $2,000 per patient lured into a National Medical hospital, and that some of the recipients of these fees were probation officers and clergymen. Jeremy was, it appears, the target of a bounty hunter.

This first category of fraud – getting patients and insurers to pay for unnecessary services – is usually accomplished without the strong-arm tactics used against Jeremy and his guardians. For example, an ophthalmologist who billed his state Medicaid program a million dollars over five years for cataract operations was convicted of operating on patients without cataracts or with cataracts too small to warrant surgery. The doctor told his patients cataracts were contagious. In one case, his unnecessary surgery on the one good eye of a 57-year-old woman left her completely blind.[45] Here's another example of the fraudulent sale of unnecessary services: HealthSpan, a large hospital chain in Minnesota, paid $3 million to settle charges by the Minnesota attorney general, a U.S. attorney, and the Department of Health and Human Services that it had sent fully equipped ambulances to carry nursing home patients to their doctors' offices when much less expensive vans would have sufficed. HealthSpan billed Medicare and Medicaid $156 to $196 per ambulance trip when it should have billed $32 to $34 for van service. According to government investigators, 36 percent of the ambulance trips provided by HealthSpan over a three-and-a-half year period should have been made by vans.[46]

The second category of fraud (billing for services that were never rendered) is generally easier to detect than the first category of fraud (billing for unnecessary services) because it is generally easier to determine that a service was not *provided* than it is to determine that the service was not *necessary*. The psychiatrist who billed Medicaid for almost 24 hours of work per day for an entire year, and the physician who billed for services for people who were dead at the time of the alleged service, were, to take two examples, easier to detect and prosecute than, for example, HealthSpan's scheme to use ambulances instead of vans.[47]

But some forms of billing for services never provided can be very difficult to detect and, therefore, very expensive. It is possible that scam artists who are not health professionals – people who don't even see patients – are billing for services never rendered at a greater rate than crooks in the health professions are.  According to government fraud investigators and private-sector insurers, the nation's insurance industry is being bilked out of perhaps billions of dollars annually by phony clinics and equipment suppliers and companies pretending to be the billing agencies for real clinics.  These fake providers and billing agencies steal patient medical records, either by going through the trash of clinics and hospitals, bribing nurses and others who have access to patient files, or burglarizing doctors' offices, and then send bills to insurance companies for treatments never delivered.  These bandits operate for a few months, then shut down, and reopen with a new name and new address.  The *New York Times* quotes Ron Poindexter, director of the fraud division of the Florida Department of Insurance, saying, "In terms of health-care fraud, this is the biggest thing on our plate.  It's out of control; it's draining our resources."[48]

The most common form of the third category of fraud – charging more than the good or service warranted – is usually accomplished by billing for a good or service that is more expensive than the actual good or service provided.  For example, federal investigators have caught suppliers of nursing homes billing Medicare and Medicaid $859 for orthotic body jackets (jackets that help frail patients stand or sit upright) when in fact what they delivered was a $50 wheelchair pad with restraining shoulder straps.

When physicians charge an insurance company too much, it is done by "upcoding," and if the upcoding was done deliberately, the action constitutes fraud. Physicians have to enter a code on the claim forms they submit to Medicare, Medicaid and other fee-for-service insurers to indicate what type of service they are billing for.  The most commonly used coding system is published in a book entitled *Current Procedural Terminology*.  The CPT, as it is known, contains codes to describe all the treatments that doctors can give patients these days.  Many conditions have several codes.  For example, removal of a small mole has one code and removal of a large mole has another.  Thus, removing a small mole but placing the code for removal of a large mole on the claim form would constitute upcoding.

Sometimes, however, this third form of fraud (inducing payers to pay too much) is accomplished by inducing two payers to pay for the same item. Suppliers of nursing homes, for example, have been known to bill both the nursing home and Medicare for the same item.[49]

So what does all this fraud cost? Because fraud is, by its nature, difficult to detect, no one knows for sure. The most commonly cited number is 10 percent. That estimate comes from a 1992 report to Congress by the U.S. General Accounting Office. The GAO noted how difficult it is to measure the cost of fraud, and then said fraud accounts for "some 10 percent" of total health-care spending.[50] According to the National Health Care Anti-Fraud Association, a coalition of private-sector insurers and law enforcement agencies, people in the insurance industry believe the figure is "at least 3 percent."[51] Whatever the true fraction, the total number of dollars lost is enormous.

## The total cost of waste

We saw in Chapters 4 and 5 that the evidence does not support the common excuses for the high cost of the U.S. health-care system. In Chapter 6 and this chapter, we reviewed the evidence supporting the statement that the U.S. health-care system is wasteful. In the last two chapters we reviewed evidence of excessive administrative costs, excess capacity, excessively high fees and prices, and fraud.

It is difficult to say what the exact total cost of this waste is, and impossible to state with any precision what portion of the difference between the per capita cost of the U.S. system and those of other countries is attributable to these four types of waste. A rigorous analysis of the cost of all types of waste combined has never been done for any one country, much less several countries at once. My educated guess is that nearly all of the difference between U.S. per capita health expenditures and those of the more expensive foreign health systems (e.g., the Swiss, German, French, and Canadian systems) can be attributed to waste. I say that because the evidence indicates these countries are not achieving their 35- to 50-percent-lower costs by sacrificing quality. (I'm not willing to make the same guess if the comparison country is one of the lower-spending countries such as Britain.) We can, however, offer some estimates for three of the waste categories (see Table 7-5). When we total these estimates, the total cost of supply-side waste comes to somewhere between 20 and 40 percent of total spending.

Administrative waste absorbs somewhere between 10 and 15 percent of total health-care spending. I base this estimate primarily on two studies – a 1991 study by the U.S. General Accounting Office, and a 2003 study by Steffie Woolhandler et al. The GAO study asked the question, How much could the U.S. save in administrative costs if we adopted a single-payer system like Canada's? (I would have preferred that the GAO had been asked to study the administrative savings achievable by expanding Medicare to cover all Americans, but for some reason that was not how the request was phrased.) The GAO estimated savings of 9.5 percent, roughly half from reduced overhead in the insurance sector and half from reduced overhead in the provider sector.[52] The research on administrative costs that we examined in Chapter 6 strongly suggests that the spread of managed care since 1991, the year the GAO used

---

**Table 7-5: America wastes 20 to 40 percent of its health-care dollar on administrative waste, excess capacity, excessively high fees and prices, and fraud**

| Type of waste | Cost as % total spending |
|---|---|
| Administrative waste | 10-15% |
|     Insurance company overhead | |
|     Provider overhead | |
| Excess capacity | ? |
| High fees and prices | 10-15%[a] |
|     High physician fees | 5-10% |
|     High drug prices | 3% |
| Fraud | 3-10% |
| Total | 20-40%[b] |

(a) To avoid suggesting that this total is precise, I rounded the lower- and upper-bound numbers to 10 and 15 percent respectively.

(b) To avoid suggesting that this total is precise, I rounded the lower-bound number to 20 percent.

for its analysis, has raised the nation's administrative costs beyond the 9.5 percent of total spending derived by the GAO. Woolhandler et al. estimated administrative costs absorbed 31 percent of total health-care spending in the U.S. in 1999 versus 17 percent for Canada, a difference of 14 percentage points.[53] I have entered in Table 7-5 a range of 10 to 15 percent as the savings achievable due to reductions in administrative costs alone under a single-payer system.

I make no attempt to estimate the waste from excess capacity because the data upon which to base such an estimate are so sparse. But to give you some idea of how much money may be wasted, consider the data from the Pennsylvania study we talked about in our discussion of the arms race between hospitals in Chapter 6. That study examined the supply and demand for lithotripters (machines which pulverize kidney stones with sound waves), as well as MRIs, cardiac catheterization labs, organ transplant facilities, and neonatal intensive care units. The authors concluded that all five types of devices were in excess supply. The authors estimated that Pennsylvania premium payers and taxpayers paid roughly $100 million annually for the excess supply of three of these devices – lithotripters, MRIs, and catheterization labs – in the early 1990s. If the rest of the nation had an excess supply equal to Pennsylvania's, the total cost to the country would have been $2 billion. Two billion dollars is a small portion of the $800 billion the U.S. was paying annually for health care back in the early 1990s. But the $2 billion represents the excess cost of just three devices. In view of the hundreds of other types of devices and facilities that might be in excess supply, we should view $2 billion as merely the tiny tip of a very large iceberg.

However, a single-payer system, properly administered, will use some of the savings it achieves by eliminating excess capacity to eliminate capacity *deficits* which exist in some parts of the country. As managed care spread, hospitals in some areas of the country shed too many buildings, beds, and machines. This was especially true of inpatient mental health beds and emergency rooms. Rectifying shortages such as these will cost money, and these expenditures will offset some of a single-payer's savings.

I estimate the total cost of excessive physician fees and drug prices to be in the range of 10 to 15 percent. We saw in Table 3-2 that expenditures on physician services account for 22 percent, and expenditures on prescription drugs account for 11 percent, of health-care spending. If U.S. physician fees were closer to those prevailing in the rest of the industrialized world, expenditures on physicians would fall by 40 percent (if German and Canadian physician incomes were the benchmark) to 65 percent (if French and Australian incomes were the benchmark; see Table 7-1).* If physician incomes in other industrialized nations are on average half what they are in the U.S. (which seems to be a conservative estimate), and roughly 20 percent of U.S. costs are attributable to expenditures on doctors, then reducing U.S. physician incomes to the level of other countries would cut approximately 10 percent off the U.S. health-care bill.

We may not want to cut physician incomes by half, however. Evidence indicates that America may have a doctor shortage within a decade or two. Evidence also indicates, however, that if this shortage materializes, it can be eliminated simply by expanding the number of students admitted by our medical schools. It appears, in other words, that we do not need to pay physicians the high fees and salaries they earn now to induce a sufficient number of Americans to become doctors. But predicting the need for physicians is difficult. In my opinion, we should err on the side of educating and retaining too many doctors. To err on the conservative side, then, I've entered a range of 5 to 10 percent as the savings achievable with reductions in payments to physicians.†

Although U.S. drug prices for brand-name drugs are roughly double those in other industrialized nations, we cannot assume that price

---

* Estimating the waste due to excessive physician fees is complicated by the fact that two-thirds of U.S. physicians are specialists compared to about half in other countries. A rigorous analysis of the savings achievable by reducing physician incomes to levels in other countries would have to determine if Americans benefit from our greater abundance of specialists and, if we did, adjust for differences in the ratio of specialists to primary care doctors. I make no attempt to do that here.

† Single-payer activists estimating savings from a single-payer at the state level should definitely use a number lower than 10 percent for savings on physician costs. Ten percent is within the realm of possibility for a national single-payer system, but is probably not possible for a single state acting alone. A 50 percent cut in physician fees in a single state would probably induce a doctor shortage in at least some areas of that state.

controls on drugs (or volume-purchasing of drugs at the state level) would cut U.S. spending on drugs in half. One reason is that the international differences in generic drug prices are much less. Another is that many large purchasers of drugs, including Medicaid programs, MCPs, and hospital chains, get discounts from drug manufacturers on the brand-name drugs they buy. An analysis of the savings California would achieve under single-payer legislation pending in the California legislature in 2004 (SB 921) concluded that prices would be cut by 39 percent for people who currently have no drug coverage, 24 percent for those who have private drug coverage, and 5 percent for those whose drugs are paid for by Medicaid.[54] Based on this research, as well as other studies showing much lower per capita spending on drugs (generic and brand-name) in other countries, I believe 30 percent is a reasonable estimate of drug savings from an American single-payer. Thirty percent of 11 percent (the portion of U.S. total spending that goes for drugs) yields a savings of about 3 percent of total spending.

As we saw in the discussion of fraud in the last chapter, estimates are soft, and range from 3 to 10 percent.

As I've indicated in Table 7-5, the total cost of the three types of waste for which I've estimated a range comes to 20 to 40 percent. This 20-to-40-percent range is, it bears repeating, a soft estimate of total waste in the system. Each of the three categories for which I made estimates (administrative waste, high fees and prices, and fraud) is difficult to measure precisely. In the case of administrative waste and excess fees and prices, estimates are complicated by counter-arguments from defenders of the system that America's high administrative costs and high fees and prices buy something of value. In the case of fraud, the problem is complex because we're measuring something that is, by design, difficult to detect.

Although this exercise in calculating waste in the U.S. system does not give us a hard estimate of total waste, it does give us some sense of how costly the waste is, whatever its true dimension. If we agree that the problem we are trying to solve is universal health insurance for no more than we're paying today, we need only eliminate the first category of waste – the administrative waste – to solve that problem. According to the GAO report I mentioned earlier, a universal health insurance system with no co-payments and deductibles would add 9 percent to total U.S. health-care spending, and a single-payer system would cut administrative costs by 9.5 percent.[55] If this estimate is correct (see further discussion in Chapter 11), then merely eliminating administrative waste in the current system would permit us to achieve universal, first-dollar coverage with no additional expenditures. Eliminating the other forms of waste would permit us to cut total health-care spending substantially or to expand coverage to services that are now poorly covered, such as long-term care.

Readers should not interpret this estimate of waste in the system as a guarantee that an American single-payer system will inevitably lead to a reduction of 20 to 40 percent in U.S. health-care expenditures. The savings a single-payer will achieve in the form of reduced administrative costs will be quite close to the 10 to 15 percent I list in Table 7-5. But the savings a single-payer will achieve in the other two waste categories for which I show estimates are harder to predict because savings in these areas will hinge on research that has not been done yet and on decisions by politicians and the people who administer the single-payer system that are impossible to predict. The reductions in excessive physician expenditures, for example, may be less than my estimate because the medical profession is powerful, and because what savings we do achieve in the form of reduced physician fees may have to be offset to some degree by subsidies and higher fees paid to physicians to work in underserved areas. The reductions in excessive expenditures on drugs may be less than my estimate because the drug industry is powerful and will fight any reduction in its prices. Finally, it is unlikely that a single-payer system will wipe out all fraud. Fraud will afflict any system of insurance, even a single-payer system. But fraud will be harder to commit under a single-payer, in part because it is more difficult to commit fraud against one insurer than multiple payers, and in part because hospitals (a source of much of today's fraud) will be working under budgets, not the current fee-for-every-little-good-or-service system which makes fraud much easier to get away with. The best we can hope for from a single-payer will be a substantial reduction in fraud, not its complete elimination. A conservative estimate of the savings a single-payer can achieve is on the order of 15 to 20 percent, enough to provide universal coverage, including long-term care coverage, and still spend no more, and probably less, than we spend now.

# Endnotes

[1] Congressional Budget Office, *Economic Implications of Rising Health Care Costs*, Washington, DC, 1992, 8.

[2] "How doctors have ruined health care," *Financial World*, February 9, 1990, 48.

[3] Alain Enthoven and Richard Kronick, "A consumer-choice health plan for the 1990s," *New England Journal of Medicine* 1989;320:29-37, 30.

[4] Kaiser Family Foundation, *Trends and Indicators in the Changing Marketplace*, Exhibit 6.4, http://www.kff.org/insurance/7031/ti2004-6-4.cfm, accessed June 12, 2005.

[5] Glenn Howatt, "Study: Allina heart docs do less for more," Minneapolis *Star Tribune*, July 17, 2005, A1.

[6] Congressional Budget Office, op cit., 16.

[7] Victor R. Fuchs and James S. Hahn, "How does Canada do it? A comparison of expenditures for physicians' services in the United States and Canada," *New England Journal of Medicine* 1990;323:884-890.

[8] Congressional Budget Office, op cit., 16.

[9] Diana Jean Schemo, "Medical school applications dip sharply; minorities' rise slightly," *New York Times*, October 27, 2000, A18.

[10] Barbara Barzanksy and Sylvia I. Etzel, "Educational programs in U.S. medical schools, 2001-2002," *Journal of the American Medical Association* 2002;288:1067-1072.

[11] Donald G. McNeil, Jr., "Indian company offers to supply AIDS drugs at low cost in Africa," *New York Times*, February 7, 2001, A1.

[12] Pharmaceutical Research and Manufacturers of America, *Why Do Prescription Drugs Cost So Much and Other Questions About Your Medicines*, http://www.phrma.org/publications/publications/brochure/questions/badpricecontrols.cfm, accessed June 18, 2005.

[13] Merrill Goozner, *The $800 Million Pill: The Truth Behind the Cost of New Drugs*, University of California Press, Berkeley, CA, 2004, 7.

[14] The Third Gore-Bush Debate, October 17, 2000, Commission on Presidential Debates, http://www.debates.org/pages/trans2000c.html, accessed July 30, 2005.

[15] "Drug companies can cut their costs," Minneapolis *Star Tribune*, September 22, 2000, A23.

[16] Steffie Woolhandler and David U. Himmelstein, "Administrative costs in U.S. hospitals," *New England Journal of Medicine* 1993;329:400-403.

[17] National Science Foundation, *Research and Development in Industry: 2000*, National Science Foundation, Division of Science Resources Statistics, Arlington, VA, 2003, 3, http://www.nsf.gov/statistics/nsf05308/pdf/secta.pdf, accessed June 18, 2005.

[18] Ibid., Table A-20.

[19] James Love, *Evidence Regarding Research and Development Investments in Innovative and Non-Innovative Medicines*, Consumer Project on Technology, Washington, DC, September 2003, Table RND 3.0-2, http://www.cptech.org/ip/health/rnd/evidenceregardingrnd.pdf, accessed June 19, 2005.

[20] National Institute for Health Care Management Foundation, *Changing Patterns of Pharmaceutical Innovation*, Washington, DC, 2002, http://www.nihcm.org/innovations.pdf, accessed June 19, 2005.

[21] Love, op cit.

[22] Donald W. Light and Joel Lexchin, "Foreign 'free riders' and the high prices of U.S. patented drugs," unpublished paper.

[23] Gardiner Harris, "Drug firms, stymied in the lab, become marketing machines," *Wall Street Journal*, July 6, 2000, A1.

[24] "Medical progress depends on research," *Patient Matters*, Spring 1998, Pharmaceutical Research and Manufacturers of America, Washington, DC, 1.

[25] Jeff Gerth and Sheryl Gay Stolberg, "Drug firms reap profits on tax-backed research," *New York Times*, April 23, 2000, A1, A20.

[26] Arnold S. Relman and Marcia Angell, "America's other drug problem," *The New Republic*, December 16, 2002, 27-41.

[27] Ibid.

[28] Bill Frist, "Federal funding for biomedical research: Commitment and benefits," *Journal of the American Medical Association* 2002;287:1722-1724, 1722.

[29] "U.S. R and D spending continues fairly brisk," *Wall Street Journal*, August 19, 1996, A1.

[30] Thomas Bodenheimer, "Uneasy alliance: Clinical investigators and the pharmaceutical industry," *New England Journal of Medicine* 2000;342:1539-1544; Melody Petersen, "Madison Avenue plays growing role in the business of drug research," *New York Times*, November 22, 2002, A1.

[31] Philip J. Hilts, "U.S. weighs changes in rules on drug research conflicts," *New York Times*, August 16, 2000, A6.

[32] Richard Smith, "Medical journals and pharmaceutical companies: Uneasy bedfellows," *British Medical Journal* 2003;326:1202-1205; and Lisa Bero and Drummond Rennie, "Influences on the quality of published drug studies," *International Journal of Technology Assessment in Health Care*, 1996;12:209-237.

[33] Paula A. Rochon et al., "A study of manufacturer-supported trials of Nonsteroidal Anti-inflammatory Drugs in the treatment of arthritis," *Archives of Internal Medicine* 1994;154:157-163, 161.

[34] Dorothy S. Zinberg, "Why we exist," *Science* 1996;273, 411, http://www.doctorsintegrity.org/exist/dong/dong_science.htm, accessed June 21, 2005.

[35] Lawrence K. Altman, "Inside medical journals, a rising quest for profits," *New York Times*, August 24, 1999, D7.

[36] Anna Wilde Mathews, "In debate over antidepressants, FDA weighed risk of false alarm," *Wall Street Journal*, May 25, 2004, A1.

[37] "Senator says FDA put pressure on staffer over antidepressants," *Wall Street Journal*, June 17, 2004, A2.

[38] Anna Wilde Mathews, "FDA revisits issue of antidepressants for youths," *Wall Street Journal*, August 5, 2004, A1.

[39] Gardiner Harris, "Lawmaker says FDA held back drug data," *New York Times*, September 10, 2004, A17.

[40] Michael Scherer, "The side effects of truth," *Mother Jones*, May-June 2005, http://www.motherjones.com/news/feature/2005/05/david_graham.html, accessed June 21, 2005.

[41] Gardiner Harris, "Drug regulators are trying to quash study, senator says," *New York Times*, February 12, 2005, A11.

[42] "Most people uncomfortable with profit motive in health care," Harris Interactive, December 4, 2003, http://www.harrisinteractive.com/news/newsletters_wsj.asp, accessed August 6, 2005.

[43] Geoffrey Cowley et al., "Money madness," *Newsweek*, November 4, 1991, 50, 50-51.

[44] Sonia L. Nazario, "Allegations of fraud, malpractice still haunt operator of hospitals: National Medical profit push is alleged to have led to unneeded treatment," *Wall Street Journal*, January 8, 1993, A1.

[45] Paul Jesilow et al., "Fraud by physicians against Medicaid," *Journal of the American Medical Association* 1991;266:3318-3322.

[46] David Shaffer, "HealthSpan to pay $3 million: Government alleged fraudulent billings," *St. Paul Pioneer Press*, July 8, 1993, C1.

[47] Jesilow, et al., op cit.

[48] Kurt Eichenwald, "Unwitting doctors and patients exploited in a vast billing fraud," *New York Times*, February 6, 1998, A1.

[49] "Feds: Nursing home residents hit by medical-supply fraud," *American Medical News*, August 28, 1995, 4.

[50] U.S. General Accounting Office, *Health Insurance: Vulnerable Payers Lose Billions to Fraud and Abuse*, May 1992, Washington, DC, 8.

[51] National Health Care Anti-fraud Association, http://www.nhcaa.org/pdf/all_about_hcf.pdf, accessed January 23, 2004.

[52] U.S. General Accounting Office, *Canadian Health Insurance: Lessons for the United States*, Washington, DC, 1991, 63, Table 5.1.

[53] Steffie Woolhandler et al., "Costs of health care administration in the United States and Canada," *New England Journal of Medicine* 2003;349:768-775.

[54] John F. Sheils and Randall A. Haught, *The Health Care For All Californians Act: Cost and Economic Impacts Analysis*, The Lewin Group, January 2005, 23.

[55] U.S. General Accounting Office, *Canadian Health Insurance*, Washington, DC, 1991.

# 8

# The Clash Between Public and Expert Opinion

## Overview of diagnoses and prescriptions

In the last four chapters, I have reviewed the various explanations – the true and the bogus – for why U.S. health-care costs are so high. In the three chapters that follow, I will examine the three health-care reform proposals now under debate – managed competition, high-deductible policies, and a single-payer system. In this chapter, I will review the evidence that the public shares my perception of the problem and of the solution, and that the public's perceptions contrast sharply with those of experts. The public does not buy the experts' claim that volume of services is excessive, and, therefore, the public does not buy the experts' argument that the solution to the health-care crisis must include mechanisms to cut back on the volume of services. The public sees supply-side waste as the main problem, and, logically enough, is sympathetic to a single-payer system. For anyone who wants to build a new American health-care system, this difference between public and expert opinion is critical. The health-care crisis won't be solved with a system that contradicts the values of most Americans.

To illustrate the health policy battlefield, I have arrayed in Table 8-1 the various explanations for the high cost of U.S. health care that I reviewed in the last four chapters. In the top half of the table you see

## Table 8-1: The ten explanations reviewed so far

| Explanation | Culprit |
|---|---|
| The six common excuses | |
| | |
| (1) Americans get too many medical services | |
|     (a) because doctors order too many services | Doctors |
|     (b) because patients demand too many services | Patients |
| (2) Americans are older | Patients |
| (3) Americans have worse lifestyles | Patients |
| (4) Americans sue for malpractice too often | Patients |
| (5) Americans are more violent | Patients, attackers |
| (6) US quality is superior | (not applicable) |
| | |
| The four categories of waste | |
| | |
| (1) Administrative waste | Insurance industry |
| (2) Excess capacity | Hospitals, doctors |
| (3) Excessively high fees and prices | Health-care industry |
| (4) Fraud | Health-care industry |

the six common excuses for high costs that I examined in Chapters 4 and 5. In the bottom half you see the four categories of waste I reviewed in Chapters 6 and 7. These ten explanations fall roughly into two categories – explanations that blame *patients* and *doctors* for inflating the *volume* of medical services sold, and explanations that blame the *health-care industry* for inefficiency, fraud, and overcharging, all of which force the *price* of medical services and health insurance to rise.

With the exception of the malpractice excuse, the public rejects, or gives low priority to, the patient-is-to-blame, volume-is-to-blame justifications for the high cost of America's health-care system. The public does not see unnecessary services as a big issue and is, therefore, opposed to attacking volume of services with either the managed-care meat ax or the large-deductible meat ax. The public sees waste in the system, and the high prices generated by waste, as the primary problem. But the opinion of experts – the politicians, big business execs, pundits, and think-tank types who dominate the health-care reform debate – is inconsistent with public opinion. The experts think volume of services is the main problem. The only significant division of opinion among experts is whether the alleged overuse of medical services is primarily the fault of doctors or of patients. Experts partial to managed-care insurers think doctors are to blame for overuse, while experts partial to high-deductible insurers think patients are to blame.

## Evidence of the clash between ordinary people and experts

The gap between expert and public opinion began to emerge about the time the current health-care reform debate began, which is to say in the late 1980s. The gap was obvious by the early 1990s. The spread of managed-care plans (MCPs) in the late 1980s and early 1990s, and the inflation lull of the mid-1990s, gave experts the sensation that their biases in favor of managed care were warranted. However, the spread of MCPs during that period gave a rapidly growing portion of the public real-life experiences with managed care, and the public developed an entirely different assessment of managed care. As the data in Table 8-2 indicate, polling data as early as 1990 revealed public distaste for managed care, the great hope of experts. Other polls, including the 1993 poll shown in Table 5-2, demonstrated that majorities of Americans believed that waste, fraud and overcharging by doctors, hospitals and drug companies, not "overuse" of health care, were the most important causes of health-care inflation. Americans still think that way. A 2005 poll taken by the Kaiser Family Foundation demonstrated that Americans listed "high profits made by drug companies" (named by 69 percent) and "greed and waste" (named by 62 percent) as the number one and two causes of health-care inflation, while "absence of incentives to hunt for lower-cost doctors and services" (39 percent) ranked last among six factors listed.[1] Waste, fraud and abuse, however, are not the favorite topics of the experts.

The earliest analysis of the expert-public opinion split that I know of was published in April 1992 by the Public Agenda Foundation, a think tank founded by pollster Daniel Yankelovich and former Secretary of State Cyrus Vance. The Foundation asked experts and ordinary people to identify the health-care system's main problems. The Foundation's report indicates the Foundation assumed experts must be right, and any

## Table 8-2: Americans have never approved of managed care: Results of polls

**Before 1993 (the year the White House endorsed managed competition)**

A 1990 Gallup poll found that 75 percent of Americans supported a national health insurance program but only 30 percent did so if the program limited their choice of physician.

A 1992 Gallup poll found that only 20 percent of the population agreed that control of health-care inflation requires "limits on what health care is available to the average person."

The same Gallup poll reported that 61 percent disagree that insurance companies should be able to decide which services they will pay for.

A 1992 poll conducted by Robert Blendon at Harvard demonstrated that "about half of all Americans feel that joining a health plan that restricts their choice of physicians ... is not a desirable method of controlling high health costs."

**After 1993**

A 1994 *Newsweek* poll found 76 percent of Americans were unwilling to accept restrictions on their choice of doctor or hospital even if such restrictions would bring down health-care costs.

A 1995 poll of Minnesotans conducted by the Minnesota Health Data Institute found that traditional health plans outscored HMOs on four quality-of-care measures.

A 1996 Yankelovich poll of insured Californians found that 55 percent thought quality of care had declined.

A 1997 Lou Harris poll found that 54 percent of Americans believed the spread of managed care was harmful to them.

A 1997 poll funded by the Kaiser Foundation and others found that 55 percent thought that managed-care plans are more interested in saving money than providing the best care, and two thirds of these based their opinion on their own experiences or on the comments of family members and friends, not on media stories.

A 1998 *Washington Post*-ABC News poll found that 60 percent of American adults favored "tougher government regulation of managed-care programs like HMOs," and of these, 63 percent still favored tougher regulation even if "it raised [their] own health-care costs." Only 27 percent of adults opposed tougher regulation.

divergence of public opinion from expert opinion must reflect stupidity on the part of the public. The report, entitled *Faulty Diagnosis: Public Misconceptions About Health Care Reform*, concluded that the experts believed overuse of health services was the main problem, and the public was wrong for not capitulating to this point of view.

> The American public believes that the country's health-care system is riddled with waste and greed. Consequently, they are not eager to talk about hard choices, or to consider solutions that will increase their own costs or reduce the services they get. Nor are they ready to relinquish the miracles of modern medicine.[2]
>
> Until these differences [between expert and public opinion] are fully understood, and until leadership and media take steps to address them, the debate on health care will likely result in continued political gridlock – with the public and leaders talking past each other....[3]

In November 1992, Knight Ridder Newspapers ran an article about the Public Agenda study as well as polls by Harris and Gallup. The article began:

> Policy makers and the public are worlds apart on the most controversial element of health-care change: limiting the medical services that people can receive. Most government, business and health industry leaders believe it will be impossible to control costs ... unless people with insurance sacrifice some choices. Yet the public roundly rejects limits.

The article defined policy makers to include "major insurers, hospital chief executives, physician leaders, state officials, federal regulators, key congressional staff, members of Congress, corporate executives, and union leaders." According to the article, the Harris poll indicated that 63 percent of these "policy makers believe high-tech medical services must eventually be rationed," but the Gallup survey found "that only 20 percent of the public believes there should be limits on the care an average person can receive." Interestingly, the Harris poll showed that the subset of "policy makers" that was most likely to endorse rationing was "major insurers"; 95 percent of this group thought care must be rationed, compared to 50 percent for "union leaders," the least likely of the policy-maker groups to support rationing.[4] But even the 50-percent figure for union leaders was way above the 20 percent figure for the general public.

In a 1995 article for *Health Affairs*, Yankelovich attributed the defeat of the Clinton plan to the gap in expert and public opinion and to Clinton's failure to engage ordinary people in the formulation of his plan. "President Clinton's reform plan was not shaped by discussion with citizens ... ," wrote Yankelovich. "The plan was the product of experts and experts alone. Technical experts designed it, special interests argued it, political leaders sold it, journalists more interested in its political ramifications than its contents kibitzed it, advertising attacked it."[5] Yankelovich didn't say so, but precisely the same could have beeen said of the entire managed-care project from its inception. Paul Ellwood and other experts designed it, Ted Kennedy and Richard Nixon sold it to Congress, HMOs sold it to employers, employers forced or cajoled their employees into enrolling in HMOs, and reporters lay asleep at the switch until they were awakened by the HMO backlash. Ordinary citizens were never asked by policy makers if they thought turning the health-care system over to MCPs was a good idea. When, in the late 1980s, ordinary people were finally asked by pollsters for their opinion, they said clearly they were not happy with managed care.*

Yankelovich went on to say, however, that even if the Clintons had done a good job of engaging the public in a discussion of their plan, the public would have rejected it because public perceptions of the problem are so different from the perceptions of the experts who designed the Clintons' bill. "What really angers Americans," wrote Yankelovich, "are the causes of rising health costs, as they perceive them." Citing his own polls, Yankelovich said the public perceives "hospital costs, ...

---

* To be precise, what the polls conducted prior to the HMO backlash indicated was that people were not happy with the tools managed care uses, e.g., restrictions on their choice of doctor, financial incentives for doctors, and utilization review. Prior to the backlash, polls which used the phrase "managed care" instead of a phrase depicting one of managed care's tools tended to evoke a less critical, more ambivalent reaction.

malpractice suits … , physician fees … , fraud and abuse in the health-care system … , and the costs of medications" as the primary causes of health-care inflation.

> Given this perception, it is not surprising that most Americans resist making sacrifices…. The vast majority rejects the idea that the explosion of health costs must lead … to "limits on what health care is available to the average person." Only 20 percent of adults nationwide endorse this view, *while an impressive 77 percent major-ity insists that the cure to rising costs is "to cut the waste, high profits, and fraud in medicine."* … Since the public blames the system, not itself, it understandably rejects calls for sacrifice…. This perspective puts the public on a collision course with the majority of experts. In the experts' view, the two main causes of rising costs are the aging of the population and the explosive costs of new technologies and medical advances. The majority of the public brushes aside both of these explanations (empha-sis added).[6]

The chasm between expert and public views continued into the late 1990s, several years after it had become apparent that managed care was a bust. "Health policy experts are constantly talking about ration-ing and setting limits and balancing costs and the benefits of care, but for the average American those are just ridiculous notions," said Larry Levitt, an analyst at the Kaiser Family Foundation, in a 1999 interview with the *Washington Post*.[7]

Although the experts no longer celebrate managed care in its original incarnation (financial incentives and utilization review implemented by MCPs), they still cling to the most fundamental of managed-care's as-sumptions – that overuse is the primary driver of health-care inflation (a notion the public disagrees with) and that some third party must "man-age" this overuse somehow – and they still cling to the hope expressed by the first advocates of HMOs that report cards will somehow lead us to the promised land. The newer and ostensibly kinder and gentler version of managed care – let's call it managed care 2.0 – imagines that the iron fists of managed care 1.0 – bonuses for cutting services and utilization review – can be replaced with the velvet glove of report cards and "pay for performance" as measured by report cards. Managed care 2.0 calls for government agencies to develop report cards on doctors and hospitals and for all purchasers (government programs, employers, MCPs, and patients) to reward providers who get good grades on report cards and punish those who get bad grades. Because publishing report cards requires standards of care against which to measure provider performance, proponents of managed care 2.0 insist that some third party, typically the government, must develop standards of care for thousands of medical treatments. Because the great majority of report cards require that provider scores be adjusted to reflect the health status of patients seen by particular providers, advocates of managed care 2.0 demand easy access to the medical records of all Americans. To establish easy access to all medical records, proponents of managed care 2.0 demand that providers convert all medical records from paper to computerized files, and that these files be dumped into huge regional or national databases in which report-card publishers will be free to roam.

I will discuss this latest version of managed care, and why it will fail, in more detail in the next chapter. For now, it's important to observe only that the endorsement of this version of managed care by the experts does not close the gap between expert and public opinion. The public does not accept the overuse diagnosis, and polling data and focus-group research indicate the public is at best ambivalent about report cards and is strongly opposed to allowing third parties to see medical records.

Support among the experts for high deductibles has never approached the level of support experts used to give to managed care and now give to managed care 2.0. In fact, the preponderance of opinion within the American health policy community is against high deductibles. Among politicians, Democrats split sharply with Republicans over this issue. Because there is no consensus among experts and policy makers on high deductibles, the difference between expert and public opinion on this issue is much harder to perceive.

## The public supports single-payer

The data we have just reviewed indicate Americans perceive waste and price-gouging as the primary causes of health-care inflation, and reject the claim that excessive use of medical services is the problem. Those perceptions suggest the public would support a single-payer system. We have less reliable data on what *solutions* the public supports than we have on the public's perception of the *causes* of the crisis, but the data we have tell us a large majority of Americans will support a single-payer over other options if they are exposed to a fair debate among proponents of those options. I base this conclusion primarily on polling data and the results of a few focus groups and "citizens juries," and secondarily on my own experience talking to thousands of Minnesotans over the last 15 years.

Table 8-3 shows the results of six polls, three of which were taken in the late 1980s and early 1990s before managed competition became the darling of the chattering classes and before single-payer was driven into the wilderness. These polls indicate that roughly two-thirds of

## Table 8-3: Majorities favor single-payer in polls

|  | For single-payer | Opposed to single-payer |
|---|---|---|
| Harvard University poll (1988) | 61% | 37% |
| *Wall Street Journal*-NBC poll (1991) | 69% | 20% |
| CBS-*New York Times* poll (1993) | 59% | not asked |
| *NEJM* poll (medical school faculty and students) (1999) | 57% | not asked |
| ABC News poll (2003) | 62% | not asked |
| *Arch Int Med* poll (doctors) (2004) | 64% | not asked |

Sources: Robert J. Blendon, "Three systems: A comparative survey," *Health Management Quarterly* 1989;11(1):2-10, Exhibit 5, 5, for Harvard poll; *Wall Street Journal*, June 28, 1991, A4, for *Wall Street Journal*-NBC poll; *American Health Line*, April 19, 1993 for CBS-*New York Times* results; Steven R. Simon et al., "Views of managed care: A survey of students, residents, faculty, and deans of medical schools in the United States," *New England Journal of Medicine* 1999;340:928-936, 929, for medical school poll; ABC News Poll Vault, http://abcnews.go.com/images/pdf/935g3HealthCare.pdf, accessed July 30, 2005, for ABC News poll; and Danny McCormick et al., "Single-payer national health insurance: Physicians' views," *Archives of Internal Medicine* 2004;164:300-304.

Americans supported a single-payer then. The 1988 Harvard poll asked Americans if they would be willing to swap the U.S. system for the Canadian system; 61 percent said they would. The 1991 *Wall Street Journal*-NBC poll described single-payer in general terms; 69 percent of Americans said they would endorse a single-payer. The last three polls shown in the table were taken after the HMO backlash began circa 1996. The respondents in two of these were physicians. In 1999, the *New England Journal of Medicine* reported, "Overall, 57.1 percent [of the doctors surveyed] thought that a single-payer system with universal coverage was the best health-care system for the most people.... A total of 21.7 percent favored managed care, and 18.7 percent preferred a fee-for-service system (2.5 percent did not state a preference)."[8] The other poll surveying physicians found that 64 percent of Massachusetts doctors endorse single-payer.

The third post-HMO-backlash poll listed in Table 8-3, conducted by ABC News, asked respondents how they felt about "a universal health insurance program, in which everyone is covered under a program like Medicare that's run by the government and financed by taxpayers." Sixty-two percent said they would prefer such a system over the current system, described as one in which people got their coverage through employers and some people are uninsured.

The widespread support for Medicare is an indication of American support for a single-payer system. As I noted earlier, Medicare resembles a single-payer because it is the sole source of financing for medical care for the nation's elderly and disabled, and because it sets limits on what doctors and hospitals can charge. Surveys which find high levels of public support for Medicare are numerous. For example, in 2000, 88 percent of nonelderly American adults said it was "important" to them that Medicare "will still be providing health coverage for seniors" when they retire;[9] and in 2001, 70 percent of adults wanted more money spent on Medicare, 26 wanted spending kept where it was, and only 2 percent supported a cut.[10]

But polls are not the most reliable evidence available on public opinion about how to solve the health-care crisis. Polls that don't describe single-payer accurately, particularly those that use loaded phrases to describe it, have reported support for single-payer in the 40-to-50-percent range. But survey evidence is not the only evidence available.

The most compelling evidence in favor of my claim that a majority of Americans would support a single-payer system if they were exposed to a fair debate are the results of a few public hearings and "citizens juries" at which participants were exposed to presentations on single-payer, managed competition, and other proposals. These events include town hall meetings in the fall of 1993 in Minnesota and New York, a citizens jury sponsored by the Jefferson Center in 1993, and the 1996 Minneapolis *Star Tribune*-KTCA citizens jury I described at the beginning of this book. Single-payer won by landslides at all of these events.

In the Twin Cities, the *Star Tribune* sponsored "roundtables" in more than 100 neighborhoods in November 1993 to discuss the managed-competition bills introduced by President Clinton and Senator David Durenberger (R-MN), the late Senator Paul Wellstone's (D-MN) single-payer bill, and the Heritage Foundation's version of the Medical Savings Account (MSA) proposal. More than 1,000 people participated. To facilitate discussion at these meetings, the *Star Tribune* published a 36-page insert which contained information on the health-care crisis plus arguments for each of the four major plans. The *Star Tribune* stacked the deck against single-payer; it was the only proposal for which the *Star Tribune* published a rebuttal, in this case, from the Health Insurance Association of America. Nevertheless, when the votes of the 220 participants who filled out questionnaires were counted, single-payer won handily with 43 percent of the vote. In distant second place was Clinton's plan at 16 percent. The MSA proposal got 15 percent, and something the *Star Tribune* called "pure managed competition" (presumably Durenberger's proposal) got 4 percent.[11]

A series of less structured town hall meetings took place in New York at about the same time as the *Star Tribune* was conducting its roundtables. The New York meetings were hosted by a state task force chaired by New York's Commissioner of Health, Mark Chassin (yes, the same guy who used to do appropriateness studies for the Rand Corporation) and New York's Commissioner of Social Services. In its December 12, 1993 edition, *Newsday* reported the hearings revealed widespread hostility to Clinton's plan and "overwhelming" support for single-payer. "Consumers, doctors, hospital chiefs and insurers have a message for Governor Mario Cuomo about President Clinton's health-care plan: New York can find its own better way," *Newsday* reported. *Newsday* said the supporters of a single-payer plan among consumers constituted "an overwhelming majority" of those who spoke. Dr. Chassin was quoted saying, "It's pretty remarkable that almost unanimously the consumer representatives described their support for a single-payer approach. I was surprised by the magnitude of that proportion."[12]

At the beginning of this book, I described my role in a 1996 citizens jury experiment in Minnesota in which single-payer won eight votes, managed competition three votes, and MSAs no votes. A similar vote took place on a citizens jury convened three years earlier in Washington, DC, by the Jefferson Center, a nonprofit organization that had been experimenting with citizens juries since the late 1970s. The Jefferson Center would expose a representative group of Americans to proponents of various solutions to a problem, and then publish the jury's conclusions. The Center convened a meeting of 24 Americans from 15 states to discuss health policy during the week of October 10 to 14, 1993, less than a month after Bill Clinton had presented his managed competition plan to Congress on national television. The jurors included, among others, a grain handler from New Jersey, a court clerk from New York, a retired insurance agent from Florida, a retired nurse from Louisiana, a carpenter from Wisconsin, a janitor from Minnesota, a legal secretary from Texas, an electrical contractor from Nevada, and an antique dealer from California.

Although the Jefferson Center's goal was to give ordinary people a voice in the debates about significant issues facing the country, the agenda the Center imposed on the jury was stacked against single-payer. For starters, the jury was told its sole purpose was to discuss two questions: "Do we need health-care reform in America?" and "Is the Clinton plan the way to get the health-care reform we need?" There would be no vote on single-payer, the Republican version of managed competition, MSAs, or anything other than Clinton's plan. Ned Crosby, the founder of the Center and co-moderator of the proceedings, later told Mike Casper, Wellstone's former policy advisor, that he framed the question for the jury narrowly in order to "gain legitimacy" in Washington and to ensure that Clinton administration officials would participate (former U.S. Representative Toby Moffett, Clinton's point man to the jury, had apparently warned Crosby he would not participate if single-payer were on the agenda).[13] A second obstacle to single-payer was the witness list

– it consisted almost entirely of proponents of either the Clinton plan or one of the Republican plans. Of the 28 witnesses listed in the Jefferson Center report on this jury, only two had indicated support for single-payer – Gail Shearer of Consumers Union (Consumers Union publishes *Consumer Reports*, which endorsed a single-payer system in 1992), and Senator Wellstone.[14]

But despite the handicaps imposed on the single-payer proposal, it wound up getting a thorough hearing because the jurors demanded it. The demand came after Senator Wellstone presented the case for his single-payer legislation. Wellstone was one of three Senators who testified. The others were Senator Durenberger, who presented the Republican-and-conservative-Democrat version of managed competition (known as "Clinton lite"), and Senator Don Nickels (R-OK) who argued for MSAs. As William Raspberry reported in the *Washington Post*, the Durenberger and Nickels proposals were "dismissed without a vote."[15] "[O]nly the single-payer approach led [the jury] to want to hear more," reported the Jefferson Center's newsletter. "By votes of 22-0, the jurors invited Wellstone back for two more question periods."[16]

By the jury's fifth and last day of deliberation, it was clear that most jurors were not happy with the Clinton plan and that many would like to vote on single-payer. But the jurors were reluctant to embarrass their hosts by rewriting the agenda, and so they concluded their formal deliberations by voting only on the two questions put to them by the Jefferson Center. On the question of whether America needed health-care reform, the jury voted unanimously in the affirmative. On the question of whether the Clinton plan was the way to get the necessary health-care reform, 19 jurors said no and 5 said yes. Immediately after the close of the jury's proceedings, Roger Mudd, a reporter then with ABC News who had been hired to produce a documentary on the jury, observed that a majority of the jurors seemed to support single-payer. He then asked the jurors, "Why the hell didn't you have a formal vote on the Wellstone plan?" Kathleen Hall Jamieson, a professor at the University of Pennsylvania's Annenberg School of Communications who had co-moderated with Crosby, then asked the jurors, "How many would have voted for the Wellstone plan?" Seventeen raised their hands.[17]

The jury clearly understood what they were rejecting and what they were endorsing. They agreed on 25 criteria they wanted any health reform plan to meet. These criteria included comprehensive coverage for all Americans, freedom to choose one's doctor, minimal "bureaucracy and paperwork," "use [of] price guidelines to hold down costs," and reduction in "fraud, waste and abuse." These criteria said nary a word about competition. The jury obviously didn't believe the Clinton and Republican claims that overuse was the main problem and that competition would reduce prices and protect patients.

As Dr. Chassin was impressed by the extent of the support for single-payer in New York, so Jefferson Center staff expressed amazement at their jury's support for single-payer. "The whole damn world seems to think the Clinton plan is the way to go," said Bob Meeks, president of the Jefferson Center. "Yet they [the jurors] like the single-payer system, which isn't even getting considered in Washington."[18] I got a similar reaction from Laurie Sether, the woman who asked me to participate in the 1996 *Star Tribune*-KTCA TV citizen forum that I described in Chapter 1. "Were you surprised by the vote?" she asked me as the forum was breaking up. I said I was surprised only that people were willing to make a decision after a few hours of debate. I was not surprised that most of the forum participants favored single-payer.

## Conclusions

The surprise that people experience when they learn of the public's support for single-payer is due (a) to the great chasm between the opinion of experts and the opinion of average people, and (b) to the great differences in power between the relatively small group of experts and the large but unorganized public. The experts think excessive volume of services – overuse – is the problem, and that either managed-care plans or large deductibles are the solution. The public, on the other hand, thinks price, and the waste and fraud that drive price up, are the primary culprits, and, therefore, there is no need for patients to suffer the deprivations inflicted by managed care and large deductibles. Because the experts have money and media access, they have enormous power to frame the debate that the public does not have. Therefore, anyone who attempts to comprehend the U.S. health policy debate by listening to the mainstream media is easily fooled into thinking the experts are correct and reflect public opinion. The evidence I presented in Chapters 4 through 7 indicates the experts are incorrect. The evidence in this chapter indicates the experts do not represent public opinion.

## Endnotes

[1] "Why are health care costs rising," *American Medical News*, March 28, 2005, 8.

[2] Haynes Johnson and David S. Broder, *The System: The American Way of Politics at the Breaking Point*, Little Brown, Boston, MA, 1996, 91.

[3] Ibid., 90.

[4] R. A. Zaldivar, "Limits on services at crux of health care debate," *St. Paul Pioneer Press*, November 29, 1992, 21A.

[5] Daniel Yankelovich, "The debate that wasn't: The public and the Clinton plan," *Health Affairs* 1995;14(1):7-23, 8-9.

[6] Ibid., 13-14.

[7] Amy Goldstein, "How HMOs became the enemy: From nonprofit ideals to corporate horror stories," *Washington Post*, October 10, 1999, A1, A8.

[8] Steven R. Simon et al., "Views of managed care: A survey of students, residents, faculty, and deans of medical schools in the United States," *New England Journal of Medicine* 1999;340:928-936.

[9] Kaiser Family Foundation, *Health Care and Other Elder Care Issues Survey*, June 2000, http://roperweb.ropercenter.uconn.edu/cgi-bin/hsrun.exe/roperweb/HPOLL_new/StateId/SI-BGrk7Y-nqwrapF9dAP6qDM4/HAHTpage/Summary_Link?qstn_id=432672, accessed October 30, 2002.

[10] Pew Research Center, *News Interest Index Poll*, April 2001, http://www.ropercenter.uconn.edu/cgi-bin/hsrun.exe/roperweb/HPOLL/StateId/SI-BGrk7Y-nqwrapF9dAP6qDM4/HAHTpage/Summary_Link?qstn_id=442447, accessed October 30, 2002.

[11] Jeremy Iggers, "People agree they disagree on health care: Universal coverage is common ground," Minneapolis *Star Tribune*, November 15, 1993, 1B.

[12] *Newsday*, December 12, 1993, quoted in *American Health Line*, December 20, 1993, 8-9.

[13] Barry M. Casper, *Lost in Washington: Finding the Way Back to Democracy in America*, University of Massachusetts Press, Amherst, MA, 2000, 235.

[14] Jefferson Center, *Citizens Jury Update*, December 1993, Minneapolis, MN, 6-7.

[15] William Raspberry, "Citizens Jury won over by merits of Wellstone's single-payer plan," Minneapolis *Star Tribune*, October 21, 1993, 23A.

[16] Ibid., 4.

[17] Casper, op cit., 236.

[18] Patrick Howe, "'Citizens Jury' supports Wellstone's health care proposal over Clinton plan," Minneapolis *Star Tribune*, October 15, 1993, 10A.

# 9

# Why Managed Competition Can't Work

## Introduction

In the remaining three chapters of this book, I examine the three contenders in the modern health-care reform debate in more detail than I did in Chapters 1 and 2. The three contenders, again, are managed competition, high deductibles, and single-payer. I have saved this task for the end for an obvious reason: Your ability to evaluate any proposal to solve the health-care crisis depends on your ability to identify the causes of the crisis. If you don't understand what's driving the crisis, you're in a poor position to decide what the best solution is. But if you have plowed through Chapters 4 through 7 with me, you have a good understanding of what is and is not causing the crisis. You understand that the overuse excuse and other common explanations for the crisis have little or no explanatory power, and that the real cause of the crisis is supply-side waste. And if you read Chapter 8, you know Americans are in general agreement with the supply-side-waste diagnosis and are supportive of single-payer, especially when they're exposed to a fair debate about single-payer and the other two contenders.

In this chapter, I examine the theory of managed competition. I demonstrate that managed-care plans (MCPs), the centerpiece of managed competition, are incapable of containing cost because they cannot address the waste I described in Chapters 6 and 7, and they cannot stop themselves from damaging quality and privacy. I demonstrate, moreover, that publishing report cards on plans and providers, the most prominent feature of managed care 2.0, cannot make managed care and managed competition work.

Some readers may wonder why this chapter is necessary. Isn't the performance of the current MCP-dominated system evidence enough of its inferiority and incorrigibility? For the average American, the answer is probably yes. But some very influential groups and individuals are still attracted to managed competition, even if they no longer use the phrase to denote what it is they advocate. George W. Bush and congressional Republicans still want to turn Medicare into a showcase for managed competition, many large employers still subscribe to the notion that someone has to tell doctors what services can and cannot be ordered, and many within the health policy community continue to deny managed care has done harm to quality of care. For example, a conference of leading health policy experts convened by the Institute of Medicine (an agency within the National Academy of Sciences) in late 1997 (which is to say, well after the HMO backlash materialized) concluded that managed care was not only not a problem but in fact deserved some credit for improving quality of care. In a report on the conference, two experts present at the conference wrote:

> The workshop participants agreed.... [i]t is ... probably impossible ... to "fix" one component of health-care organizations without addressing systems as a whole – or, as one speaker remonstrated, "trying to fix the parts when the whole chassis is broken." The "broken chassis" in question, moreover, is not managed care. The patterns of practice we contend with today were largely established under fee-for-practice [*sic*] medicine, and the transition to managed care has generally held quality constant or, in some instances, has improved it.[1]

Managed competition, the theory that competition among MCPs can be made more vigorous with some "managing," has taken a dreadful beating, but it is not dead yet. Although its proponents are way out of line with public thinking, they are powerful enough to force us all to continue debating whether the current system is as bad as I and many others say it is, and whether the system's defects can be eliminated with a little tweaking. It is essential, therefore, that anyone who seeks to understand the modern health-care reform debate understand the arguments for managed care and managed competition.

## The assumptions underlying managed competition

"Health maintenance strategy" is the phrase Paul Ellwood used to describe his proposal to Nixon in the early 1970s. "Managed competition" is the name given to the theory developed by Stanford professor Alain Enthoven in the 1980s and endorsed by Ellwood and others in the early 1990s. Managed competition was a more elaborate version of Ellwood's health maintenance strategy. Ellwood's health maintenance strategy and Enthoven's managed-competition theory both started with the assumption that volume of health services is the main problem. They also shared the assumption that HMOs are better than other types of insurance companies at reducing volume because HMO doctors are exposed to financial incentives that induce them to cut out unnecessary services (and never necessary services) and to place more emphasis on preventive services. Ellwood's proposal and managed-competition theory also shared the assumption that report cards on HMOs and other insurers that use managed-care tactics are essential to protect consumers against abuse, and that such report cards are technologically and financially feasible. Finally, both Ellwood's proposal and managed competition shared the unspoken premise that the administrative costs created by managed care are insignificant.

The theory of managed competition appeared when it did – in the late 1980s – because by then it was clear to everyone, even HMO advocates, that the spread of HMOs and the conversion of many traditional insurers to MCPs was having no effect on inflation. Obviously, something more than a takeover of the insurance industry by MCPs was needed. In a pair of articles for the *New England Journal of Medicine* published in 1989, Enthoven and his colleague Richard Kronick argued that HMOs and managed care were wonderful inventions, but their mere appearance was insufficient to bring inflation under control. What was needed, they argued, was stronger competition within the insurance industry. Competition could be strengthened, they said, if it were "managed."

They argued, in essence, that two features had to be added to Ellwood's simple strategy of subsidizing HMOs and publishing report cards. First, they argued that a majority of insured Americans were staying away from HMOs, even though HMO premiums were relatively low, and were instead buying insurance from traditional insurers because Americans were not sufficiently motivated to seek out the lowest-cost insurance. This lack of "cost consciousness," they said, could be fixed with two reforms. First, federal tax law had to be amended to eliminate the subsidy employees received when their employer paid for all or some of their health insurance. Because federal law says employees don't have to report premium payments by their employer as income, employees don't pay income and payroll taxes on those premium payments. The unpaid tax is, in effect, a subsidy from the government for the purchase of health insurance. Second, argued Enthoven and Kronick, employers should require employees to pay a higher share of their premiums if employees chose more expensive (less tightly managed) policies. If these two reforms were implemented, they claimed, Americans would get even madder than they already were about the high cost of health insurance, and would be even more motivated to abandon traditional insurers and MCPs that were relatively unaggressive at managing doctors, and would enroll with cheaper HMOs and more aggressive MCPs.

Purchasing coalitions was the second reform Enthoven and Kronick added to Ellwood's strategy. If consumers were bunched into big buying coalitions, they would have a lot more bargaining power with the big insurance companies.

Like Ellwood before them, Enthoven and Kronick also endorsed MCP report cards. Like Ellwood, they offered no information on how report cards would be produced, whether they could be used, and what they would cost.

To sum up, here are the assumptions, some explicit and some implicit, that Enthoven and Kronick made:

(1) Volume, not price, is the main problem;
(2) Capitation and bonuses for denying care will save money without harming patients because capitation and bonuses cause

doctors to want to keep patients healthy, and doctors will cut volume by eliminating unnecessary services and increasing preventive services;

(3) Even if capitation and bonuses do threaten quality, quality will not decline because someone will some day concoct, and consumers will then use, mammoth report cards on the quality of thousands of medical services provided by MCP doctors;

(4) Administrative costs will remain unaffected by the spread of managed care, and by the need to construct report cards;

(5) Many more consumers will enroll in HMOs and more tightly managed MCPs if their tax subsidies are eliminated and they are required to pay out of their own pocket for the privilege of avoiding HMOs, which will save money because we all know managed care saves money; and

(6) Consumers would have more power to negotiate lower premiums if they were represented by huge buying coalitions.

The first four of these assumptions were also endorsed by Ellwood and the early disciples of HMOs. Assumptions 5 and 6 were added by Enthoven and Kronick. The six assumptions together constitute managed competition. Assumption 1 (that volume is the main problem) is not irrational; it's just wrong – it's not supported by the evidence (see Chapter 4). But assumptions 2, 3, and 4 are worse than wrong; they defy common sense. Assumption 5 (higher out-of-pocket costs for premiums will make consumers more willing to enroll in HMOs) is actually rational, but it is bad policy. Only assumption 6 (purchasing coalitions) holds any promise, but this promise is limited to the inflation problem; huge buying coalitions can do little to stop the degradation of quality and privacy caused by the current system.

The flabbiness of the first four premises meant MCPs and managed competition had to fail. But why wasn't this obvious in 1970, or even 1990? How do we explain the fact that "managed competition was the cost control vehicle of choice [in 1993 and 1994], appearing in nearly every major proposal advanced during the 103rd Congress," as one expert put it?[2] Why were so many intelligent people seduced by the claims made for HMOs and managed competition? Why didn't policy makers and reporters question the assumptions underlying HMO propaganda long before HMOs and MCPs took control of the system? In this chapter, I will concentrate on the three most important factors that permitted MCPs to escape criticism until it was too late. In the course of discussing these factors, I will examine the defects in managed care and managed competition that guaranteed their failure.

The first factor is what I'll call the "HMO halo" conferred upon the nation's earliest HMOs by the support HMOs got from populist organizations and unions and, conversely, by the hostility directed at HMOs by the American Medical Association. This halo seduced many policy makers and reporters into thinking HMOs were run by people who were more altruistic than the people who ran traditional insurance companies, and that this altruism would survive once HMOs were transformed from a few small, community-controlled organizations into hundreds of huge corporations accountable primarily to large employers and to Wall Street.

The second factor that contributed to uncritical thinking about HMOs, and eventually all MCPs, was the ability of HMOs and many MCPs to keep their premiums 5 to 10 percent below those of traditional insurers. At first glance, this fact would seem to constitute proof that MCPs were capable of rolling back health-care inflation. But this impression was an illusion. MCPs, it turned out, could keep their premiums slightly lower only because they had three advantages over traditional insurers that had nothing to do with efficiency. First, they enrolled healthier people. Second, they rationed health care (by which I mean they denied *necessary* services), something traditional insurers couldn't do because they didn't have control over doctors as MCPs did.* Third, MCPs shifted costs onto other payers, including traditional insurers, taxpayers, and patients and their families, using methods that were less available or completely unavailable to traditional insurers (such as extracting large

---

* "Rationing," as I use the word here, refers to the denial of necessary medical services. It does not refer to decisions by insurers that certain types of medical goods and services fall outside the coverage authorized by law (in the case of public insurers) or by the contract between the insurer and the employer or individual enrollee (in the case of private-sector insurance companies). If, for example, I buy an insurance policy that does not cover mental health services, my insurer is not guilty of rationing if it refuses to reimburse me for the cost of a visit to a psychiatrist.

discounts from hospitals, which forced the hospitals to raise their rates for less powerful payers including the uninsured). These three HMO advantages – healthier enrollees, the power to ration, and the ability to shift costs – were not obvious to casual observers (a class into which many so-called experts fall), and, of course, MCP supporters did not go out of their way to call attention to these advantages.

The third factor which seduced a lot of smart people into thinking MCPs could perform as advertised was the unusually steep decline in health-care inflation that occurred during the mid-1990s, just as MCPs were completing their takeover of the market. This inflation lull did not last, of course, but for a few years in the 1990s the lull was hailed by MCP advocates as solid evidence that MCPs really were more efficient than traditional insurers.

These three factors – the HMO halo effect, lower HMO premiums, and the mid-1990s inflation lull – created a willingness among policy makers, academics, and reporters to accept uncritically the strange assumptions articulated by HMO and managed-competition proponents. Of course, as the MCP industry grew and accrued more and more economic and political power, it became increasingly difficult for critics of the industry to be heard above the din of industry propaganda. The cumulative effect of the HMO halo, lower HMO premiums, the mid-1990s inflation lull, and oceans of MCP money thrown behind the effort to promote managed competition proved to be overwhelming. With all that going for them, it is little wonder that managed-competition theorists managed to pull off a great illusion – for awhile, anyway. In the following sections, I examine in more detail the HMO halo, lower HMO premiums, and the 1990s inflation lull.

## The origin of the HMO halo

Managed competition would not have been developed (or, if it had been, it would never have become famous) if there had been no HMO industry; there probably would have been no HMO industry if there had been no HMO Act of 1973; and there almost certainly would have been no HMO Act of 1973 if there had been no HMOs for the proponents of the HMO Act of 1973 to brag about. HMOs and other types of MCPs were the centerpiece of managed competition. So we begin our inquiry into the first phase of the evolution of managed competition with an analysis of the track record of the 30 to 40 HMOs that existed in 1970, the year Paul Ellwood convinced the Nixon administration to support legislation subsidizing the creation of an HMO industry.*

Today, promotion of MCPs is associated primarily with the Republican Party. Since 1994, Republicans in Congress have successfully fought off legislation to protect patients from MCPs (the first patient protection bill was introduced by Senator Paul Wellstone in 1994). Since 1995, Republicans have promoted the notion that Medicare can save money if seniors are pushed, with financial pressure, into HMOs (former House Speaker Newt Gingrich was promoting this idea by 1995). Thus, newcomers to the health-care reform debate may be shocked to learn that the HMO concept was passionately supported during the 1930s by union workers, poor farmers, consumers, and a few altruistic doctors, many of whom drew their inspiration from the populist and co-op movements of the late 1800s and early 1900s. Dr. Michael Shadid, who started one of the earliest HMOs in Elk City, Oklahoma, in 1927, and who did some consulting for the founders of Group Health Cooperative of Puget Sound in Seattle, was a member of the Socialist Party.[3] Maurice McKay, the director of Group Health in the Twin Cities, was a labor union representative before joining Group Health; his father was an organizer for the Industrial Workers of the World.[4] (Someone told me 15 years ago that Maurice McKay was known as "the commie from Como," an allusion to the fact that Group Health's headquarters were on Como Avenue in St. Paul.) For many liberals and progressives, the role that populist groups played in establishing the early HMOs created a halo over the HMO concept. By the same token, the hatred of HMOs exhibited by the American Medical Association added luster to this halo.

Community groups, unions, and farm groups supported the formation of HMOs, called "prepaid group practices" prior to 1970, for the same reason they supported food co-ops, milk co-ops, and electricity

---

* Joseph Falkson put the number of HMOs operating in the U.S. in 1970 at 39 (*HMOs and the Politics of Health System Reform*, American Hospital Association, Chicago, IL, 1980, 197). Mayer and Mayer put the number at "between 28 and 39" (Thomas R. Mayer and Gloria Gilbert Mayer, "HMOs: Origins and development," *New England Journal of Medicine* 1985;312:590-594).

co-ops, namely, to meet a basic human need with a community-controlled enterprise. They most definitely were not in it to make big bucks. Dr. Shadid organized the cooperative in Oklahoma to provide hospital services for the same reason Baylor University Hospital developed the first hospital insurance program two years later – to make it feasible for ordinary people, many of whom were poor, to get medical care when they needed it. There was a significant difference, however, between Shadid's co-op and the Baylor University insurance plan: Shadid's co-op was controlled by the townspeople and farmers who bought a share in the co-op, whereas the teachers who paid $6 in annual premiums to the Baylor plan gained no voice in the running of the hospital nor the insurance company that took their money.

Group Health Cooperative of Puget Sound, which merged with Kaiser Permanente in 1997, was formed in 1945 by unions, co-ops, and the Washington Grange (a populist farm organization). The motive was not moolah, power or market share. The spark leading to the creation of this HMO was the refusal of Washington's doctor-owned Blue Shield plan to pay for treatment of what even then were called "pre-existing conditions" (diseases and illnesses that existed before the patient signed up for insurance). As the following excerpts indicate, the preamble to Group Health's bylaws expressed classic populist values:

> The Cooperative shall endeavor:
> (a) to develop some of the most outstanding hospitals and medical centers to be found anywhere, with special attention devoted to preventive medicine.
> (b) to serve the greatest possible number of people under consumer cooperative principles without discrimination.... [and]
> (f) to educate the public as to the value of the cooperative method of health protection, and to promote other projects in the interest of public health.[5]

I love the sentiments expressed in this preamble. I know I would have enjoyed working with the people who wrote it.

The nation's first urban HMO, Group Health Association of Washington, DC, founded in 1937, was organized by employees of the

Home Owner's Loan Corporation because these employees were acutely aware that many of their customers had incurred huge medical bills during the Depression, and that these bills forced people out of their homes when they could no longer keep up their mortgage payments.

Large employers in rural areas also played a significant role in the creation of the first generation of prepaid group practices in the first half of the 20th Century. As one observer put it,

> One of the most powerful forces leading to these arrangements was the practice of recruiting people to work in isolated areas such as sugar and pineapple plantations in Hawaii; lumber camps in Michigan, Wisconsin, and Washington State; mines on the iron ranges of northern Minnesota; and railroads just about anywhere.[6]

The most famous of these early, company-formed, prepaid group practices were those started by Henry Kaiser, the construction and ship-building magnate who made his millions during the Depression and the Second World War. Kaiser used prepaid group practices during the Depression to provide medical care to workers building an aqueduct in the Southern California desert (its purpose was to bring water from the Colorado River to Los Angeles). He did so again to provide medical care to workers who built the Grand Coulee Dam in Washington, and yet again to provide care to 90,000 workers employed at his shipbuilding plants in San Francisco during World War II. The San Francisco prepaid group practice eventually became Kaiser-Permanente Health Care Program, for decades the nation's largest HMO and, along with Group Health of Puget Sound, one of the most respected HMOs in the country. Kaiser's original goal was not to make money on his HMO, to become the CEO of a great big corporation, nor to become famous on Wall Street. His goals were quite pragmatic: to make sure his workers had access to doctors when they needed them.

Thus, when Paul Ellwood began to peddle HMOs in the early 1970s, he was proposing an idea that had the endorsement not only of groups representing America's dispossessed, but some employers as well. These endorsements created the impression that HMOs were unique in the insurance world – public-spirited organizations that were adept at protecting patients from unnecessary services and delivering preventive services that doctors in the fee-for-service sector wouldn't think of providing.

## Lower premiums and the illusion of greater HMO efficiency

The ability of most HMOs to keep their premiums slightly below those of traditional insurers was another significant factor that contributed to the widespread acceptance of the strange assumptions underlying Ellwood's HMO fantasies and the theory of managed competition. Whether HMO premiums were always lower than those of traditional insurers is not clear. I have seen reports suggesting that HMO premiums prior to the 1980s were often equal to those of traditional insurers. But I have no doubt that the typical HMO's premium eventually fell below that of the typical traditional insurer (this probably occurred in the early 1980s), and that many non-HMO MCPs were also able to charge less than traditional insurers. I'm positive of this because I know a majority of Americans never liked managed care. That means there was no way HMOs could have made such huge inroads into the health insurance market if their premiums had not eventually fallen below those of traditional insurers. The great majority of Americans who enrolled in HMOs did so for one reason, and one reason only: to save money.

The HMOs' ability to keep their premiums low was not due, as HMO advocates would have us believe, to greater HMO efficiency. (It is possible HMOs were even less efficient than traditional insurers. As we have seen, the spread of HMOs drove up administrative costs for providers, and it might have driven up overhead for insurers as well.) HMOs were able to keep their premiums below those of traditional indemnity insurers because they enjoyed "favorable selection" (which means they enrolled healthier people), they shifted costs to other payers, and they rationed.

The possibility that HMOs enjoyed two of these advantages – favorable selection and the ability to ration – was acknowledged as early as 1978. That year, in an article for the *New England Journal of Medicine*, Harold Luft, who would subsequently become a fan of managed care, reviewed all the studies published in professional journals over the previous 25 years on the subject of how HMOs save money. He found only five solid studies, most of which reported data from the 1960s. On the basis of these studies, all of which compared Kaiser-Permanente to traditional insurers, Luft concluded that HMOs did indeed have lower total costs (defined as premiums plus out-of-pocket costs incurred by patients, both for treatment in the HMO and outside of it), and that HMOs achieved their savings primarily via reduced hospitalizations and, to a minor extent, by not having to pay for services that patients sought outside of the HMO. Citing other studies (that is, other than the five involving Kaiser), Luft concluded that out-of-plan use "ranges from less than 1 percent in some studies to about 8 percent." (I assume Luft meant 1 to 8 percent of the *dollar value* of all services was obtained out-of-plan, but it's possible he meant 1 to 8 percent of HMO *enrollees* sought services outside the HMOs' network of providers.)

Luft concluded that HMOs were cutting their total costs by 10 to 40 percent compared with traditional insurers, but he warned that these savings might be illusory because they could reflect "undertreatment," and because they could simply reflect the better health status of people who enroll in HMOs.[7] Interestingly, Luft said nothing about the possibility that HMOs were shifting costs by extracting large discounts from doctors and hospitals or engaging in other practices that shifted costs to other payers. Luft did comment on the possibility that frustrated enrollees might have sought services outside Kaiser, but he implied this form of cost-shifting was minimal. Luft's inattention to cost-shifting may be evidence that Kaiser was engaging in little cost-shifting prior to the 1970s, or it might represent an oversight by Luft.

Luft's conclusion that HMOs might cut total costs by 10 to 40 percent was widely quoted over the next decade by managed-care advocates, but without Luft's caveats about favorable selection, undertreatment, and out-of-plan visits. Alain Enthoven was one of the worst abusers of Luft's conclusion. In a 1978 article, he claimed that Luft's assessment was based on "many comparison studies" (there were only five, all involving Kaiser), and that Luft had concluded HMO savings could not be explained by other factors such as "out-of-plan utilization, differences in age and sex composition, previous health status, or government subsidies."[8] Enthoven's remarks were wildly inaccurate; Luft's paper said nothing of the sort (Luft didn't even discuss "government subsidies"). Enthoven repeated this false characterization of Luft's study in subsequent papers, including his widely read 1989 paper laying out his theory of managed competition[9] and a 1993 article purporting to explain why the spread of HMOs had done nothing to reduce inflation.[10] Because Enthoven's inexcusable distortions of Luft's work appeared in prominent journals, they played an important role in convincing policy makers, reporters, and other health policy experts that HMOs' slightly lower premiums constituted evidence that HMOs were more efficient than traditional insurers.

## The evidence that HMOs and other MCPs enroll healthier people

Subsequent research indicated that Luft was justified in warning his readers that HMOs might be saving money by enrolling healthier people. In a review of the literature in 1987, Fred Hellinger concluded that HMOs clearly benefited from favorable selection.[11] In another review published in 1995, Hellinger confirmed this conclusion for both HMOs and non-HMO MCPs.[12] A 1996 report by what used to be called the Physician Payment Review Commission (PPRC, now called the Medicare Payment Advisory Commission), an agency that advises Congress on health-care issues, concluded that the research firmly establishes that seniors who leave the traditional fee-for-service (FFS) Medicare program to enroll in Medicare HMOs are much healthier than seniors who stay in traditional FFS Medicare.

The differences in health status reported by some of these studies are huge. Original research by the PPRC demonstrated that seniors who enroll in HMOs cost those HMOs only 56 percent of what it costs Medicare to take care of the sicker seniors who stay with traditional Medicare.[13] Another study, which examined data on more than 400,000 seniors, reported that seniors who enrolled in Florida Medicare HMOs during the period 1990-93 were half as expensive to care for as seniors who stayed in traditional FFS Medicare. Specifically, this study found that HMO seniors incurred only $693 in hospital costs in the year before they joined an HMO compared with $1,260 incurred by seniors who stayed in traditional Medicare. To make matters worse, the study found that those seniors who enrolled in HMOs tended to stay enrolled only as long as they were healthy. When they got sick, they disenrolled and returned to traditional Medicare, thus saving their HMOs lots of money and driving up the cost of traditional Medicare. This study was entitled, appropriately enough, "The Medicare-HMO revolving door – The healthy go in and the sick go out."[14]

We don't have any studies indicating how much money favorable selection has saved the average HMO serving the *non*elderly (we know only that the nonelderly who enroll in HMOs are healthier). The studies comparing *seniors* who enroll in Medicare HMOs with seniors who stay in traditional Medicare indicate Medicare overpaid HMOs somewhere between 15 to 40 percent during the last two decades of the last century thanks to favorable selection. What we can say is that by the 1980s, and possibly much earlier, favorable selection was helping HMOs and non-HMO MCPs in the nonelderly market keep their premiums at or below the levels of traditional insurers, and that, in a market where a difference between premiums of even a few percentage points can swing big chunks of market share to lower-priced insurers, favorable selection played a very important role in permitting MCPs to take over the U.S. insurance market.

## The evidence that MCPs benefited from cost-shifting

Although managed-competition advocates argued that excessive volume was the main cause of inflation, and although they had virtually nothing to say about excessive prices charged by doctors, hospitals, drug companies, and equipment manufacturers, in fact HMOs and other MCPs used their market power to extract low prices from providers, drug companies, and equipment suppliers. Because large market share is needed to extract big discounts,[15] it is unlikely that HMOs were extracting these hefty discounts in the 1970s when they were small and just beginning to spread. During the 1970s, favorable selection and denial of services were probably the HMOs' most important advantages over traditional insurers.

But between the early 1980s, by which time many HMOs had acquired substantial market share within their local markets, and the mid-1990s, by which time extracting discounts had become more difficult because virtually every insurer was doing it, discounts contributed significantly to the ability of MCPs to keep their premiums below those of traditional insurers. This practice resulted in cost-shifting. Doctors, hospitals, and drug companies would make up for the revenues they gave away to MCPs by charging higher prices to less powerful payers, including traditional insurers and the uninsured.[16] But by the mid-1990s, cost-shifting was more difficult because the entire health insurance industry had fallen under the control of large MCPs, all of which were demanding discounts. Finding a weak buyer upon which to shift costs was now much more difficult. Another factor which made cost-shifting more difficult by the mid-1990s was the great consolidation among providers which had occurred by then. Merger madness had given many doctors and hospitals so much negotiating clout they could ignore or minimize MCPs' demands for more discounts.

The size of the discounts extracted by MCPs is hard to ascertain because MCPs are so secretive; most contracts between MCPs and providers require the providers to stay mum about how much they're being paid. But the few studies available indicate MCPs extracted enormous discounts in the 1980s and early 1990s when they were taking over the industry. Table 9-1 shows the discounts Twin Cities hospitals gave to three types of payers (Medicare, Medicaid, and HMOs) compared to the average for all payers in 1981 and 1982, and to four types of payers (Medicare, Medicaid, HMOs, and all other payers) in 1990. You can see that HMOs got much larger discounts than traditional private-sector insurers did in all three years. This is clearest in the 1990 data because those data break out the non-HMO, private-sector insurers from all other payers. HMOs forced the hospitals to cut their rates by 38 percent while all other private-sector payers got an average discount of only 3 percent. Table 9-2 indicates that one year later HMOs nationally were forcing *drug manufacturers* to charge only 72 percent of the list price for drugs.

But discounting was not the only method MCPs used to shift costs off themselves and onto others. Other tactics included using financial incentives that encourage HMO doctors to classify injured enrollees as injured on the job so that their expenses could be billed to workers compensation programs;[17] avoiding their share of research expenses,[18] charity care,[19] and graduate medical expenses even while being subsidized by Medicare for graduate medical expenses; billing Medicare for billions of dollars (equal to approximately 5 to 10 percent of total Medicare payments to HMOs) in administrative costs that should have been billed

## Table 9-1: Discounts offered to four types of payers by Twin Cities hospitals, 1990: HMOs extracted large discounts from hospitals, traditional insurers got almost no discount

|  | Discount* | | |
| --- | --- | --- | --- |
| Payer | 1981 | 1982 | 1990 |
| Medicaid | 12.8% | 15.7% | 54.1% |
| HMOs | 8.6% | 10.2% | 37.6% |
| Medicare | 10.6% | 15.7% | 36.3% |
| All other payers | | | 3.2% |
| All payers | 6.5% | 9.4% | |

* The 1981 and 1982 discounts are for 26 Twin Cities hospitals, whereas the discounts shown for 1990 are for four Minneapolis hospitals.

Sources: 1981 and 1982 figures from Allan N. Johnson et al., "Cost-shifting: The discount dilemma," *Journal of Health Politics, Policy and Law* 1984;9(2):251-260; 1990 figures from Katherine Hiduchenko, "Do Health Maintenance Organizations control costs or shift costs?" *New England Journal of Medicine*, letter, 1993;328:971.

to private payers;[20] and failing to reimburse Veterans Affairs Hospitals for services rendered by VA hospitals to Medicare HMO enrollees.[21]

Provoking enrollees to go out-of-network for their services is another form of cost-shifting. Since this is probably accomplished most of the time by rationing, this issue could be classified as evidence of rationing and discussed in the next section on rationing. But because the consequences so clearly amount to cost-shifting, I discuss this problem here under the rubric of cost-shifting.

In the preceding section on favorable selection, I discussed Harold Luft's 1978 estimate that HMO enrollees sought 1 to 8 percent of the services they needed outside of their HMO network. That figure was either low for its time, or the percent of HMO enrollees seeking care outside their HMO rose dramatically during the 1980s and early 1990s. A 1995 study by Davis et al. found that "17 percent of managed-care

## Table 9-2: Prices paid by various types of prescription drug purchasers, 1991: MCPs extract large discounts from drug manufacturers

| | |
|---|---|
| Average wholesale price | $1.00 |
| Independent pharmacies | .87 |
| Chain pharmacies | .78 |
| Managed-care plans | .72 |
| Hospitals | .60 |
| Government programs | .50 |

Source: *Prescription Drug Study: A Report to the Minnesota Legislature on the Prescription Drug Market*, Minnesota Department of Health, 1994, Figure 2.10.

enrollees reported using services outside of their plan in the past twelve months" and that these out-of-plan users reported "an average of four out-of-plan visits within the past year for services not covered by their plan."[22] A 1996 survey by *Consumer Reports* found that 18 percent of enrollees in MCPs reported seeking medical services outside their plans (the magazine didn't say over what period).[23] Common sense indicates out-of-plan use is evidence of dissatisfaction. The study by Davis et al. specifically made that finding. This means that HMOs are not simply the passive beneficiaries of patient out-of-network care-seeking. It means HMOs are doing something to provoke it, such as refusing to pay for joint-replacement surgery for people who need it.

A study by Morgan and colleagues, several of whom were co-authors of the "revolving door" study on seniors who enroll in Medicare HMOs, lent credence to this conclusion that HMO enrollees who seek care outside their HMO do so because they are dissatisfied. Morgan et al. found that seniors in HMOs who needed hip or knee replacement surgery returned to traditional Medicare about the time they decided to undergo this surgery because their HMO refused to pay for the surgery. Specifically, the study reported that Florida HMO disenrollees were four times as likely as seniors who enrolled in traditional Medicare to have hip and knee replacements in the three months after they left their HMOs. The authors concluded, "These data provide indirect evidence

that Medicare HMOs ... are rationing [hip and knee replacement sur-
gery] and that beneficiaries respond by returning to the FFS [Medicare]
system to seek care."[24]

## The evidence that managed-care plans ration care

In addition to favorable selection and cost-shifting, the evidence
indicates MCPs have enjoyed a third advantage over traditional insurers
– they save money by rationing. The MCP industry denies this. MCPs
do not dispute the fact they deny many more services to their enrollees
than traditional insurers do. In fact, MCP representatives trumpet
that fact to employers and policy makers to justify their claim that they
are the solution to the health-care crisis. But the MCP industry does
dispute the claim by its critics that a substantial portion of the services
it denies are necessary services, that is, that MCPs routinely engage
in rationing. They argue, as we have seen, that overuse of health care
services occurs at epidemic levels and that they are merely cutting out
overuse.

It may well be that MCPs have reduced some overuse of the system.
But the evidence that MCPs ration, and thereby harm patients, is now
overwhelming. That evidence falls into three categories: anecdotal
evidence (aka "HMO horror stories"), polling and focus group data,
and scientific studies of the quality of MCP care versus care provided
by doctors paid by traditional FFS insurers.

The anecdotal evidence grew rapidly in the 1990s as more Americans
enrolled in MCPs. By 1995, media coverage of MCPs, which had been
unduly positive, turned decidedly negative, and "HMO horror stories"
were the primary type of evidence reported. *Time*'s cover story "The
soul of an HMO," *Glamour*'s "What killed Karin Smith?" and a column
in the *New York Times* entitled "Torture by HMO," all published in
1996, were typical of the terrible stories told about MCPs in 1996 and
subsequent years. In July 1996, the *New York Times* described the MCP
industry's publicity as "a hailstorm of stories about necessary care being
denied, about so-called gag rules that prevent physicians from telling
patients about alternative and usually more expensive treatment, and
about 24-hour 'drive through' maternity stays."[25] In early 1997, John
Iglehart, editor of *Health Affairs* and a member of the Jackson Hole
Group, observed that the managed-care industry's publicity was by then

"continuously and overwhelmingly negative."[26] In 1998, the *New York Times* declared in a headline on the front page, "Reality of the HMO system doesn't live up to the dream."[27]

By 1996 the media was describing the appearance of an "HMO backlash." Here are some typical headlines: "HMO backlash" (*St. Paul Pioneer Press*, 1996), "Managed care: National leap of faith" (*Chicago Tribune*, 1996), and "Backlash against HMOs" (*Time*, 1997). The most immediate and visible manifestation of the backlash was the explosion in "patient protection" bills introduced in Congress and state legislatures. "In 1996 alone," reported Tom Bodenheimer in an article for the *New England Journal of Medicine*, "1,000 pieces of legislation attempting to regulate or weaken HMOs were introduced in state legislatures, and 56 laws were passed in 35 states."[28] Many of these early patient protection bills dealt with "drive-through deliveries" (delivery of newborns with only one day of hospitalization). Many states passed laws requiring MCPs to let new mothers stay in the hospital for at least 48 hours. Other problems addressed by patient protection laws were retaliation by MCPs against doctors for advocating for their patients, and refusal to pay for emergency services because the MCP, with the benefit of hindsight, decided the patient did not need ER services. By the late 1990s, the question of whether patients had the right to sue MCPs dominated the patient protection debate. By 1999, lawsuits against MCPs on behalf of doctors were also drawing headlines.

Another manifestation of the HMO backlash was the appearance of hostile statements about MCPs and managed care in media of all forms – in op-eds, statements by politicians, news stories, TV dramas and sitcoms, best-selling novels, movies, cartoons, and jokes heard at work, on the Internet, and on late-night TV talk shows.* One of the most frequently cited manifestations of public anger at MCPs was the reac-

---

* The joke below circulated on the Internet throughout the late 1990s and early 2000s. I received it several times, the last time in January 2004.

INFORMATION TO HELP YOU CHOOSE YOUR NEXT HEALTH PLAN

Question. What does HMO stand for?
Answer: This is actually a variation of the phrase, "Hey Moe." Its roots go back to a concept pioneered by Moe of the Three Stooges, who discovered that

tion of movie-goers to a furious comment about HMOs by the actress Helen Hunt in the 1997 movie, "As Good as It Gets." Hunt played the role of a single mother being courted by a screwball fiction writer played by Jack Nicholson. In an early scene in the movie, we see Hunt in her kitchen explaining her anger at her HMO's refusal to pay for treatments for her son's asthma. "HMO bastards pieces of crap," she shouted (Hunt actually used another four-letter word for "crap"). According to several columnists who saw the movie, audiences applauded Hunt's blue streak. "Justified or not, anger with managed care has penetrated American culture so deeply that it drowned out long and well-funded protests by insurance and business lobbyists," reported the *Washington Post* in a 1999 article entitled, "How HMOs became the enemy: From nonprofit ideals to corporate horror stories." "Even in a country with

---

a patient could be made to forget about the pain in his foot if he was poked hard enough in the eyes.

Q. I just joined an HMO. How difficult will it be to choose a doctor?

A. Just slightly more difficult than choosing your parents. Your insurer will provide you with a book listing all the doctors in the plan. These doctors basically fall into two categories: those who are no longer accepting new patients, and those who will see you but are no longer participating in the plan. But don't worry; the remaining doctor who is still in the plan and accepting new patients has an office just a half-day's drive away and has a diploma from a Third World Country.

Q. Do all diagnostic procedures require pre-certification?

A. No. Only those you need.

Q. Can I get coverage for my pre-existing conditions?

A. Certainly, as long as they don't require any treatment.

Q. What happens if I want to try alternative forms of medicine?

A. You'll need to find alternative forms of payment.

Q. My pharmacy plan only covers generic drugs, but I need the name brand. I tried the generic, but it gave me a stomach ache. What should I do?

A. Poke yourself in the eye.

Q. What if I'm away from home and I get sick?

A. You really shouldn't do that.

Q. I think I need to see a specialist, but my doctor insists he can handle my problem. Can a general practitioner really perform a heart transplant right in his office?

A. Hard to say, but considering that all you're risking is the $15 co-payment, there's no harm in giving him a shot at it.

ebbing faith in many of its basic institutions, managed care holds an exceptionally low berth in public esteem," said the article.[29]

In the early years of the backlash, the MCP industry and its supporters blamed everyone but themselves for the industry's awful publicity. They denied that HMO horror stories were as numerous as reporters, politicians, and the public claimed. Instead, they blamed doctors allegedly disgruntled about loss of income (as opposed to loss of authority to do right by their patients), consumers who had allegedly been pampered by the former fee-for-service system, politicians looking for attention, and reporters making mountains out of molehills. Ellwood, for example, denounced "HMO bashing" in a 1996 interview with *Modern Healthcare*,[30] and "attack by anecdote" in a 1996 interview with the *New York Times Magazine*.[31] In the summer of 1996, *Modern Healthcare* reported one of the strangest events in the modern healthcare reform debate:

> Officials of the Health Insurance Association of America [the trade group at the time for the insurers that had adopted some managed-care tactics but had not morphed completely into HMOs] and the Blue Cross and Blue Shield Association summoned reporters to a press briefing in Washington. But it wasn't to answer questions. They wanted reporters to tell them why the managed-care industry is getting such bad press.[32]

The horrendous publicity MCPs were getting by 1996 was not due to a conspiracy among reporters. The bad publicity and the public backlash against MCPs was inspired by widespread meddling in the physician-patient relationship by MCPs, much of it leading to rationing.

The second category of evidence indicating that MCPs ration – data on consumer attitudes – is also extensive. We reviewed some of the polling data in Chapter 8; those data indicate that Americans did not approve of managed-care tactics before or after MCPs became dominant. Several surveys done annually during the 1990s documented the increase in the proportion of Americans who believed that MCPs were damaging quality of care. For example, the Harris Poll reported that the percentage of Americans who thought managed care harmed the quality of medical care rose from 39 to 59 percent between 1995 and 2000.[33] A 2004 survey of Americans indicated that American perceptions of the quality of our system continues to deteriorate. The survey found that 55 percent were dissatisfied with the quality of health care, up from 44 percent in 2000.[34]

Focus-group data confirmed the polling data. One of the most rigorously done studies of consumer perceptions of the new system was conducted by the Picker Institute for the American Hospital Association. Based on discussions with more than 300 adults in 31 focus groups in 12 states between May and September 1996, the Picker Institute reached these conclusions:

> Few people ... perceive there to be a planned system of health care that operates in their behalf.... If a system is in operation at all, it is seen as one designed to block access, reduce quality, and limit spending for care at the *expense* of patients. What's more, this impression comes *not* from sensational media accounts or the scare campaigns of special interest lobbying groups, but largely from personal experience. Patient after patient tells stories of their struggles to get past the many "gatekeepers" in the system or to get insurance or managed care approval for the care they and their doctors think they need. They talk about how assertive they must be to get answers and the frustrations of trying to coordinate care among many different specialists – and many of them worry about what will happen if and when they are too sick to manage such things on their own behalf. And they describe a feeling of being abandoned when they are released from the hospital – like "jumping off into nowhere," as one patient described it (emphasis in original).[35]

The third category of evidence – scientific studies – provides compelling evidence that MCPs ration. Patchy evidence suggests that MCPs began to ration much more aggressively in the 1990s. If this in fact occurred, I believe it happened then because MCPs were losing their favorable-selection and discounting advantages at about that time. The MCP industry's ability to cherry-pick their enrollees began to disappear as the industry's market share grew. When the industry was small, it was easier to avoid sick people. But by the mid-1990s, when the industry's market share had grown to encompass 95 percent of the nonelderly insured population, avoiding the sick was much more difficult. Similarly, extracting large discounts from providers was easier for the HMOs in the 1980s when they were the only ones doing it than it was for the MCPs of the 1990s. By the 1990s, nearly the entire insurance industry was engaging in the practice of demanding discounts, and doctors and hospitals, with no one left to shift costs to, were becoming increasingly unwilling to provide discounts. By the 1990s, the ability to ration was probably more important to MCPs than either cherry-picking or discounting. If this theory is correct, it would, along with the huge market share achieved by MCPs by the early 1990s, explain the appearance of the "HMO backlash" in 1995 and 1996.

We have already reviewed two scientific studies that strongly suggested that HMOs ration – the "Medicare revolving door" study and the joint-replacement study, both of which examined HMO behavior between 1990 and 1993. Other studies confirmed that MCPs cut services aggressively, and many of these services were necessary services. Tables 9-3 and 9-4 present data from a study of a national MCP that operated in 47 states. Table 9-3 indicates that hospital services were cut in the 1990s not by denying *admission* (MCPs had already cut admission rates during the preceding two decades), but by cutting down on the *number of days* patients could stay once they had been admitted. We see that nearly all (97 percent) of patients for whom requests were made were allowed to be admitted to the hospital by the MCP's utilization-review gnomes. This MCP achieved its savings by refusing to authorize a large portion of the days-in-hospital that the patients' doctors asked for. You can see that mental health patients suffered the biggest cutbacks in hospital days; only 54 percent of the total mental health days requested by doctors were approved by the MCP. My jaw dropped when I saw the data in Table 9-4. This table shows that total days authorized by utilization reviewers working for this MCP dropped substantially between 1990 and 1993. The drop was enormous for mental health patients. In

**Table 9-3: Utilization review reduced hospital services primarily by reducing the number of days patients could stay in the hospital, not by denying hospital care completely: Outcome of physician requests to a national MCP for hospitalization, January 1989 through December 1993**

| | |
|---|---|
| Request for admission denied | 0.4% |
| Outpatient care or case mgmt authorized instead | 3.1% |
| Inpatient care authorized | 96.6% |
| Percent of inpatient days authorized for | |
|     Obstetric admissions | 92.9% |
|     Medical admissions | 86.0% |
|     Surgical admissions | 83.4% |
|     Mental health admissions | 54.0% |

Source: Thomas M. Wickizer and Daniel Lessler, "Effects of utilization management on patterns of hospital care among privately insured adult patients," *Medical Care* 1998;36:1545-1554, Table 1.

1993, the average number of hospital days authorized for mental health patients was 10.88, down from 20.72 in 1990.

The MCP industry's aggressive effort to limit hospital use, and the belt-tightening by hospitals that ensued, unquestionably damaged the quality of care in U.S. hospitals. A number of studies attest to this conclusion. For example, in a subsequent article, Wickizer and Lessler, the authors of the study presented in Tables 9-3 and 9-4, sought to determine what impact shortened length-of-stay had on readmission rates for patients with cardiovascular disease who underwent surgery. They reported an association between (a) reductions in length-of-stay below those requested by the patients' physician and (b) 60-day readmission rates. The authors reported that when utilization reviewers reduced the length-of-stay by two or more days, the patient's odds of being readmitted to the hospital within 60 days was 2.6 times that of patients who were permitted to stay in the hospital as long as their doctor recommended.[36]

---

**Table 9-4: MCPs reduced lengths of stay substantially between 1990 and 1993, especially for mental health patients: Number of hospital days authorized by a national MCP, 1990 and 1993**

|      | Obstetric | Medical  | Surgical | Mental health |
|------|-----------|----------|----------|---------------|
| 1990 | 2.82 days | 6.81 days | 4.66 days | 20.72 days |
| 1993 | 2.38 days | 5.22 days | 3.99 days | 10.88 days |

Source: Thomas M. Wickizer and Daniel Lessler, "Effects of utilization management on patterns of hospital care among privately insured adult patients," *Medical Care* 1998;36:1545-1554, Table 5.

---

Studies comparing the volume of *non-hospital* services MCP and fee-for-service (FFS) patients got also suggested that many of the Americans who migrated from FFS to MCP plans in the early 1990s encountered a lot more resistance to their demands for health care than they had been used to. Table 9-5 presents data on utilization of physician services by depressed patients during the late 1980s and early 1990s. The data indicate that depressed HMO and FFS patients were equally likely to have at least one visit to a mental health professional, but that FFS patients got many more visits than HMO patients did (14 versus 9 over six months). Table 9-6 indicates Medicare patients insured in HMOs received only 13 home health visits after being hospitalized compared with 19 for patients who stayed in traditional FFS Medicare. The study cited in Table 9-6 found that the difference in the number of visits damaged the health of the HMO patients. The HMO patients were less likely to recover numerous functions (including the ability to bathe, eat, and manage medications by themselves) than were FFS beneficiaries. By cutting back on home health visits, HMOs saved themselves about $400 per patient.

Even preventive services, services which MCPs were supposed to be so good at providing, apparently took a hit during the late 1980s or early 1990s. According to a study which compared the rate at which HMOs and FFS plans provided preventive services to women (including breast

**Table 9-5: Fee-for-service patients get more mental health visits: Probability and number of mental health visits by depressed HMO and fee-for-service patients[a]**

|     | Probability of mental health visit in 6 months[b] | No. visits among those with visits[c] | Psychological health prior to start of study[d] |
| --- | --- | --- | --- |
| HMO | 50% | 9 | .34 |
| FFS | 56% | 14 | .32 |

(a) The data for this study were collected over a two-year period that occurred some time between 1986 and 1991. The authors did not indicate which two years.

(b) The difference between these scores was statistically significant.

(c) The difference between these scores was statistically significant, and was due primarily to higher utilization rates by patients of psychiatrists. There were only minor differences in utilization rates of patients of general medical providers (family practice and internal medicine doctors).

(d) These scores are a composite measure of psychological health. A higher score is worse. The difference between these scores was not statistically significant (in other words, HMO and FFS patients were equally sick).

Source: Roland Sturm et al., "Mental health care utilization in prepaid and fee-for-service plans among depressed patients in the Medical Outcomes Study," *Health Services Research* 1995;30:319-340.

exams and Pap smears), HMOs provided more such services in 1987 but had "lost this comparative advantage" by 1992. By 1992, HMOs and FFS plans were providing equal amounts of preventive services.[37]

In 1999, I published an article in the *American Journal of Public Health* in which I reviewed the scientific literature comparing the quality of care offered by HMOs and traditional FFS plans. I reported finding a total of 34 rigorously conducted studies done between 1980 and 1996. These 34 studies reported a total of 44 comparisons of HMO and FFS doctors. Table 9-7 shows the results. You see that HMO doctors outperformed FFS doctors in only four of the comparisons but were worse in 21. Thirty-four studies over 16 years is not a lot of research, but it confirmed the anecdotal and survey data – the advent of HMOs reduced the quality of care American patients receive.

**Table 9-6: Fee-for-service patients get many more home health-care visits: Number of home health-care visits received by hospitalized fee-for-service and HMO Medicare patients within 60 days after discharge from the hospital during period 1989 to 1991**

| | |
|---|---|
| FFS patients: | 18.8 visits |
| HMO patients: | 12.7 visits |

Source: Peter W. Shaughnessy et al., "Home health care outcomes under capitated and fee-for-service payment," *Health Care Financing Review* 1994;16(1):187-222.

**Table 9-7: Scientific data: A review of the scientific literature indicates HMOs rarely offer better care and frequently offer inferior care**

Number of comparisons in which

| | |
|---|---|
| HMO care was better than FFS care | 4 |
| HMO and FFS care were equivalent | 19 |
| HMO care was worse than FFS care | 21 |
| Total number of comparisons | 44 |

Source: Kip Sullivan, "Managed care plan performance since 1980: Another look at two literature reviews," *American Journal of Public Health* 1999;89:1003-1008.

Several of the studies I reviewed drew substantial coverage from the media when they were published. One of these was by John Ware, Jr. and his colleagues which appeared in the *Journal of the American Medical Association* in 1996. The study was unusually well done. It had a large sample size drawn from three cities – Boston, Chicago, and Los Angeles. The study found that elderly patients were *twice* as likely to suffer deterioration in their health over a *four-year* period (not a decade or a lifetime) if they were enrolled in an HMO than if they were enrolled in traditional FFS Medicare.[38*]

Unlike most of the studies comparing the quality of HMO with FFS care, which did not attempt to determine the effect of any single component of managed care, studies of drug formularies do tend to focus exclusively on one managed-care tool, in this case, formularies. These studies confirm the negative picture of managed care painted by the studies comparing HMO and FFS quality in general. Here is an excerpt from a 1996 study that examined the effect of formularies on patients with five diseases (arthritis, asthma, epigastric pain/ulcer, hypertension, and otitis media): "For all conditions except otitis media, formulary limitations on drug availability were significantly positively related to higher rates of emergency department visits and hospital admissions...."[39] In other words, because patients couldn't get the drugs their doctors wanted them to have, or they took a drug on a formulary that their doctor suspected they would react badly to, they got so sick they required treatment in hospitals at greater rates than patients not subject to formularies. The authors of this study cited seven studies of Medicaid HMOs that reached similar conclusions. Here's how they described those studies: "A causal relationship between stricter HMO cost-containment practices and increased resource use also is supported by previous studies reporting shifts to more expensive resources when restrictions are placed on the availability of drugs in Medicaid programs."[40]

These three types of data – the anecdotal reports, the opinion surveys and focus groups, and scientific studies – support the conclusion that MCPs do not cut out only unnecessary services. The data indicate, rather, that MCPs deny necessary medical care to substantial numbers of patients. This ability to ration helped MCPs keep their premiums relatively low and take market share from traditional insurers. That MCPs would ration should come as no surprise. The instruments available to MCPs to cut back on volume of service are terribly blunt. Financial incentives and utilization review may lead to some reduction in unnecessary services, but

---

* Research comparing the quality of care offered by doctors under the influence of managed care with doctors who are not became difficult to do by the mid-1990s because managed care had become so widespread by then.

they must inevitably cut out necessary care as well. The tools of managed care resemble a hatchet more than a scalpel.

## The mid-1990s inflation lull

During the 1970s and early 1980s, the HMO halo effect was the primary cause of the myth that MCPs save money. By at least the 1980s, MCPs' lower premiums, caused by favorable selection, cost-shifting, and rationing, constituted a second factor fueling the myth of MCP efficiency and fooling smart people into thinking the premises of managed care and managed competition were sound. Around 1992, a third factor appeared which, for a few years, totally seduced the nation's policy makers and pundits into accepting the argument that MCPs save money. That was the appearance of an unusually steep and prolonged decline in health-care inflation. The decline was obvious whether one measured inflation by gauging year-to-year changes in premiums paid by employers, or changes in total U.S. health-care spending.

Throughout the late 1980s and early 1990s, health-care inflation had been torrid despite the fact that a majority of Americans under 65 were insured by MCPs. Even managed-care advocates were admitting publicly that the spread of MCPs had not reduced health-care inflation. As late as 1993, Alain Enthoven published an article in *Health Affairs* entitled, "Why managed care has failed to contain health costs."[41] In 1993 and 1994, the Congressional Budget Office released studies saying that managed-competition bills introduced by President Clinton and Representative Jim Cooper (D-TN) would *raise*, not lower, total spending on health care.[42]

But a slowdown in premium inflation began in 1992, and it turned out to be unusually sharp and prolonged. The rate fell sharply, from 10.9 percent in 1992 to 0.5 percent in 1996.[43] The five years over which this inflation lull lasted was also unusually long; prior to 1992, premium inflation tended to fluctuate in three-year cycles – inflation would be high for three years, then low for the next three years. But this cooling of inflation in the mid-1990s had little to do with managed care. The slowdown was caused by several other factors, the most important of which were a halving of the general, underlying inflation rate beginning in 1991, and a merger avalanche that began in 1990 and continued throughout the slowdown. In Minnesota, where merger madness struck about a year before it hit most states, the market share of the largest four health insurers rose from 64 percent in 1992 to 80 percent in 1994.[44]

Tables 9-8 and 9-9 present data on consolidation at the national level over the decade 1987-1997 for the insurer and provider sectors respectively. You can see that consolidation accelerated in 1990, then soared in 1993, the year Bill Clinton, many other state and federal politicians, and numerous large employers endorsed managed-competition legislation. Anticipating that they might soon be forced, either by employers or by managed-competition legislation, to join or become a huge MCP or provider network (such as a hospital or clinic chain), insurers and providers all over the country set off on a feverish quest for size. If you were an insurer, you wanted large size in order to maximize your ability to squash provider fees and force doctors to ration services. If you were a provider, you sought large size in order to be attractive to MCPs (MCPs disdain solo practitioners because they have so little "market share") and to have some negotiating power with them. You could acquire size either by attracting more "customers" or by being

---

## Table 9-8: Merger madness struck the insurance industry just as the 1992-1996 inflation lull began: Value of HMO mergers and acquisitions, 1987-1997, millions of dollars

| 1987: | $17 |
|-------|------|
| 1988: | 72 |
| 1989: | 1 |
| 1990: | 12 |
| 1991: | 309 |
| 1992: | 2,285 |
| 1993: | 1,317 |
| 1994: | 4,426 |
| 1995: | 1,327 |
| 1996: | 13,318 |
| 1997: | 3,269 |

Source: Srija Srinivasan et al., "Wall Street's love affair with health care," *Health Affairs* 1998;17(4):126-131.

---

## Table 9-9: Merger madness struck the provider sector just as the 1992-1996 inflation lull began: Value of health services\* mergers and acquisitions, 1987-1997, millions of dollars

| | |
|---|---|
| 1987: | $4,247 |
| 1988: | 8,501 |
| 1989: | 5,560 |
| 1990: | 1,298 |
| 1991: | 2,048 |
| 1992: | 6,096 |
| 1993: | 17,535 |
| 1994: | 21,240 |
| 1995: | 14,582 |
| 1996: | 26,924 |
| 1997: | 19,296 |

\* The authors of this study defined "health services companies" as follows: "offices and clinics of doctors of medicine or osteopathy, dentists, or other health-care providers; nursing and personal care facilities; hospitals' medical and dental laboratories; home health-care services, and miscellaneous health and allied services."

Source: Srija Srinivasan et al., "Wall Street's love affair with health care," *Health Affairs* 1998;17(4):126-131.

part of a merger. Both tactics, especially drawing "customers" away from competitors quickly, require artificially low prices. These prices couldn't last forever, however, and they didn't. Losses became intolerable throughout the health-care industry in 1996, and by 1997 insurers were jacking up premiums even though the underlying inflation rate remained very low.\*

One consequence of the merger avalanche was increased consolidation among providers, especially among hospitals. That reduced the

---

\* I invite readers to consult an article I wrote for *Health Affairs* in which I presented the evidence for my conclusion that the 1990s inflation lull had nothing to do with managed care ("On the 'efficiency' of managed care plans," *Health Affairs* 2000;19(4):139-148).

power of MCPs to extract discounts from providers and to tell doctors how to practice medicine. The health-care inflation we have seen since 1997 was, therefore, caused not only by MCPs raising premiums to make up for losses sustained during the 1992-1996 inflation lull, but by clinics and hospitals using their newfound market power to extract higher reimbursements from MCPs.

The resumption of high inflation after 1996 was not foreseen by MCP advocates in 1995 and 1996. By 1995, many MCP proponents had convinced themselves that the inflation lull signified a permanent reduction in inflation which had been caused by the spread of managed-care tactics. By 1997, Enthoven, who only four years earlier had conceded managed care wasn't saving money, was asserting, "Since the early 1990s cost pressures have moderated significantly, and there is no explanation except competitive markets and managed care."[45] The argument that the spread of managed care explained the 1992-1996 slowdown was quickly accepted among experts and reporters as well. But, as we saw in Chapter 2, that happy consensus was short-lived. By 2000, when premium inflation was back to double digits, a noticeable change in elite opinion had materialized. Employers, most Democrats, some Republicans, and many within the health-policy community ceased claiming that the mid-1990s inflation lull was evidence of MCP efficiency. Only the MCP industry and some Republicans at the national level persisted in claiming that MCPs could save money.

## Managed competition and managed care cannot be rescued

The HMO halo effect, MCPs' generally lower premiums, and the 1992-1996 inflation lull helped conceal the irrationality of the assumptions underlying Ellwood's health maintenance strategy and Enthoven's managed-competition theory. But the illusion could not last forever. By the mid-1990s, MCPs had lost their cherry-picking and cost-shifting advantages. Moreover, their reliance on rationing, which appears to have increased in the early 1990s, had created great hostility among Americans by 1995. And by the late 1990s, it was clear that the cooling of inflation that began in 1992 had only been temporary. The contrast between what MCP advocates promised and what they delivered was now painfully obvious. By 2000, as we saw in Chapter 2, experts all over the country were saying managed care had failed. Even executives within the insurance industry are conceding the great HMO experiment has failed. At the annual meeting of the National Managed Health Care Congress held in Washington, DC, in March 2005, Dr. Robert S. London, who served in the top ranks of three of the nation's largest MCPs, announced that HMOs had failed on both cost and quality grounds and, as a result, the nation was witnessing "the demise of the HMO." Dr. London made these announcements as a member of a panel for a session entitled, "Is Selling HMO Product Dead?"[46]

It is not possible to close the gap between what MCP advocates promised and what they delivered, either with respect to cost or quality. Let's look at cost first. MCPs are incapable of reducing any of the four categories of waste I discussed in Chapters 6 and 7, with the possible exception of high physician fees and high drug prices. I say "with the *possible* exception" because, although it is clear MCPs, especially large ones, can force clinics, hospitals and drug companies to cut their prices, providers and drug companies recoup from weaker payers at least a portion of the discounts they give to MCPs. In other words, MCPs may be able to reduce the prices doctors and drug companies charge *them*, but they are incapable of making significant reductions in *system-wide* prices. As we saw in Chapter 7, physician incomes and drug prices in the U.S. remained very high in the 1990s by international standards despite the dominance of MCPs in that decade.

The fact of the matter is that the options available to MCPs to cut costs are quite limited. MCPs can attempt to cut costs at the expense of *patients* by rationing more aggressively; they can attempt to cut costs at the expense of *providers* by demanding even bigger discounts; or they can attempt cut costs at their *own* expense by cutting back on administrative costs. But none of these strategies is feasible. Public hostility to MCP rationing, and the threat of patient protection legislation and lawsuits, will prohibit more aggressive rationing. Anger among doctors and hospital administrators, and greater consolidation among providers, will make further cuts in provider reimbursements very difficult to achieve. And MCPs have little leeway to cut back on administrative costs. If they reduce marketing expenditures, their sales decline. If they reduce activities required to "manage care," their medical costs rise.

Similarly, the gap between what MCP advocates said would happen to *quality* and what in fact happened cannot be closed. The argument that financial rewards for doctors who cut costs would somehow turn doctors into better doctors by inducing them to cut unnecessary services (and *only* unnecessary services) and increase preventive services had neither logic nor evidence behind it, and nothing can turn that sow's ear into silk now. The notion that utilization review – the second-guessing of doctors by people who have no contact with the patient – would cut out only unnecessary services and leave necessary services alone was also illogical, and nothing can fix that logic now. Moreover, financial rewards for cost-cutting and utilization review can do little or nothing to ameliorate the underuse problem; they can, obviously, do a lot to aggravate it.

Because managed care formed the centerpiece of managed-competition theory, the destruction of managed *care's* reputation in the late 1990s meant the destruction of managed *competition*. Managed competition is rarely discussed these days. But the battering that managed care and managed competition have taken does not mean that managed care has disappeared and cannot make a comeback. MCPs still use utilization review and financial incentives, although to a lesser degree than in the past. The powerful groups and individuals who brought us managed care and managed competition are still promoting the fundamental assumptions of managed care (that overuse is the main problem, and doctors and patients need overseers to improve their ability to make good decisions), and they continue to promote the secondary features of managed competition – purchasing coalitions, elimination of tax subsidies for insurance, and, above all, report cards – but usually as separate proposals rather than as part of a comprehensive package.

But if MCPs cannot function as advertised, establishing the secondary features of managed competition will not make managed competition work. In fact, implementing those secondary features might even make the health-care crisis worse. The argument that the current system can't control inflation until consumers are stripped of their tax subsidy is absurd. Consumers are already furious about the high cost of health insurance, and have reluctantly enrolled in ostensibly lower-cost MCPs by the tens of millions over the last three decades, and still inflation runs wild. All the loss of the tax subsidy will do is torque consumer frustration with the current system to a higher level.* Given the enormous power and the great consolidation of the MCP industry, even the most infuriated consumer will be unable to make a dent in health insurance premiums. It is possible that bunching consumers into large purchasing groups (another plank in the managed-competition platform) could make a dent in premium inflation, but if that happened it would almost certainly come at the expense of quality of care as long as MCPs control the system. Because there are so many ways to short-change patients that are hard to detect, and because even visible acts of rationing can be difficult for sick patients to resist, rationing will be a relatively easy way for MCPs to cut their cost if they are forced by large purchasing coalitions to reduce their premiums.

Because managed care developed such an awful reputation in the 1990s, MCPs and their allies have lately begun to promote a softer and more sophisticated version of managed care, a version I referred to in the last chapter as managed care 2.0. The most important change in the message delivered these days by managed-care supporters and former managed-competition advocates is a new emphasis on report cards. Whereas managed-care advocates in the past saw report cards as but one plank in the managed-competition platform, today's managed-care advocates speak of report cards as if they can solve the health-care crisis single-handedly. Whereas Ellwood, Enthoven and other managed-care advocates in the past said almost nothing about how report cards were to be constructed, distributed, and paid for, today's managed-care advocates promote more elaborate plans for constructing and paying for report cards, plans which include a prominent role for the federal government and which call for spending untold billions on electronic medical records and virtual medical records depots into which all Americans' medical records will be funneled. Whereas Ellwood et al. envisioned report cards being used by *employers* and *individuals* to select the best MCPs, today's managed-care proponents envision report cards being used mainly by *insurers* (including Medicare) to reward and punish doctors.

---

* Eliminating the tax subsidy for health insurance is a good idea on tax fairness grounds. Treating employer payments for employee health insurance as non-taxable confers greater benefits on higher-income employees than it does on lower-income employees.

Paying doctors according to how well they perform on report cards became such a hot topic within the American health policy community in the late 1990s that it was given a name – "pay for performance." In 2002, the Centers for Medicare and Medicaid Services announced, per instructions from Congress, it would conduct a three-year pay-for-performance demonstration project (starting in 2003),[47] and the Integrated Healthcare Association, a coalition of seven California plans, announced a pay-for-performance project.[48] Minnesota's three largest plans – Blue Cross and Blue Shield, Medica, and HealthPartners – have all announced pay-for-performance programs.[49] "Pay for performance" was a hot topic at the 2005 National Managed Health Care Congress meeting I just mentioned.

But report cards and pay-for-performance are going to fail as abjectly as utilization review and capitation did, and for the same fundamental reason: It is extremely difficult for third parties to distinguish good care from bad care, and necessary services from unnecessary services, day in and day out. Accurate report cards will require an astronomical expenditure on data collection, and even then the probability that quality of care will improve is low, and the probability that costs will drop is zero.

## Why report cards will fail

Beginning with Paul Ellwood, report card promoters have routinely minimized the difficulties of measuring the quality of medical care. They are fond of saying, for example, that Americans know more about the cars and other consumer products they buy than they know about their doctors.[*] Here is an example of such talk from researchers affiliated with the Rand Corporation: "More information is available on the quality of airlines, restaurants, cars and VCRs than on the quality of health care."[50] The implication of this glib analogy is that the quality of physicians is as easy to ascertain as the quality of automobiles and restaurants, and that Americans are fools for not demanding *Consumer Reports*-style report cards on doctors. But like so many other assumptions underlying

---

[*] Today's report card advocates want report cards to apply to hospitals and nursing homes, not just doctors. Some report card advocates want insurance companies subjected to report cards as well. For the sake of brevity, I will refer only to physician report cards here.

managed-care theology, the assumption that the quality of health care is as easy to measure as the quality of cars and restaurants is nonsense. Human beings are far more complex than cars and prepared meals, and what physicians and other health-care professionals do for patients is far more complex than what Ford or Toyota employees do to assemble cars or what chefs do to cook meals. The differences in complexity are so vast I feel confident in predicting that we will never see accurate report cards on the great majority of medical services sold today.

To understand the debate about report cards, you must first understand the distinction between *process* measures of quality and *outcome* measures. A process measure grades doctors on how well they comply with a medical guideline. An *outcome* measure grades the effect of treatment on patients. The percent of a clinic's diabetics who have had their cholesterol checked in the last year is an example of a process measure of quality, while the percent of diabetics who have their cholesterol under control is an example of an outcome measure. Similarly, the percent of a hospital's or doctor's heart attack patients who are discharged with a prescription for beta-blockers is an example of a process measure, while the percent of heart attack patients who live more than one year after their heart attack is an example of an outcome measure.

Both types of quality measures are difficult to prepare. Process measures require, first of all, a standard of care against which to measure doctors' performance. For simpler types of services, especially preventive services, guidelines are easy to develop. Flu shots once a year for all elderly people is an example of a very simple, easy-to-prepare guideline. But for the great majority of illnesses and conditions to which human flesh is heir, precise guidelines against which doctors can be measured are very difficult to construct. The guideline for treatment of inner ear infections in children that we discussed in Chapter 4 illustrates the difficulty of laying down a standard that applies to all patients and yet is specific enough to be useful to report card publishers. For thousands of other diagnoses, guidelines, precise or imprecise, based on solid science just don't exist. The proportion of medical services for which a science-based standard of care exists is apparently no more than 15 to 20 percent.* According to a group of experts writing in the *Journal*

---

* "In fact, several studies estimate that only 15 to 20 percent of medical practices can be justified on the basis of rigorous scientific data establishing

*of the American Medical Association*, "[F]ew medical specialties have an evidence base that is robust and comprehensive enough to support PCPA [physician clinical performance assessment]."[51]

But finding a reliable guideline is only the first of two gigantic hurdles producers of process measures have to get over. The second big hurdle is the fact that patients differ in a variety of ways that affect a doctor's ability to score well on a process measure. Patients who are in poorer health, who have lower incomes, and who have worse insurance coverage are less likely to make visits to their doctor and to comply with their doctor's recommendations.[52] A clinic that treats a disproportionate number of diabetics without insurance, for example, is going to have a much harder time scoring well on many process measures than a clinic with a disproportionately low number of uninsured diabetics. The best doctors in the world cannot force uninsured diabetics to visit them and pay not only for the visit but for a cholesterol test, a blood sugar test, and other tests and examinations that diabetes guidelines call for. Experts agree that any report card comparing one clinic to another, or one doctor to another, must adjust scores so that doctors are not punished for factors outside their control, such as patient health, income and health-insurance status. A report card that failed to do that would be neither fair to doctors nor useful to consumers "shopping" for doctors and MCPs seeking to reward good doctors and punish inferior doctors.

The need to adjust scores for factors outside physician control also applies to outcome measures. It is neither fair nor useful to compare, for example, the 30-day mortality rate among patients of a heart surgeon whose patients are all over 80 and have serious comorbidities (like cancer and diabetes) with the mortality rate of another surgeon who treats only patients in their 50s who have no serious health problems other than their heart condition. The surgeon treating the older and sicker patients may actually be the better surgeon, but he or she will inevitably look bad on a report card that uses raw, unadjusted mortality rates.

---

their effectiveness. For most conditions, something other than rigorous data on efficacy or effectiveness must be used to determine criteria of appropriateness" (Paul G. Shekelle et al., "The reproducibility of a method to identify the overuse and underuse of medical procedures," *New England Journal of Medicine* 1998;338:1888-1895, 1888).

But adjusting scores on outcome and process measures to reflect differences in patient health, income, insurance status and other factors beyond doctor control, a process known as "risk adjustment," is a complex and expensive process. Adjusting for health differences requires collecting data from medical files, an expensive project in itself. Adjusting for socioeconomic differences may be even more expensive because the typical medical file does not indicate what a patient's income is or whether the patient has only a sixth grade education and has trouble following instructions from doctors and nurses. Gathering data on these factors may require hiring researchers to interview individual patients and their family members and to examine their insurance policies and their tax returns.

To give you some idea of how expensive report cards can be, consider the cost of the nation's most highly regarded report card, the New York Department of Health's annual report card on coronary artery bypass graft (CABG) surgeons and the 36 hospitals where they operate. The report card is highly regarded among health policy experts because its risk-adjustment methodology is unusually sophisticated. It adjusts post-surgery mortality rates with 72 measures of patient health. But because the risk adjustment is so thorough, the report card is very expensive. It requires approximately 40 full-time employees. These include five full-time staff at the Department of Health to maintain a database, as well as a "utilization review agent ... to audit a sample of 50 cases from half the hospitals each year." Moreover, each of the hospitals graded by the report card must hire a "data coordinator," typically full-time, "to collect and maintain their databases."[53] If each of these 40 staff cost $50,000 a year in salaries and fringe benefits, the cost of staff alone for this one report card is $2 million annually. That $2 million might buy 30 nurses annually; it could insure perhaps 400 adults. And this estimate is only for the *human* resources required. The computers and software needed to do all that data collection add more costs. The annual cost of even a few hundred report cards as sophisticated as the New York CABG report card that cover the entire nation will run into billions, probably tens of billions, of dollars annually.

But despite the cost and reputation of the New York report card, it has been shown to damage quality of care for sicker patients. This has happened because surgeons do not believe the report card is accurate. Surgeons believe, in other words, that the post-surgery death of a patient who was in below-average health prior to surgery will not be sufficiently discounted by the New York Department of Health's risk-adjustment method, and, therefore, their report card score will suffer unfairly as a result. Surgeons respond to their doubts about the accuracy of the report card by refusing to operate on older and sicker patients. The strongest evidence that sicker patients are losing access to New York cardiac surgeons as a result of the report card appeared in 2003 in the *Journal of Political Economy*. The paper (co-authored by Mark McClellan, the current director of the Centers for Medicare and Medicaid Services), concluded, "Taken together, our results show that [CABG] report cards led to ... marginal health benefits for healthy patients, and major adverse health consequences for sicker patients."[54] The authors noted that their findings contradicted two earlier studies which found a decline in CABG-associated mortality rates in New York following the publication of the first CABG report card. They attributed the difference to the fact that their study examined all patients eligible for CABG surgery whereas the earlier studies had examined only those patients who actually received CABG surgery. "[O]bserved mortality [in the earlier studies] declined as a result of a shift in the incidence of CABG surgeries toward healthier patients, not because CABG report cards improved the outcomes of care for individuals with heart disease," they concluded.[55]

If rigorously adjusted report cards can induce physicians to reject sicker patients, it is obvious that poorly or completely unadjusted report cards will have the same effect. Research is demonstrating this obvious fact. One study, for example, found that when Maine began paying its substance abuse providers on a "pay for performance" basis with no risk adjustment of the quality measures, providers quickly rid themselves of their "greatest severity" patients "in order to improve their performance outcomes."[56]

The argument that report cards and pay-for-performance can salvage the current MCP-dominated system depends on a second assumption that is as dubious as the assumption that quality of medical care can be measured accurately at a reasonable cost. That second assumption is that improvements in quality always, or most of the time, lead to reduced cost. That is simply not so. One can think of numerous examples of quality improvement that raise rather than lower health-care spending. Diagnosing people with AIDS earlier rather than later, for example, increases the treatment time for those patients and improves their longevity, which means the system will have to incur the expenses of treating those patients over a longer period of time than if they had simply been left undiagnosed and untreated.

In addition to having to demonstrate that quality of medical care is measurable at a cost that won't bankrupt the nation, that report cards won't damage quality, and that quality improvement inevitably leads to lower costs, report card advocates must convince the public that the destruction of patient privacy that report cards entail is worth the benefits report cards will produce. Report card advocates argue that risk-adjusting performance scores would be less costly, or at least less time-consuming, if all patient medical records were converted to electronic medical records (EMRs) and dumped routinely into virtual medical-records databases without patient consent. That way, report-card publishers wouldn't have to hire nurses to paw through paper medical records to find the medical data necessary to do good risk adjustment. Therefore, those who trumpet report cards and pay-for-performance invariably also trumpet the need for EMRs. Of course, they usually pay lip service to the need to ensure that medical records depots are safe from hackers and leakers, but that of course is not possible. Moreover, the lip service ignores the fact that the very act of delivering medical records to a database violates patient privacy.

## Summary

In hindsight, it seems obvious that managed care could not reduce costs or improve quality. Even though insurers that employed managed-care tactics cut services so severely they damaged quality, they still could not cut costs because the very tactics they were using to cut services drove up administrative costs. They could not improve quality because their tools were too blunt.

And why did it take our political and economic elite so long to accept the truth about managed care? We have discussed three reasons why: the HMO halo; the fact that HMOs managed to keep their premiums low using antisocial strategies that were difficult to detect (cherry-picking, cost-shifting, and rationing); and the mid-1990s inflation lull.

But managed-care advocates have not given up. Now they tell us report cards, developed mainly by governments, and pay-for-performance, administered by insurers, will improve quality, and when that happens, costs will come down. But report cards and pay-for-performance will fail as miserably as the current version of managed care has failed. Report cards will either be inexpensive, in which case they will be crude and therefore unable to improve quality and likely to damage quality for sicker patients, or they will be very expensive, in which case they will improve quality for some patients and damage quality for a lesser number of patients but, in the end, save no money and perhaps even drive costs up. Either way, the kinder and gentler version of managed care now being peddled by MCP advocates – the version that ostensibly depends less on financial incentives and utilization review and more on report cards – will fail to make a dent in the health-care crisis, and might even aggravate it.

---

# Endnotes

[1] Molly Joel Coye and Don E. Detmer, "Quality at a crossroads," *Milbank Quarterly* 1998;76:759-773, 760.

[2] Kenneth E. Thorpe, "Managed care as victim or villain?" *Journal of Health Politics, Policy, and Law*, 1999;24:949-956, 950.

[3] Walt Crowley, *To Serve the Greatest Number: A History of the Group Health Cooperative of Puget Sound*, University of Washington Press, Seattle, WA, 1996, 4.

[4] Mary Jo and Walter Uphoff, *Group Health: An American Success Story in Prepaid Care*, Dillon Press, Minneapolis, MN, 1980, 83.

[5] Crowley, op cit., viii.

[6] Emily Friedman, "Capitation, integration, and managed care: Lessons from early experiments," *Journal of the American Medical Association* 1996;275:956-962, 956.

[7] Harold S. Luft, "How do health-maintenance organizations achieve their 'savings'?" *New England Journal of Medicine* 1978;298:1336-1343.

[8] Alain C. Enthoven, "Cutting cost without cutting the quality of care," *New England Journal of Medicine* 1978:298:1229-1238.

[9] Alain Enthoven and Richard Kronick, "A consumer-choice health plan for the 1990s: Universal health insurance in a system designed to promote quality and economy (First of two parts)," *New England Journal of Medicine* 1989;320:29-37.

[10] Alain C. Enthoven, "Why has managed care failed to contain health costs," *Health Affairs* 1993;12(3):27-43.

[11] Fred J. Hellinger, "Selection bias in health maintenance organizations: Analysis of recent evidence," *Health Care Financing Review* 1987;9:55-63.

¹² Fred J. Hellinger, "Selection bias in HMOs and PPOs: A review of the evidence," *Inquiry* 1995;32:135-142.

¹³ Physician Payment Review Commission, *Annual Report to Congress*, Washington, DC, PPRC, 1996, 255-279.

¹⁴ Robert O. Morgan et al., "The Medicare-HMO revolving door – The healthy go in and the sick go out," *New England Journal of Medicine* 1997;337:169-175.

¹⁵ John M. Brooks et al., "Hospital-insurer bargaining: An empirical investigation of appendectomy pricing," *Journal of Health Economics* 1997;16:417-434.

¹⁶ R. L. Van Horn et al., "The Impact of physician involvement in managed care on efficient use of hospital resources," *Medical Care* 1997;35:873-89.

¹⁷ R. J. Butler et al., "HMOs, moral hazard and cost shifting in workers' compensation," *Journal of Health Economics* 1997;16:191-206.

¹⁸ E. Moy et al., "Relationship between National Institutes of health research awards to U.S. medical schools and managed care market penetration," *Journal of the American Medical Association* 1997;278:217-221; J. S. Weissman et al., "Market forces and unsponsored research in academic health Centers," *Journal of the American Medical Association* 1999;281:1093-1098.

¹⁹ P. J. Cunningham et al., "Managed care and physicians' provision of charity care," *Journal of the American Medical Association* 1999;281:1087-1092.

²⁰ Robert Pear, "HMO study finds U.S. overpayment: Medicare is spending billions on 'highly inflated' fees," *New York Times*, August 11 1998, A1.

²¹ L. J. Passman et al., "Elderly veterans receiving care at a Veterans Affairs Medical Center while enrolled in Medicare-financed HMOs: Is the taxpayer paying twice?" *Journal of General Internal Medicine* 1997;12:247-249.

²² Karen Davis et al., "Choice matters: Enrollees' views of their health plans," *Health Affairs* 1995;14(2)99-112, 106.

²³ "How good is your health plan?" *Consumer Reports*, August 1996, 28-41.

²⁴ Robert O. Morgan et al., "Medicare HMO disenrollment and selective use of medical care: osteoarthritis-related joint replacement," *American Journal of Managed Care* 2000; 6:917-23.

²⁵ Milt Freudenheim, "Assessing HMOs by new standard: A patient's progress," *New York Times*, July 16, 1996, A1.

²⁶ John Iglehart, "The pursuit of commercialism," *Health Affairs* 1997:16(2):7.

²⁷ Peter T. Kilborn, "Reality of the HMO system doesn't live up to the dream," *New York Times*, October 5, 1998, A1.

²⁸ Tom Bodenheimer, "HMO backlash – righteous or reactionary?" *New England Journal of Medicine* 1996;335:1601-1604, 1601.

²⁹ Amy Goldstein, "How HMOs became the enemy: From nonprofit ideals to corporate horror stories," *Washington Post*, October 10, 1999, A1.

³⁰ "Father of the HMO mulls quality measures," *Modern Healthcare*, April 21, 1996, 33.

³¹ Lisa Belkin, "But what about quality?" *New York Times Magazine*, December 8, 1996, 68, 106.

³² "Figure it out for yourselves," *Modern Healthcare*, July 29, 1996, 24.

[33] "While managed care is still unpopular, hostility has declined," *Health Care News*, HarrisInteractive, October 21, 2002.

[34] Benedict Carey, "In the hospital, a degrading shift from person to patient," *New York Times*, August 16, 2005, A1.

[35] Picker Institute, "Eye on Patients," http://www.aha.org/PatientSafety/ EyeonPatients.asp., accessed December 10, 2001.

[36] Daniel S. Lessler and Thomas M. Wickizer, "The impact of utilization management on readmissions among patients with cardiovascular disease," *Health Services Research* 1999;34:1315-1329.

[37] Robin M. Weinick and Karen M. Beauregard, "Women's use of preventive screening services: A comparison of HMO versus fee-for-service enrollees," *Medical Care Research and Review* 1997;54:176-199.

[38] John E. Ware et al., "Differences in four-year health outcomes for elderly and poor, chronically ill patients treated in HMO and fee-for-service systems: Results from the Medical Outcomes Study," *Journal of the American Medical Association* 1996;276:1039-1047; "Some patients do poorly under managed care: Poor and the elderly fare better in traditional plans, study finds," Minneapolis *Star Tribune*, October 2, 1996, A16.

[39] Susan D. Horn et al., "Intended and unintended consequences of HMO cost-containment strategies: Results from the Managed Care Outcomes Project," *American Journal of Managed Care* 1996;2:253-264, 253.

[40] Ibid., 252.

[41] Alain C. Enthoven, "Why managed care has failed to contain health costs."

[42] Tom Hamburger, "CBO puts high price on managed competition," Minneapolis *Star Tribune*, May 5, 1994, 7A.

[43] P. J. Ginsburg and J. R. Gabel, "Tracking health care costs: What's new in 1998?" *Health Affairs* 1998;18(5):141-146.

[44] Kip Sullivan, *Strangled Competition: A Critique of Minnesota's Experiment with Managed Competition*, Minnesota COACT, St. Paul, MN, 1995.

[45] Alain C. Enthoven and Sara J. Singer, "Markets and collective action in regulating managed care," *Health Affairs* 1997;16(6):26-35, 27.

[46] Robert Kazel, "Are HMOs dead?" *American Medical News*, April 18, 2005, 12.

[47] Markian Hawryluk, "Medicare experiments with quality incentive programs," *American Medical News*, November 4, 2002, 7.

[48] Integrated Health Care Association statement, http://www.iha.org, accessed December 17, 2003.

[49] Dan McLaughlin and Brian Campion, "Pay for performance," *Minnesota Physician*, October 2003, 1; Douglas Hiza, "BCBSM launches provider incentive programs," *Minnesota Physician*, October 2003, 11.

[50] Mark A. Schuster et al., "How good is the quality of health care in the United States?" *Milbank Quarterly* 1998;76:517-563, 518.

[51] Bruce E. Landon et al., "Physician clinical performance assessment," *Journal of the American Medical Association* 2003;290:1183-1189.

[52] Carol Friedman et al., "Association between health insurance coverage of office visit and cancer screening among women," *Medical Care* 2002;11:1060-67; Peter Franks

et al., "Effects of patient and physician practice socioeconomic status on the health care of privately insured managed care patients," *Medical Care* 2003;41:842-52.

[53] Edward L. Hannan et al., "Public release of cardiac surgery outcomes data in New York: What do New York state cardiologists think of it?" *American Heart Journal* 1997;134:55-61, 62.

[54] David Dranove et al., "Is more information better? The effects of 'report cards' on health care providers," *Journal of Political Economy* 2003;111:555-588, 577.

[55] Ibid., 581.

[56] Yujing Shen, "Selection incentives in a performance-based contracting system," *Health Services Research* 2003;38:535-552, 535.

# 10

# Why High-Deductible Policies and Tax Credits Won't Work

## Introduction

In the early 1970s, the single-payer and HMO proposals were the most visible proposals in the health-care reform debate. The single-payer proposal had the support of prominent Democrats and labor unions, and the HMO proposal drew the support of the unlikely coalition of Walter Reuther, Ted Kennedy, Paul Ellwood, and Richard Nixon. A third proposal – encouraging employers to offer policies with large deductibles – surfaced back then, but it got little attention because it did not attract the support of someone as powerful as Kennedy or Nixon. Martin Feldstein, a professor of economics at Harvard and later chairman of Ronald Reagan's Council of Economic Advisers, tried to persuade Nixon to adopt this proposal, but Nixon turned him down. For the next two decades, conservatives who supported policies with large deductibles – often called "catastrophic" coverage – got little respect from the nation's political and business leaders. Managed care's star shone so bright that catastrophic coverage, like single-payer, could hardly be seen.

But conservatives never abandoned the high-deductible approach, and when health-care reform returned to the public agenda in the early 1990s, they were ready with a sweetened version of catastrophic coverage they called the "medical savings account" (MSA). By 1996 they had passed legislation authorizing the sale of MSAs on a limited basis. In 2003, Congress terminated the MSA experiment (effective at the end of 2003) and authorized an even sweeter version of the MSA called the "health savings account" (HSA). HSAs, which contain deductibles of $1,000 to $5,000 for individuals and $2,000 to $10,000 for families, went on sale on January 1, 2004. According to America's Health Insurance Plans, 1 million Americans were insured by HSAs as of March 2005.[1] One million is a tiny fraction of the 160 million Americans with employer-sponsored health insurance, and an even tinier fraction of the 300 million people who live in America. But HSA enrollment is growing rapidly. Moreover, HSAs have the support of a movement that is as powerful as the HMO movement was in the 1980s. HSAs are going to have an impact on the U.S. health insurance industry, and have already had a substantial effect on the health-care reform debate. Anyone who seeks to influence the current health policy debate has to understand HSAs.

I will begin this chapter by explaining the MSA-HSA concept and reviewing the history of the high-deductible movement. Then I'll explain why HSAs will fail as badly as HMOs have. At the end of this chapter I will look briefly at proposals that utilize tax credits to encourage more people to buy health insurance.

## Explanation of the HSA

Imagine that you run a business with 100 employees, including yourself, and that these 100 employees represent a typical slice of the nonelderly American population. Let's assume, for the sake of simplicity, that all your employees have dependents, that you provide health insurance with a $500 deductible for each employee, and you pay 100 percent of the premium. This insurance is costing you $10,000 a year (which is less than today's national average for employees with dependents). Like all employers, you are desperately looking for alternatives to 10-percent annual increases in your health insurance costs. Like the great majority of employers today, you feel that you've already exhausted other options. In the mid-1980s, you added an HMO to the insurance options your employees could choose from, and in the late 1980s you ceased offering traditional, unmanaged indemnity insurance all together. In the early 1990s, you politely forced your employees to give up choice of insurer (you were offering three MCPs up to that point) because one of the MCPs promised you slightly lower premiums if it could insure all your employees, not just a portion of them. Still premiums continued to skyrocket. You've considered dropping health insurance completely, but you have rejected that option (for now anyway) because you care about your employees' health, and you fear that if you drop health insurance you might lose some valuable employees. You are, in short, between a rock and a hard place.

Imagine now that you get a call from High Deductible Health Insurance Company offering to sell you insurance for $7,000 per employee. That is $3,000 less than the $10,000 you're currently paying, so you're definitely interested in hearing more. The catch is that this insurance is cheaper because it has a huge deductible – $5,000, or ten times the $500 deductible in your current policy. You know that getting your employees to accept a $5,000 deductible is going to be very difficult, but you feel you have to try. You call a meeting of your employees.

You begin the meeting by describing the savings in premiums that the company will enjoy if you switch to High Deductible Insurance Company's policy. You warn that making the employees pay a portion of the premiums, and dropping coverage all together, are other options you are looking at. Nevertheless, the reaction to the high-deductible policy among your employees is universally unfavorable. Even the healthiest of your employees foresee a high risk of incurring at least a few hundred dollars a year in medical bills, so even they view the high-deductible plan as the equivalent of lost income. The sicker members of your work force are even more opposed to a high-deductible policy.

So you look for a way to sweeten the deal for your employees. You come up with an obvious compromise: You'll share a portion of your premium savings with your employees. "Tell you what," you say. "I'll be saving $3,000 per employee. If you let me switch from our current policy to High Deductible Insurance, I'll give each of you a cash contribution of $1,500. Unlike my payments for health insurance on your behalf, which are not taxable, you'll have to pay income and payroll taxes on that contribution, which will cut the take-home value of my contribution by perhaps a third – to $1,000. But you can use that money to pay for the first $1,000 in medical expenses. Of course, you'll have to pay for expenses between $1,000 and $5,000 per year, but maybe you'll be lucky and won't incur expenses over $1,000."

Now a minority of your employees – the healthiest of them – are willing to consider a high-deductible policy. The healthiest 40 percent will incur bills considerably below $1,000 per year. The healthiest 20 percent will pay on average about $50 a year and the next less-healthy 20 percent will pay about $420 a year if they're reasonably lucky and don't have an accident, get pregnant, or develop a costly illness.* Although odds are good they'll save some money by accepting a High Deductible Insurance policy, all of these healthier employees place some value on the security provided by low-deductible insurance. For that reason, many of them are not thrilled about the prospect of exposing themselves to the risk of being personally liable for medical bills between $1,000 and $5,000 – the "doughnut hole" in this policy – for the sake of saving a few hundred bucks. But they understand they could be facing worse alternatives down the road (worse coverage, or no coverage at all), so they keep their minds open to your proposal.

But you would prefer to have more support for the high-deductible policy. So you rack your brain to find one more sweetener. It occurs to you that if your $1,500 cash contribution to each of your employees were tax free, more employees would accept a $5,000-deductible policy. But you realize this will take an act of Congress to fix. If Congress doesn't pass a law exempting your contribution from taxes, your employees will have to pay taxes on it. Because you happen to be well connected to the Republican Party, which favors high deductibles as the solution to the health-care crisis, you take the matter up with leaders of the party. With the help of High Deductible Health Insurance Company and other insurers interested in selling high-deductible policies, your lobbying is successful; Congress enacts a law exempting your contribution to your employees.

However, Congress attaches a condition to the exemption. It requires that employees spend your contribution only on medical goods and services. Congress bought your argument that more employees would accept high-deductible policies and, therefore, more employees would have health insurance, if employer contributions to employees

---

* I base these estimates of expenditures by healthier employees on data for 2000 reported by Consumers Union (see Table 10-2 below).

were tax-exempt. But since that was the justification for exempting your contribution from taxes, Congress wanted to make sure employees did not use their employer's contribution for food, cigarettes, vacations or other non-medical items. So the new law forbids you from just handing a $1,500 check to each of your employees. The new law requires you or your employees to open an account with a bank or insurance company and that you deposit your contribution in that account. That way, the IRS will have access to good records should it decide to audit an account to ensure that any withdrawals from the account were for medical care. Because the new law requires employees to open individual accounts, the proponents of the new law call this combination of high-deductible policies with accounts "health savings accounts." The name is slightly misleading. An accurate but longer name would be, "Health savings accounts coupled with policies with very high deductibles."

Now you return to your employees and tell them, "Now my entire $1,500 contribution is yours, not just two-thirds of it. Now what do you think?" This proposal is acceptable to an even higher proportion of your workforce. As was the case before the new law went into effect, the healthiest of your employees show more interest in your proposal while the sicker ones remain quite disinterested. But the new law exempting your $1,500 contribution from taxes has introduced another factor: Now your better paid employees are going to be more interested in your offer than your lower-paid employees. That's because they are in higher tax brackets and stand to benefit more from the new exemption. Like all tax exemptions, the exemption of the contribution deposited in HSAs rewards the rich more than the middle class, and the middle class more than the poor. As the *Wall Street Journal* put it, "The tax benefit from health savings accounts [authorized by Congress in 2003] is worth more to people in higher income-tax brackets."[2] In 2004, a married couple with two children earning less than $25,000 got absolutely no tax benefit from an HSA, while the same couple earning $500,000 derived a $721 benefit (see Table 10-1). We may characterize HSAs as policies that will attract the rich and the healthy in far greater numbers than they will attract the sick and the lower-income.

This discussion of a hypothetical employer has allowed me to illustrate the fundamental arguments for HSAs. The basic arguments are that high deductibles cut premium costs, that employers can induce their employees to accept HSAs if employers share a portion of the premium savings with them, and that some employees, especially the healthier and wealthier, stand to gain from enrolling in an HSA. Before we turn to the arguments against HSAs, I present a brief history of the high-deductible policy.

## History of the high-deductible policy

The history of the high-deductible policy resembles the history of the HMO. Like the HMO, the high-deductible policy was not developed because the public was demanding it. Like the HMO, the concept of high-deductible policies hooked to savings accounts originated with a few well-connected individuals. Like the HMO, the high deductible was heavily promoted by a handful of powerful groups and individuals, first to Congress and then, when Congress approved the concept, to employers. As Paul Ellwood, founder of his own think tank (InterStudy), was called the "father of the HMO,"[3] so John Goodman, a conservative who founded his own think tank (the National Center for Policy Analysis), has been called the "father of Medical Savings Accounts."[4]

---

## Table 10-1: Health savings accounts reward the rich more than the poor: Tax benefit of HSAs for married couples with two children at selected income levels, 2004

| Adjusted gross income ($) | Tax benefit ($) |
| --- | --- |
| $25,000 | $0* |
| 35,000 | 200 |
| 50,000 | 300 |
| 150,000 | 615 |
| 500,000 | 721 |
| 1,000,000 | 721 |

* No tax benefit because at this income level the couple owes no federal income taxes.

Source: Sarah Lueck, "Medicare law reaches the under-65 set, too," *Wall Street Journal*, December 16, 2003, D1.

---

As was the case with the early HMO advocates, high-deductible supporters make claims for their product that are not supported by the evidence
and, in some cases, defy common sense. Whereas Kaiser Permanente and
a few other HMOs served as models for the early HMO advocates and
provided private-sector leadership in the campaign for the 1973 HMO
Act, so Golden Rule Insurance Company (now owned by United Health
Group) served as a model for the early MSA advocates and spearheaded
the campaign to enact the 1996 MSA and 2003 HSA laws. Just as the
early HMOs were able to grab market share from traditional indemnity
insurers because they attracted healthier enrollees, so today's insurers offering deductibles in the thousands of dollars are grabbing market share
away from MCPs with traditional $250-to-$500 deductibles because
they are attracting healthier enrollees. Just as HMO advocates felt it
necessary to invent a misleading label for their new-fangled type of insurance, so high-deductible advocates have invented the misleading phrase
"consumer-driven plan" to describe any policy with a big deductible. Just
as there was no reason to believe doctors working for HMOs would be
better at "maintaining health" than doctors working for traditional insurance companies, so there is no reason to believe huge deductibles allow
consumers to "drive" anything.

The most important similarity between HMO and HSA advocates
is their obsession with overuse. HSA advocates see overuse everywhere
and underuse nowhere. The only difference between HMO and HSA
advocates on this score is their explanation of the cause of overuse.
Whereas HMO proponents claimed doctors were the primary cause of
overuse, HSA advocates see "overinsured" patients as the primary cause.
Here are some statements by leading MSA-HSA advocates which reveal
their preoccupation with overuse:

> The United States is the only country in the world where
> people can consume medical care almost without limit,
> unconstrained by market prices or by government ration-
> ing.[5] (John Goodman and Gerald Musgrave, 1994)

> The potential demand for health care is virtually unlim-
> ited. Even if there were a limit to what medical science
> can do (which, over time, there isn't), there is an almost

endless list of ailments that can motivate our desire to spend.... Even when the illnesses are not real, our minds have incredible power to convince that they are.[6] (John Goodman and Gerald Musgrave, 1994)

Imagine that we all carried grocery insurance. In return for a monthly premium, our grocery-insurance policy would pay for most of the things we put into our market baskets. How would this affect our food-purchasing habits? In my case, the answer is simple. Not only would I eat better, but so would my dog. In fact, if every American had grocery insurance, no grocery store in the country would sell dog food. Nothing less than steak would do. But that's just for starters. The supermarket would be stocked with expensive gourmet and specialty items, its aisles would be swarming with solicitous salespersons eagerly catering to the customer's every whim, and besides delivering groceries to our doors, some of these insurance-financed supermarkets would send along a chef to cook the meals.... Very soon, the cost of grocery insurance would begin to climb.[7] (Senator Phil Gramm, R-TX, 1994)

John E. McManus, Republican staff director on the House Ways and Means health subcommittee, was apparently so impressed with Senator Gramm's grocery insurance analogy that he had to repeat it nearly verbatim. At a health policy conference in 2002, hosted by UC Irvine's graduate school of management, McManus said Medicare beneficiaries should pay a larger share of their medical costs. Why? "Imagine if you had grocery insurance, and every time you went to the market your insurance paid 80 percent of it," he said. "You'd eat a whole lot differently – and so would your dog."[8]

Another important similarity between HMO and HSA advocates is their enthusiasm for report cards on plans and providers. HMO proponents tended to emphasize report cards on *plans* because they saw plans as the dominant force in the health-care system, while HSA advocates tend to emphasize report cards on *providers* because they claim to prefer that patients, not plans, enforce quality standards. Former Speaker Newt Gingrich, one of the more prominent HSA advocates and an opponent of single-payer systems, can become almost ecstatic about report cards. "[Y]ou want patients to have choice, and that means they have to have knowledge," Gingrich said in an interview published in *Health Affairs*. That means patients have to have report cards on providers; which requires calculating grades on providers; which requires ready access to patient medical records; which requires that providers put all medical records on computers and deposit them into databases. "So part of what we need to do," Gingrich went on, "... is to set up a system that gives providers an incentive to adopt IT [information technology]. Initially, outcome reporting should be incentivized, but within five years there ought to be a mandatory reporting of a set of indicators.... Then patients should be able to access that data."[9]

The most significant difference between the HMO movement and the high-deductible movement is that the latter was always an exclusively conservative movement whereas the HMO movement had liberal and conservative supporters from its inception. Even today, the fundamental assumptions underlying managed care (that overuse is the main problem, and that doctors need to be managed) still have bipartisan support. But the MSA-HSA movement has been a conservative movement from the beginning. Jesse Hixson, the man who apparently invented the concept of the MSA in 1974, was an economist in the Nixon administration. Patrick Rooney, the former head of Golden Rule Insurance Company, was a fundamentalist Christian and Republican who, beginning in 1989, showered Republicans, especially Newt Gingrich, with campaign donations to promote the MSA. John Goodman ("the father of the MSA") has promoted numerous right-wing causes, not just the big deductible. Other groups and individuals who played a significant role in the MSA campaign were the Cato Institute, the Heritage Foundation, the American Medical Association, former Representative Bob Michel (R-IL), and former Senator Phil Gramm.

Representative Michel introduced what may have been the first MSA legislation in 1992. By early 1994, the MSA was part of "[a]ll the leading Republican health system reform proposals," according to *American Medical News*.[10] When Republicans took control of Congress in 1995, they made enactment of MSA legislation a high priority. They got a law passed out of Congress in 1995 that would have permitted Medicare beneficiaries to leave traditional Medicare and enroll in MSAs. Because this bill also cut $270 billion from Medicare over the next seven years, President Bill Clinton vetoed it. But in 1996, Republicans succeeded in enacting a law (it was part of the Health Insurance Portability and Accountability Act of 1996) that permitted the sale of MSAs to the *nonelderly* with deductibles up to $2,250 for individuals, and another law in 1997 (it was part of the Balanced Budget Act of 1997) that permitted *Medicare beneficiaries* to enroll in MSAs with deductibles up to $6,000 for individuals. In order to get Democratic support for these bills, Republicans had to limit the number of MSAs that could be sold. The 1996 law said MSAs could only be sold to workers who were either self-employed or employed in a business with 50 or fewer employees, and the total number sold could not exceed 750,000. The 1997 law introducing MSAs into Medicare limited the number of Medicare beneficiaries who could enroll in an MSA plan to 390,000, and it required that enrollment cease on December 31, 2002.*

Neither law succeeded. No MSAs were ever sold under Medicare because no insurer could be found to sell them. And, according to the Internal Revenue Service, only 70,000 MSAs had been opened by the nonelderly by the year 2001.[11] Among the factors cited for the low level of interest in MSAs among the nonelderly were consumer distaste for high-deductible policies and the unusually tight labor market of the late 1990s. When employers are having a hard time keeping employees, they are less likely to force them to accept a complex, high-deductible policy they don't want. The traditional tendency of smaller employers (who were the only employers who could buy MSAs under the 1996

---

* The 1997 legislation authorizing MSAs for Medicare would have given seniors who enrolled in MSAs a contribution to help them defray the costs to which the large deductible exposed them. The contribution was to be the difference between what Medicare was paying per senior under the traditional Medicare program (about $6,000 by the year 2000) and the premium that an MSA company like Golden Rule would charge to insure one senior with an MSA with a deductible that could run as high as $6,000. If, for example, the premium for the MSA were $4,000, then Medicare's contribution to seniors' medical savings accounts would be $2,000. That in turn meant seniors would be exposed to the risk of paying out of pocket for medical expenditures that exceeded $2,000 a year until they hit the $6,000 cap.

law) not to offer health insurance was unquestionably another factor. The limitations on the number of MSAs that could be sold, the type of customer they could be sold to, and the limited time frame in which they could be sold were also factors in the failure of the 1996 MSA law. Many insurers concluded that selling MSAs under these limitations would be difficult and ultimately not profitable.

The failure of the 1996 and 1997 MSA laws did not discourage insurance industry entrepreneurs, business consultants, and business reporters from touting high-deductible policies as a money-saver for employers and as a solution to the health-care crisis that managed care had failed to solve. The political debate over the MSA laws that began in the mid-1990s, the HMO backlash that became front-page news in 1996, and the business community's shock over the return of double-digit premium inflation in 2000, all created fertile conditions for a new fad in health policy. By 1999, the media, especially business magazines, were buzzing about high-deductible policies that resembled MSAs but were even less attractive, from the employee's perspective, than MSAs were. Like MSAs, these policies had large deductibles plus employer contributions to employees that were much less than the deductibles. But unlike MSAs, the employer's contribution to employees was temporary; it returned to the employer if the employee didn't use it by the end of the year or if the employee left the company. These limitations permitted employers to make contributions to their employees without having to pay payroll taxes and without exposing their employees to higher income taxes. But because the employer's contribution really didn't belong to the employee, these policies had even less allure than MSAs.

These MSA-like policies were given several labels. They were at first called "defined contribution" plans, and then, within a year or two (around the year 2000), "consumer-driven" plans. Promoters of these plans justified the label "consumer-driven" on two grounds. They claimed these new plans didn't use managed-care tactics; and they said that people who enrolled in these plans would have access to lots of useful information on Web sites that would help them find the best and least expensive providers. Both of these claims were greatly exaggerated. The claim that "consumer-driven" plans do not manage care is an even greater exaggeration today because all the nation's largest MCPs have either bought out one of the early "consumer-driven" insurers or have developed their own high-deductible policies.

The year 2001 was a turning point for high-deductible plans. In March 2001, eight insurers formed a trade group called the Consumer Driven Health Care Association. The founding organizations of this group had names no one had ever heard of: Definity Health, Destiny Health, HealthAllies, HealthMarket, Lumenos, Myhealthbank, Sageo and Vivius. In April 2001, Blue Cross of California introduced the first MSA-style plan sponsored by "a major insurer," according to the *San Francisco Chronicle*.[12] In November 2001, the Pacific Business Group on Health, a coalition of 44 big California-based companies that did as much to promote managed competition as any business group in the country, announced it had decided to contract with Definity. "We believe this selection ... will change the course of how health care is delivered, not just in California but in the country," gushed a spokesman for the coalition.[13] In December 2001, the *New York Times* reported that Aetna, Humana, Cigna, United Health Group, and Wellpoint Health Networks were all preparing to market high-deductible plans.[14] By 2002, roughly 100,000 people were enrolled in these plans; by early 2003, roughly a half-million.[15]

November 2003 was another turning point for high-deductible policies. In that month, Congress enacted the Medicare Prescription Drug, Improvement and Modernization Act (George W. Bush signed it in December). That law ended the MSA experiment and authorized the sale of HSAs to the nonelderly beginning January 1, 2004. Under the new law, employers may contribute up to $2,600 a year to individuals and $5,150 to families tax free.* These contributions must be paid into an account maintained by a bank or insurance company. Employers do not pay payroll taxes and employees do not pay income taxes on these contributions, and employees pay no taxes when they withdraw the funds as long as they do so for the purpose of paying a medical bill. If

---

* The law permits individuals to contribute pre-tax money to their own HSAs as well. However, for the sake of simplicity, and because observers agree that HSAs without employer contributions are going to be difficult to sell, I describe HSAs as if only employers were contributing to HSAs. The $2,600 and $5,150 limits that I describe above as limits on employer contributions are actually limits on the total of employer and individual contributions. These limits were for 2004. They rise each year by a percent indexed to inflation.

they withdraw funds from their account for a purpose other than medical care prior to turning 65, they have to pay taxes on the withdrawn money as well as a 10 percent fine. After employees reach age 65, they can withdraw funds for *non*medical purposes and not have to pay the 10 percent fine (they still have to pay taxes).

It is safe to say HSAs are going to spread because they are more attractive to employees than MSAs as well as the "consumer-driven" policies that don't allow them to keep their unspent employer contributions, and they are much more attractive to insurers because there are no limitations on who can buy HSAs and no time limits on how long HSAs will be legal. But for three reasons, it is difficult to predict just how far HSAs will spread. First, it is difficult to estimate how much cheaper HSAs will be compared with low-deductible MCPs. Second, it is difficult to predict how many employers will be interested in HSAs that will also appeal to their employees. Even if, for example, 50 percent of employers were to offer HSAs, few will be sold if the HSAs that employers offer have deductibles at the high end of what the law allows ($5,000 for individuals and $10,000 for families) and employers make no contributions to employee accounts. Third, even if we knew how many employers would offer HSAs and how generous these HSAs were, it would still be difficult to predict precisely how many employees will prefer HSAs over lower-deductible plans or no coverage at all.

HSA advocates generally claim HSA premiums are 30 to 60 percent below the premiums of MCPs with low deductibles. However, they rarely cite research (mainly because so little is available). They cite, rather, the premiums of insurers that offer both low- and high-deductible policies or the experience of businesses that switched from a low- to a high-deductible policy. But because these anecdotes fail to take into account the health of the employees who enrolled in HSAs, we can't trust these anecdotes. It may well be that savings of up to 60 percent are possible only for those employers with unusually healthy employees. In a 2004 article that reviewed the literature on the subject of who would benefit from high-deductible plans, the author, Dwight McNeill, presented the results of his own simulation comparing a "traditional" MCP with several versions of a "'first-generation' consumer-directed" plan offered by Definity. He concluded, "This simulation ... support[s] the hypothesis that the healthy, especially young men, are the potential winners with these plans."[16]

According to the U.S. General Accounting Office (now the Government Accountability Office), insurers themselves anticipate HSAs will benefit from favorable selection, just as HMOs did when they began to compete with traditional indemnity insurers in the 1970s. According to a survey of insurance companies conducted by the GAO, health insurance companies believe high-deductible plans will attract primarily healthy people, and therefore they set their premiums below what they would be if they were insuring a more typical sample of the population. "Insurers view high-deductible plan enrollees as presenting a lower claims risk than enrollees in traditional low-deductible plans," the GAO reported. "Insurers expect relatively better health status and lower service utilization by enrollees selecting high-deductible plans and price their products accordingly."[17]

Research examining some of the first companies to offer high-deductible policies confirms that these policies enjoy favorable-selection advantages. The August 2004 edition of *Health Services Research* presented two papers which apparently constitute the first peer-reviewed, scientific evidence on the question of who enrolls in high-deductible policies. Unlike previous studies of HSAs, which had relied on assumptions about which patients would benefit from enrolling in HSAs and which would be better off staying away from HSAs, these papers looked at data on people who actually chose to enroll in HSAs. The first paper, authored by Sasso et al., examined the experience of three employers who had offered high-deductible policies to their employees by January 2002. This paper found solid evidence of favorable selection for one of the employers, and suggestive evidence for the other two. Interestingly, the employer for which solid evidence of biased selection existed was Humana, one of the nation's largest health plans. Humana made an MSA-like plan available to its employees at its St. Louis headquarters in July 2001. When Sasso et al. compared medical spending in the year prior to July 2001 by the employees who stayed with low-deductible MCPs with the employees who chose the MSA-like plan, they found that the low-deductible enrollees had medical bills that were double those of the high-deductible enrollees ($2,837 per person for the low-deductible enrollees versus $1,492 for the high-deductible enrollees).[18]

The second paper examined the experience of the University of Minnesota with high-deductible insurance offered by Definity. The authors, Parente et al., claimed to find no evidence of biased selection, but their measure of health status was crude. They asked employees if they or anyone in their family had a "chronic condition," they treated all chronic conditions as equally serious, and they lumped all employees with at least one family member with a chronic condition into the same category.[19]

Both Sasso et al. and Parente et al. reported that higher-income employees were more likely to enroll in high-deductible policies. Because upper-income people tend to be healthier than lower-income people, this finding is also evidence of biased selection favoring high-deductible plans.

I have little doubt that future research will confirm these early studies. The vast majority of chronically ill people will be financially worse off if they enroll in HSAs. Only those people who are paying a portion of their own premiums, and who are so sick their expenditures exceed their deductible year in and year out by a substantial margin, will be better off with an HSA than a low-deductible plan. (These people will be better off because their lower premiums will save them more money than their higher deductibles cost them.) Most chronically ill people do not fit this description. I am confident, therefore, that any future study which purports to show that the chronically ill are enrolling in HSAs will turn out to be sloppily done, or it will demonstrate that some chronically ill people don't understand what they were getting into when they choose an HSA.

On the basis of existing evidence, we may conclude that the claim that HSA premiums are much lower than low-deductible premiums is exaggerated because it fails to account for selection favoring HSAs. I predict that the gap between low-deductible and high-deductible premiums will shrink as HSAs capture a larger and larger share of the market, including a rising share of the nation's sick people. But because high-deductibles always save insurers more money than low-deductibles, the gap will never go away.

But lower premiums are not the only factor essential to the HSA's success. The willingness of employers to offer HSAs with relatively small "doughnut holes," and the reaction of employees to this new form of insurance, will also play a role. "[T]he average citizen hates high-deductible coverage," reported *American Medical News*, paraphrasing

Robert Blendon, a nationally known expert and pollster early in the MSA debate.[20] If most employers offer HSAs with big "doughnut holes" – that is, if they offer HSAs with very high deductibles and pass on little of their premium savings in the form of contributions to workers' accounts – few HSAs are going to be sold.

Although it is unclear how enthusiastic employers and employees will be about HSAs, it is clear that *insurers* are much more enthusiastic about HSAs than they were about MSAs. Unlike the 1996 MSA law, the 2003 HSA law puts no limits on the size of employers who can buy them nor on the number that may be sold. For this reason primarily, insurers are much more optimistic about HSAs than they were about MSAs.

So what's a good guess on the number of HSAs that will ultimately be sold? According to an edition of the *Wall Street Journal* published just days after the HSA law was signed, "Congressional tax analysts estimate that the number of people holding [health savings accounts] could reach about 3 million in 2013."[21] I suspect total HSA sales will be much higher than that within a few years.

But we don't need to know how many HSAs will be sold in order to predict with confidence that HSAs will fail to solve the health-care mess. If few HSAs are sold, they will fail, obviously, because they will have affected only a small percent of the population. But HSAs are going to fail even if they take over the health insurance industry as MCPs did. They will fail for two reasons: they focus on overuse when supply-side waste is the real problem; and they damage quality of care for at least some patients, which in at least some instances drives up costs. I take up each of these problems in the next two sections.

## The obsession with overuse and the failure to address supply-side waste

As the statements from HSA advocates quoted a few pages ago indicate, HSAs are based on the premise that the average American overuses health care. Those statements offered not one word about the high price of medical service, nor about the problem of under-treatment even for insured people. All the blame is laid on volume of services (it's excessive), and "overinsured" patients are the cause. Patients with low-deductible insurance are like idiots in a grocery store spending someone else's money. We are gluttons for medical care, so much so that we even invent a substantial portion of our afflictions in order to savor the experience of undergoing unnecessary medical treatments. We rush around the medical supermarket filling our carts with services we don't need and then, like the fat heads we are, we wonder why our "grocery insurance" premiums are so high.

One does not need a PhD in economics to understand that food is very different from medical care. The most obvious difference is that most forms of food are pleasurable to consume. The same cannot be said of medical care. People who do not have cancer will not undergo surgery, radiation and chemotherapy, for example, even if you paid them. Similarly, people who do not have decay in their teeth will not undergo drilling by a dentist; people who have no reason to think they need heart surgery will not rush to the hospital to have their chest cut open; women who do not need their uterus cut out will not have it done; men who do not need their prostate rubbed will not demand that it be done. Even medical services that are not painful do not have the allure of food. Most human beings have had an extra helping of food they didn't need, but most people do not want to waste time in a clinic or hospital getting a test or examination they don't need. In fact, as we saw in Chapter 4, Americans are more likely to underuse health care than they are to overuse it.

Because high-deductible proponents think overuse is the main problem, they claim reductions in overuse will be the primary method by which HSAs lead to lower costs. Few HSA advocates explicitly make the additional claim that high deductibles will somehow give consumers the power to force providers and drug companies to lower their prices, and those who do make this claim typically do so outside the peer-reviewed literature. Here are examples of the "HSAs will cut volume" explanation from high-deductible advocates.

> The real benefit, to citizens and to the economy, comes from lower spending on medical care, which will occur when people have the opportunity to choose between medical care and other goods and services.... (Mark Pauly and John Goodman, 1995)[22]

> HSAs marry real insurance (that is, coverage for high
> and unpredictable costs) with contributions to a savings
> account that can be "rolled over" from year to year. In
> other words, individuals, not insurance companies, "ra-
> tion" most of their own health care.... (Editorial, *Wall
> Street Journal*, 2004)[23]

> Higher coinsurance and deductibles, by making con-
> sumers more aware of the true cost of medical services,
> will reduce health-care utilization. (Susan Lee, 2004)[24]

Most HSA advocates concede, in other words, that if HSAs save any money it will be in the form of reduced volume of services, not reduced fees or prices or some other type of supply-side waste.

But this argument that HSAs will cause patients to demand fewer medical services, so central to HSA ideology, is vastly overstated. HSAs will never affect the bulk of health-care spending. There are several reasons, the most important of which is that approximately 80 percent of total health-care spending is attributable to the sickest 20 percent of the population, and the patients in this sickest 20 percent spend far more per year than the $2,000 to $3,000 annual deductible for individuals that HSA advocates propose. In other words, even if all Americans were forced into HSAs, 80 percent of total spending would still not be influenced by HSA deductibles. This logic seems crystal clear to me, but since it does not seem clear to HSA advocates, let me take another paragraph to explain.

As HSA advocates themselves never tire of pointing out, patients are not motivated to self-ration if their deductible (or the unspent portion of it) is lower than the price of the good or service their doctor has ordered for them. If my deductible is $300, for example, and I need stroke rehabilitation services worth $10,000, I have no motivation to deny myself any of those services because any savings will merely accrue to the insurance company. (Nor do I have any incentive to haggle over the price of rehab services with my provider.) Patients will be motivated to cut back on the amount of medical care they buy only if the services they need cost less than their deductible. HSA advocates claim that raising the average deductible from the current level of $250-to-

$300 for individuals into the $2,000-to-$3,000 range will encourage more self-rationing. Strictly speaking, this is true. But when we ask *how much* self-rationing can we expect to see, the answer is, Very little compared with total health-care spending. HSAs with deductibles in the neighborhood of $2,000 will influence less than 20 percent of total health-care spending.

The "twenty-eighty" rule – the rule that the sickest 20 percent of us account for 80 percent of spending – has been well established for several decades. Two of the latest studies on this issue were done by The Lewin Group at the request of Consumers Union. One study examined the distribution of health-care spending across the entire population, the other examined spending only within the population covered by employer-sponsored insurance. The results are shown in Table 10-2. The table indicates that the distribution of spending is almost identical whether we examine all Americans or just those covered by employer-sponsored insurance. We see that in 2000 the sickest 20 percent, or quintile, of Americans accounted for 82 percent of total spending, while the sickest quintile of Americans with employer coverage accounted for 79 percent of total spending by that group. We see as well that the people in the sickest quintile are spending more than $10,000 per person annually, which is way beyond $2,000, the typical individual HSA deductible today.* In fact, we have to go deep into the fourth-sickest quintile in both groups before we encounter people who spend less than $2,000 annually. The data in Table 10-2 don't allow us to determine at exactly what percentile we reach this point, but the 75th percentile is a

---

* The average deductible in high-deductible plans sold as of 2004 was probably below $2,000. According to one of the early surveys of insurers selling MSA-like policies in 2002, the average individual deductible was $1,645 and the average employer contribution was $824 (Meredith Rosenthal and Arnold Milstein, "Awakening consumer stewardship of health benefits: Prevalence and differentiation of new health plan models," *Health Services Research* 2004;39:1055-1079). According to a survey of the health insurance industry conducted by America's Health Insurance Plans (AHIP), the typical HSA deductible appears to be less than $2,000. AHIP reported that the average deductible for the "best-selling" HSAs for individuals was $1,607 in the large-employer (over 50 employees) market, $1,850 in the small-employer market, and $2,970 in the individual market. The deductibles for families were about double those for individuals. Since most families consist of more than two individuals, factoring in the family deductibles

conservative guess. This means that a $2,000 deductible would affect even less than 20 percent of total spending today.[*]

In addition to the "twenty-eighty" rule, there are three other reasons to predict that HSAs with deductibles of $2,000 or so per individual will influence less than 20 percent of total spending. First, the calculation we just went through to determine that 20 percent or less of spending will be affected by HSAs assumed that 100 percent of the U.S. population will choose HSAs or be forced into them. But no one, not even the HSA's most ardent supporters, proposes that or predicts that.

Second, some HSA insurers and advocates propose exempting certain services (e.g., preventive and emergency services) from exposure to the deductible. Destiny Health, for example, offers an HSA that divides drug costs into "controllable" and "uncontrollable" categories. "If you have any of 110 or so chronic medical conditions that are deemed as having 'uncontrollable' costs – like diabetes, heart disease, asthma or high cholesterol – the cost of medication for them comes out of insurance instead of your personal account," reports the *New York Times*.[25] In their book

---

means the average deductible for all HSA policies is lower than the figures AHIP reported for one-person HSAs (America's Health Insurance Plans, *Number of HSA Plans Exceeded One Million in March 2005*, http://www.ahipresearch.org/pdfs/ HSAExceedMillion050405_full.pdf, accessed July 15, 2005).

[*] Earlier studies reached similar conclusions. In its evaluation of Representative Michel's 1992 MSA bill, the Congressional Budget Office reported that only 15 percent of the U.S. population had medical expenditures above $2,500, but these people accounted for 83 percent of total national health-care expenditures (Congressional Budget Office, *Analysis of Subtitle C (Medical Savings Accounts) of HR 5325, introduced by the Honorable Bob Michel (R-IL)*, cited in Minnesota Department of Health, *Medical Savings Accounts: A Feasibility Study for the Minnesota Legislature*, 1994, St. Paul, MN, 17). The CBO was saying, in other words, that the incentive for patients to be "prudent" about medical expenditures would have applied to just 17 percent of all health-care spending in 1992 if all Americans had been forced into MSAs with $2,500 deductibles. Paul Fronstin found that only 22 percent of adults aged 18 to 64 insured through an employer spent more than $2,000 on health care in 1998, and this 22 percent accounted for 77 percent of this population's health-care expenditures. In other words, the incentive created by a $2,000 deductible to be "prudent" would apply to just 23 percent of total health-care spending (Paul Fronstin, "Can 'consumerism' slow the rate of health benefit cost increases?" *Health Care Focus*, Figure 9, https:// www.healthnet.com/brokers/ pdf/13040_ Oct_ 2002_HCare _Focus_Vol2_I3.pdf, accessed October 2002).

---

## Table 10-2: The sickest fifth account for four-fifths of spending: Average annual health-care expenditures by quintiles and percent of total spending for the entire U.S. population and the population with employer-sponsored insurance, 2000

| | Entire population | | Employer-sponsored population | |
| --- | --- | --- | --- | --- |
| | Avg amount | % of total | Avg amount | % of total |
| Healthiest quintile (1-20%) | $14 | 0% | $30 | 0% |
| Second quintile (21-40%) | 224 | 1 | 264 | 2 |
| Third quintile (41-60%) | 695 | 4 | 694 | 5 |
| Fourth quintile (61-80%) | 1,992 | 12 | 1,766 | 13 |
| Sickest quintile (81-100%)* | 13,764 | 82 | 10,375 | 79 |
| Average | 3,338 | | 2,628 | |

\* Shearer (see sources below) actually reported figures for the two deciles within this sickest quintile; I list in this table the average of those two deciles. For the people in the 81-90 percent decile, the figures Shearer reported were $4,949 and $4,040 for the entire population and the employer-sponsored population respectively. For the people in the sickest decile (91-100 percent), Shearer reported figures of $22,578 and $16,710 respectively.

Sources: For average amounts for the entire population, Gail Shearer, *The Health Care Divide: Unfair Financial Burdens*, Consumers Union, Washington, DC, August 2000, Chart 1, 7; for average amounts for population with employer-sponsored coverage, *Testimony of Gail Shearer before the Joint Economic Committee*, February 25, 2004, unnumbered figure, http://www.consumersunion.org/pdf/consumertest-0204.pdf, accessed July 15, 2005; percents of total are my calculations using Shearer's figures.

---

*Patient Power* touting MSAs, Goodman and Musgrave conceded that people "with recurring large medical bills over many years" would lose money if they were insured by an MSA. "[M]ost of those people would be disadvantaged...," they wrote. The solution, they argued, is "a per-condition deductible, which would be paid only once for an extended illness."[26] "With a per-condition deductible," they explained, "a person diagnosed with cancer would pay the deductible only once, and insurance would pay all of the remaining costs of the cancer treatments, even if those costs were incurred over many years."[27] If numerous medical goods and services are protected with first-dollar or low-deductible coverage, the motivation to self-ration and "shop" is going to be less extensive than it would be if no exceptions were made.

The third reason that HSAs are likely to influence less than 20 percent of total spending (in addition to the twenty-eighty rule) is that the average per-person deductible may turn out to be less than $2,000.

To sum up: HSAs are likely to influence 20 percent or less of total spending because of the twenty-eighty rule, because fewer than 100 percent of Americans will sign up for HSAs, because many high-deductible policies will exempt some services from exposure to the deductible, and because the typical per-person deductible will be less than $2,000.

Even if HSAs could influence a portion of health spending far in excess of 20 percent, they would still have little or no effect on supply-side waste. The angriest, most "cost-conscious" consumers in the world cannot force America's multiple-payer system to spend less money on administration. Nor can they force hospitals and clinics to stop buying excessive amounts of equipment, force providers and drug companies to stop overcharging them, and force providers, insurers, and con artists to stop committing fraud. High-deductible advocates rarely argue otherwise. As we have already seen, most HSA supporters don't feel they have to argue that high deductibles will reduce supply-side waste. They're convinced that overuse is rampant and that HSAs will save gobs of money by cutting overuse. Why raise the hackles of insurers, specialists, hospitals and drug companies by even suggesting that something should be done to reduce supply-side waste?[*]

I do occasionally come across undocumented arguments by HSA advocates that administrative costs will fall if HSAs spread because HSA enrollees will not file claims for services that cost less than their

---

[*] Some HSA advocates do refer now and again to high physician fees, hospital charges and drug prices, but only for the purpose of claiming that when "consumers" are motivated by high deductibles we will "shop" for medical services and drugs and this will somehow force providers and drug companies to lower their prices. But this claim is made infrequently, and when it is, it is made without any citations to supportive studies. It is possible patients will have modest success reducing the price of medical services *for which they "shop"* if

deductible. And I occasionally hear the argument that HSAs will drive administrative costs down because HSA insurers will forego managed-care cost-control tactics because they won't need them (because patients will ration themselves). Both arguments are exaggerated. Moreover, these arguments fail to examine the cost of two other "reforms" HSA advocates support – report cards, and risk-adjustment of premiums – which will drive up administrative costs. I review all four of these issues in the remainder of this section.

Michael Tanner, an analyst on the staff of the Cato Institute, is one of the few high-deductible supporters who argues publicly that high-deductible policies will reduce administrative costs. Tanner implies that administrative costs will fall because patients will not send in claims for medical bills under their deductible.[28] That is simply wrong. If patients didn't send in documentation of medicals bills they paid (because they were below their deductible), how would they ever persuade their insurer that they've spent past their deductible and it's time for the insurance company to start paying the bills?

But even those expenditures paid for out of HSA accounts are not cost-free. Banks and other financial institutions usually charge an initial fee plus a fee for maintaining these accounts, plus another fee for closing them.[*] Moreover, patients must treat the bills they pay out of their HSAs the same way they treat any other expenditure they want to deduct from their taxes – they have to keep records if they want to survive an IRS audit. IRS audits (which will be done on a small fraction

---

the following conditions are met: (1) the service is not an emergency service; (2) the patient is of sound mind and has the energy and the means to "shop" for the best price, or the patient has caretakers who are willing to do that; (3) the medical service is relatively uncomplicated and is used frequently (e.g., pediatric services and dental care) and, conversely, is not a once-in-a-lifetime purchase (e.g., a hysterectomy); and (4) the providers of these services are not consolidated into a few huge networks or corporations, but, are, rather, small and numerous. But only a small portion of the market for health goods and services meets these four criteria. But as we have seen, the percent of patients exposed to high deductibles who will be motivated to shop will be considerably below 100 percent.

[*] According to the *Wall Street Journal*, "First-year fees for [MSA] accountholders can range from a low of $12 to as much as $105" (George Anders, "Medical savings accounts are proving a tough sell," *Wall Street Journal*, May 22, 1997, A16). *American Medical News* quotes an expert saying HSAs have a

of HSA enrollees to ensure that HSA account money is being spent on medical care, not entertainment or some other non-medical item) will also cost money. Thus, even though it's true that many medical bills will not result in claims filed with insurers, it is not true that these bills will generate zero administrative costs.

Since the mid-1990s, advocates of high deductibles have professed to be hostile toward managed care and have repeatedly said high-deductible insurers wouldn't think of using managed care. For example, in their 1994 book promoting MSAs, John Goodman and Gerald Musgrave were very critical of managed care – they called it a "bureaucratic solution" and derisively referred to utilization review as "corporate approval" – and they described MSAs as an alternative to managed care.[29] Goodman and Musgrave even entitled their book *Patient Power* to emphasize their message that patients would regain their authority to make decisions that was taken from them by MCPs. Here are three more examples of large-deductible advocates professing to disdain managed care:

> MSAs help to restore the patient/physician relationship, while managed care weakens those relationships…. All … parties have come to realize that the reasons managed care has not worked as a national policy in addressing the concerns of cost, access, quality and patient satisfaction are the same reasons Medical Savings Accounts and other consumer-driven programs are attractive. (Greg Scandlen, National Center for Policy Analysis, 2001)[30]

---

"set up fee" ranging from $10 to $25, and a monthly administrative fee of about $2 to $5 (Katherine Vogt, "Doctors looking at details as interest in HSAs grows," December 20, 2004, 16). Some HSA account managers charge as much as $140 the first year and more than $100 thereafter (Kaja Whitehouse, "Health-savings-account fees draw scrutiny of consumers," *Wall Street Journal*, July 20, 2005, D2). The total cost of HSA-account fees will be large in absolute terms, but small compared with total health spending. If the average fee were $50 a year, and all 100 million U.S. households opened an HSA, the bank fees would come to $5 billion. These fees will be offset to some extent by interest paid on account balances. But interest payments will be negligible for people who receive small contributions from their employers and/or who spend most of their employer contributions every year.

> You don't have to fight with the insurance company or HMO to get treatment. (Brian McManus, Golden Rule Insurance Company, 2004, describing HSAs)[31]

> The path to better health and more cost-effective health benefits can be found here at Definity Health. We've left behind the managed-care principles of restrictions, red tape and bureaucracy and embraced the power of freedom, education and support to create a totally new health benefit. We call it Consumer-Driven Healthcare – and it works. (Definity's Web site, 2005)[32]

This deliberately cultivated impression that large-deductible plans don't use managed care is probably the most important reason the American Medical Association and many doctors support MSAs and HSAs. As *American Medical News* put it, critics of MSAs "suspect that the opportunity to sabotage managed care is what's turned so many doctors into avid MSA backers."[33]

Because insurers that sell high-deductible plans are infrequently forthright about how managed their policies are, it is difficult to know how extensively they rely on managed care to control doctor-patient decision making. It is crystal clear, however, that many of the new high-deductible plans are using managed care. The close relations between MCPs and companies that sell HSAs is the most obvious evidence that this is so. Definity Health, which I just quoted, was purchased in 2004 by United Health Group, a huge insurance company that aggressively promoted managed care when it was fashionable to do so. Destiny Health, a "consumer-driven" plan headquartered in Chicago, relies on a company called Caremark to run its drug formulary, and on United Behavioral Health (UBH) to manage its mental health and substance abuse services.[34] (UBH, a subsidiary of United Health Group, is the company that withheld medical care from the depressed woman with an eating disorder whose case I describe in Appendix A.) Golden Rule, the insurance company credited with turning MSAs into the centerpiece of Republican health policy, was purchased by United Health Group in November 2003. United has been evasive in the past about how tightly it manages its doctors and will no doubt be coy about whether it uses managed-care tactics to save money at the expense of its HSA-insured patients. In 1996, when United announced it would start selling an allegedly less restrictive form of MCPs known as a "preferred provider organizations," one official describing the new plan said, "It looks and feels like a PPO and yet underneath the hood is our HMO management and cost containment."[35]

Finding out what cost-containment tools lie beneath the hood of HSAs can be very difficult. At my request HealthPartners, Minnesota's third largest health insurance company and the MCP in which my wife and I are enrolled, sent me a promotional packet on its new HSA entitled Empower Midwest Choice Plan. The packet indicated that enrollees in HealthPartners' HSA would be subject to all the managed-care tools HMOs pioneered, including utilization review, "case management," financial incentives for doctors, a drug formulary, and financial incentives for enrollees to use "in-network" providers. Oddly, the packet also claimed, "HealthPartners does not employ incentives that encourage barriers to care and service." When I called HealthPartners' sales department and asked for details about the financial incentives used on doctors, I was assured HealthPartners would never harm patients. When I persisted in learning the details of the financial incentives, I was given the name of another person to call. After several phone calls and an e-mail exchange, I learned that doctors who treat patients enrolled in HealthPartners' HSA get a bonus if they keep the services they order at or below 110 percent of the average of medical services "throughout that specific community," whatever that means.[36]

To sum up, we have excellent reason to reject both of the arguments used to support the infrequently made claim that HSAs will reduce administrative costs. Those arguments are: patients will submit fewer claims, and HSA insurers will not use managed care.

Now let's look at the possibility that HSAs will *increase* administrative costs. Most high-deductible advocates support report cards, and many high-deductible advocates support risk-adjusting premiums in order to prevent favorable selection from wiping out low-deductible plans. Both of these projects will be very expensive.

I discussed the cost and complexity of report cards in Chapter 9. Here I'll just give you an example of a statement by an HSA advocate that indicates HSA proponents are as excited about report cards as managed-care advocates have been.

> Consumer-directed health care supposes a new formulation – one driven by consumers with cash-in-hand, demanding to know for themselves who is the best urologist in town, what are my treatment alternatives, ... how do I get the most value for the money I'm spending? Information systems to support this movement will grow exponentially. But the information is only ammunition. It is not an end to itself. The real revolution will come when health-care consumers use that information to reward higher quality and punish the mediocre....[37]

The author of this paean to report cards, Greg Scandlen, director of the Galen Institute (one of numerous right-wing think tanks that push HSAs), offered no proof that his high expectations of report cards would ever be met. And, like all other report card enthusiasts, Scandlen indicated no interest in the cost of report cards, either in terms of dollars or damage to quality of care and to privacy.

Most advocates of high-deductible policies admit that these policies will attract more than their share of healthy people, and that if this favorable selection is not stopped, low-deductible insurers will either be bankrupted or forced to raise their deductibles and thereby shift costs to their sicker enrollees, which could force sicker enrollees to disenroll. When healthy people migrate to one plan or one type of plan and leave the sick in another plan or type of plan, a "death spiral" will occur if the plans enjoying favorable selection are not required to subsidize the plans suffering from adverse selection. The plan suffering adverse selection, in this case, the low-deductible plan, will have to raise its premiums when the first wave of healthy enrollees leaves it, this will drive another wave of disproportionately healthy people away, this will force the plan to raise its premiums yet again, and around the vicious cycle goes until the plan's premiums are so high no one can afford them and the plan is bankrupted. To avoid the death spiral and bankruptcy, low-deductible plans faced with competition from high-deductible plans will stop offering low-deductible plans rather than raise their premiums endlessly. When this happens system-wide, chronically ill people will have nowhere to turn – they'll either have to buy health insurance with huge deductibles, or go without insurance all together.

The only solution is to risk-adjust premiums, which, in practice, means to funnel more money to insurers who get stuck with sick people and less money to insurers with primarily healthy enrollees. Some argue this should be done with subsidies to *insurers* so that insurers can keep their premiums low and thereby avoid mass disenrollments. Others say the subsidies should go to *sick people* so they can afford the higher premiums that adverse selection will force upon low-deductible plans. Either scheme will obviously require an enormous bureaucracy to determine who qualifies as sick, not-so-sick, and healthy, to determine which plan these people signed up with, and to distribute subsidies accordingly. But high-deductible advocates are extremely vague about how these adjustments to insurance-company revenues are supposed to be done, who will do them, and what this process will cost.

To document that some high-deductible buffs view the problem of favorable selection as a serious one, and yet are spectacularly glib about how easy it's going to be to adjust insurance company revenues to prevent favorable selection, I quote three prominent high-deductible advocates at length.

> Some critics fear that increased use of catastrophic insurance coverage protected by MSAs will worsen a serious social problem of risk segmentation and adverse selection in the private health insurance market. A similar argument has been made over the years against all innovative forms of private insurance, most especially against … HMOs – which do seem, in some circumstances, to be attractive to low risks. The natural tendency in competitive insurance markets is for premiums to reflect risks. To the degree that this process creates unreasonable burdens for some people, government interventions such as tax-financed risk pools or risk-related tax credits for unusually high risks are the correct solutions…. A full treatment of this exceedingly complex and confus-

ing issue is beyond the scope of this paper. (Mark Pauly
and John Goodman, *Health Affairs*, 1995)[38]

Moving to a more market-based system, some contend,
will make it impossible for sick employees to afford
health insurance. The insurers … will offer attractive
deals to the healthy and charge astronomical prices to
the ill. But this scenario assumes that employers will
continue to make the same contribution for all employees, regardless of their health status. In fact, one of the
tenets of consumer-driven health care is that premiums
must be adjusted for risk. (Regina E. Herzlinger, *Harvard Business Review*, 2002)[39]

By varying payments according to individual employees'
care requirements, insurers and providers will be motivated to develop new offerings – for example, multiyear
policies that promote the health of people suffering from
chronic diseases. Because insurers will earn more money
for policies for the sick, they will have a strong incentive
to create plans that attract people with chronic diseases.
To avoid concerns about invasion of privacy or job-re-
lated discrimination, companies can use neutral third-
party intermediaries like Minneapolis-based eBenX to
make the risk adjustments. (Herzlinger)[40]

Pauly and Goodman, in the quote above, tell us risk-adjustment
should be done by "government" but refuse to tell us how "government"
will do this and at what cost, all on the ground that this "exceedingly
complex and confusing issue is beyond the scope of [their] paper." (I
submit that accurate risk-adjustment of the premiums of all or even most
health insurance policies in the U.S. is beyond more than the scope of
Pauly and Goodman's little paper; it is beyond the realm of the humanly
possible.) Herzlinger asserts that risk-adjustment is so important to
HSA advocates that it is actually "one of the tenets of consumer-driven
health care," but she offers not a word about how risk-adjustment is to
be done. She merely tells us that employers should pay for it, and that

private-sector firms like eBenX should do it in the interest of protecting privacy, as if eBenX employees snooping through medical records does not constitute an invasion of privacy.

The complexity and cost of a scheme that risk-adjusts premiums for all insurance policies boggles the mind for the same reasons widespread production of report cards is complex and boggles the mind. Both projects require measuring the health status of hundreds of millions of patients, which in turn means extracting relevant medical data from the medical records of hundreds of millions of patients, entering it into computers, and crunching the data to derive the necessary adjustments. As we saw in the discussion of report cards, this would be very expensive to do even once, never mind year in and year out. Yet Pauly, Goodman, and Herzlinger, like all other published high-deductible advocates who support risk-adjustment of premiums, blithely skip over the question of how much it will cost to risk-adjust premiums for 300 million Americans, or even a substantial portion of them.

## Research on whether high-deductible policies can save money

I have now discussed two reasons why HSAs are not going to cut costs: (1) they will influence only 20 percent or less of total spending, and (2) they will have little impact on administrative costs and the other forms of supply-side waste, and they will drive up administrative costs if report cards or risk-adjustment of premiums is implemented on a large scale as many HSA buffs recommend. In this section I review studies that sought to determine whether high-deductible policies can save money at the system level, that is, for the entire health-care system or for public programs like Medicare. There is no question that healthy individuals and groups can save money if they switch to HSAs. The question is whether George Bush and other advocates of HSAs are correct when they say the introduction of HSAs into the American health-care system will lower costs for everyone, not just the healthy. Given the evidence I've discussed already, you won't be surprised to learn that the reliable research indicates high-deductible policies cannot save money for society as a whole, or for businesses and public programs that insure a mix of healthy and sick enrollees.

Research measuring system-wide savings from MSAs and HSAs has had to estimate what insurers and patients would do in the future if high-deductible policies became widespread. The reliable research done so far says high-deductible policies cannot reduce costs system-wide, and might increase costs because employers or taxpayers will be giving away a lot of money to healthy people (in the form of contributions to their accounts that don't get spent on health care). None of the research I review here sought to determine the change in administrative costs we just discussed (the alleged decline in the number of claims filed, the cost of opening millions of bank accounts, the cost of IRS audits, and the cost of report cards and risk-adjustment of premiums). All of the reliable research I have seen assumes that high deductibles reduce costs only by reducing the volume, not the price, of medical services.

The most comprehensive study of the effect of high-deductible policies on total spending appeared in the *Journal of the American Medical Association* in 1996. It examined the effect of MSAs on total spending by the insured population under 65. The study concluded that if this entire population, including those who would clearly lose financially with an MSA, were *forced* into MSAs, total expenditures for this group would fall between 0 and 13 percent. However, the study found that if people were given a choice about whether to switch to an MSA, the change in total health spending would range between plus 1 percent and minus 2 percent.[41]

The conclusions of the *JAMA* study are consistent with three studies on the impact of the 1997 legislation adding MSAs to Medicare. Studies by the Congressional Budget Office and Lewin-VHI (now called The Lewin Group) concluded MSAs would raise, not lower, Medicare costs.[42] Lewin-VHI projected that MSAs would increase Medicare costs by $15.3 billion over a seven-year period solely because of the effects of adverse selection and overpayments to the healthier seniors who would enroll in Medicare MSAs.[43] According to a third study by Kendix and Lubitz, "There is no scenario in our simulations where Medicare saves money when private insurers offer MSAs to Medicare beneficiaries."[44] Kendix and Lubitz noted moreover that "none of our calculations includes cost of administration."[45]

Because conservatives in Canada have taken up the call for high-deductible policies, peer-reviewed Canadian journals have begun to publish papers examining the claims made by big-deductible advocates. Scholars at the University of Manitoba published a paper in 2002 which reported that MSAs would not reduce costs and could well drive costs up if sick people were forced into them. "Our results suggest that MSAs will not save money, but will instead, under most formulations, lead to an increase in spending on the healthiest members of the population," they concluded.[46]

The reliable literature, then, supports the conclusion that high-deductible plans cannot save society as a whole any money and may in fact increase system-wide expenditures. Even if compulsion were some day used and the chronically ill and low-income were pushed into high-deductible plans, the savings achieved by patient self-rationing would almost certainly be overwhelmed by the cost of subsidies for the sick and low-income (it's hard to imagine even the most heartless high-deductible advocate proposing that these populations enter the brave new world of HSAs without subsidies) plus the increased administrative costs we've just discussed – the costs associated with maintaining and auditing tens of millions of individual bank accounts, risk-adjusting premiums, and preparing report cards.

There is one other type of cost that HSAs may inflict on society – the cost of providing health care to people who got sick because their HSA induced them to forgo necessary health care. I take up that subject in the next section.

## The impact of high-deductibles on quality

In this section I address the question, Do high deductibles damage quality of care? I will not discuss further the damage to quality caused by the use of managed-care tactics by high-deductible insurers. I urge readers not to forget that high-deductible insurers are using managed-care tactics, their propaganda notwithstanding.

High-deductible advocates expect that big deductibles will cut the volume of services consumed. This expectation is certainly reasonable: Numerous studies indicate that raising deductibles and co-payments reduces use of services, including preventive services, especially among low-income people. The problem is that the eliminated services include both necessary services and unnecessary services. Robert Brook, the Rand researcher we met during the discussion of appropriateness studies, criticized MSA deductibles for discouraging appropriate medical services. "Economic incentives do change behavior," he told *American Medical News*, "but they reduce appropriate and inappropriate care equally."[47]

A large body of scientific literature supports Brook's assessment that when people are exposed to out-of-pocket costs, they cut back on both necessary and unnecessary medical care. This is especially true for low- and moderate-income people – people below roughly 200 percent of the federal poverty guideline. Let me quote several papers which reviewed the literature on this question:

> The research consistently demonstrates that the low-income population is particularly sensitive to out-of-pocket costs ... even low levels of cost-sharing can have adverse effects on ... health outcomes. Research has shown that, in many communities, an income at 200 percent of the federal poverty line is not adequate to meet ... basic needs, much less health care.... [T]he national median income necessary to meet basic needs in 1999 was $33,511, which is roughly twice the poverty level of $17,463. (Julie Hudman and Molly O'Malley, Kaiser Commission on Medicaid and the Uninsured, 2003)[48]

> The Commission believes that individuals should share in the responsibility of paying for health services.... But the Commission ... recommends that ... people whose income is up to at least 200 percent of poverty be provided with subsidies.... There is some evidence that a family's income must be 250 percent of poverty before discretionary income is available to spend on health care. (U.S. Bipartisan Commission on Comprehensive Health Care, 1990)[49]

But out-of-pocket payments can damage quality of care even for employed people making reasonably good incomes. Solanki et al. found that cost-sharing for employees of a large corporation for preventive counseling, Pap smears, and mammograms "reduces the probability that adults will receive these recommended preventive services."[50]* A study by the Rand Corporation based on claims data for employees working for 25 large corporations found that doubling co-payments for prescription drugs from $5 to $10 caused a 22 percent drop in drug spending by these employees.[51] Huskamp et al. reported in the *New England Journal of Medicine* that when co-payments for ACE inhibitors (drugs that lower blood pressure) and statins (cholesterol-lowering drugs) were doubled (from $7 to about $15) by a large American company, 16 percent of employees with an ACE inhibitor prescription stopped taking that drug and 21 percent of employees on statins stopped taking their statin. Huskamp et al. did not study those patients who stopped refilling their prescriptions to see if their health was damaged. But, they noted, "The discontinuation of the use of ... statins and ACE inhibitors that are needed for the treatment of chronic illnesses raises important questions about potentially harmful effects of ... changes in co-payments."[52]

One of the few studies that did attempt to determine the impact of rising drug co-payments on health was done, ironically, by a large American corporation that had previously subscribed to the high-deductible crowd's logic that raising out-of-pocket costs saves money. This study was reported in the *Wall Street Journal*, not a medical journal. Pitney Bowes, a self-insured Fortune 500 company that makes the ubiquitous postage-stamping machine, among other things, raised co-payments on prescription drugs for its 35,000 employees in 2001. That year, the co-payments rose from a small fixed sum to percentages of the cost of the drug, percentages as high as 50 percent. But beginning in 2002, Pitney Bowes *cut* co-payments on diabetes and asthma drugs to a maximum of 10 percent of the drug's cost. This change cost the corporation $1 million. But the loss in co-payments from employees turned out to be well worth it. By the end of 2003, it was clear Pitney Bowes' total costs of caring for its asthmatic and diabetic employees and dependents had fallen dramatically. Costs for doctor visits, emergency room visits, and hospital stays had all dropped. Even

---

* Preventive counseling was defined as "counseling services about ... exercise, nutrition, smoking, injury prevention, motor vehicle safety, alcohol and substance abuse, and sexually transmitted diseases."

spending on asthmatic and diabetic drugs dropped, by about 10 percent for each of those first two years of the experiment compared with an 11 percent annual *increase* for the rest of the employee population. This seems a bit perplexing given that the lower co-payments for the diabetes and asthma drugs caused patients to take these drugs more often. According to the *Wall Street Journal*, one explanation for this paradox is that Pitney Bowes had to spend less money on "rescue medications, such as albuterol, a drug administered to stabilize a person who has suffered a severe asthma attack."[53]  Pitney Bowes estimated a net savings of at least $1 million for 2004.

Nine days after reporting the Pitney Bowes story, the *Wall Street Journal* reported on yet another study that punched holes in the claims of HSA advocates. "[A] new study indicates that when [drug] co-payments rise, the health of patients with certain chronic illnesses can suffer," the paper reported.  "Even modest increases in co-payments can lead to health setbacks for these people, according to the study ... in the *Journal of the American Medical Association*.  The study ... found that when co-payments doubled, the use of prescription drugs fell between 17 percent and 23 percent among patients with diabetes, asthma and gastric acid disease.  Meanwhile, visits to emergency rooms rose 17 percent for people with those conditions, and hospital stays increased 10 percent."[54]

High-deductible advocates have no answers to the argument that high deductibles will cause many people, especially lower-income people, to deny themselves necessary medical care.  In their book with the cloying title *Patient Power*, Goodman and Musgrave ask the question, "How do we know people would not forgo needed medical care...?" Here is their answer:

> We don't.  The theory behind medical savings accounts is that people should have a store of personal funds with which to purchase medical care.  And because the money they spent would be their own, they would have strong incentives to make prudent decisions.  Undoubtedly, some of their decisions would be wrong.  But many decisions made under the current system also are wrong.[55]

There you have it: The wrongs of the current system justify replacing it with an equally dangerous system. "Patient power," according to Goodman and Musgrave, means the power to hurt yourself.

Some high-deductible proponents, no doubt recognizing that the Goodman-Musgrave admission that high deductibles cause damage to patients is not good PR, take a different tack: They make the false claim that scientific evidence exists proving that high deductibles won't damage the health of patients. Given the large body of scientific literature on this question and the consistent message of this literature – that exposure to out-of-pocket costs causes people to forgo necessary medical care which in turn damages health – it takes gall to state that the literature finds deductibles and co-payments to be harmless.

Those who argue that high deductibles do not harm patients always cite, inappropriately, one paper – a paper by Manning et al. – out of more than a dozen generated by an expensive study conducted in the late 1970s and early 1980s by the Rand Corporation entitled the Health Insurance Experiment. The Cato Institute's Michael Tanner, for example, wrote, "Critics say consumers will forgo necessary or preventive care to save money in their medical savings accounts, but studies show that MSAs do not deter preventive care. Rather, savings result from reduced use of optional services and cost-based selection among competing providers."[56] Tanner went on to cite the Rand study. I won't attempt to explain in detail here how it is that high-deductible advocates get so confused by the Rand study. I'll just refer you back to the statement I quoted earlier by Robert Brook who was a co-author of papers generated by the Rand study: *Out-of-pocket payments "reduce appropriate and inappropriate care equally."* And I'll quote an expert who perceives, as I do, that high-deductible advocates routinely misrepresent the Rand study: "Sometimes the HIE [Health Insurance Experiment] has been characterized as finding no adverse effect on health status, but a closer reading of the results shows that there were adverse effects on health for lower-income and high-risk individuals."[57]

HSA proponents who claim science has demonstrated that gigantic deductibles don't hurt anyone are not only misrepresenting the Rand study, they are willfully turning away from the mountain of peer-reviewed literature published in the quarter-century that has elapsed since the Rand study which demonstrates that even small out-of-pocket payments cause people to forgo necessary medical care, and a smaller body of literature which demonstrates that when people forgo necessary medical care their health suffers. The high deductible, like managed care, is a meat ax, not a scalpel. It will damage quality of care for some people, and that damage may lead to higher medical costs in the long run.

## Predicting the future

Will HSAs succeed in driving low-deductible policies from the market as MCPs were successful in driving traditional indemnity insurers from the market? Consumer resistance to HSAs may prove to be more effective than it was to MCPs for the simple reason that the main defect in HSAs – the huge deductible – is much more obvious to consumers than the defects in MCPs. However, I'm not holding my breath. Because health insurance is so expensive, and because employers are beginning to shift more of the cost to employees, it is conceivable that large numbers of healthy employees will be willing to accept high deductibles in exchange for even 10-percent cuts in their premium and a chance to make some money off their employer contributions.

The critical question is how employers, especially large employers, respond. Support for HMOs from large employers was essential to the rise of managed care, and so it will be for HSAs. A substantial number of large employers and the managed-care wing of the insurance industry supported managed care in its early years, and a similar alliance – employers and the high-deductible wing of the insurance industry – has emerged to support high-deductible plans. As the power of the employer-insurance-industry alliance guaranteed the nation had to suffer through a doomed experiment with managed care, so the power of the new employer-HSA-plan alliance means the nation will have to suffer through a doomed experiment with high deductibles. I pray the high-deductible experiment will be a lot shorter, and lot less painful, than the HMO experiment was.

## A short history of tax credits

I include a brief analysis of tax credits in this chapter because support for tax credits comes primarily, although not exclusively, from the same people who support high deductibles, namely, the insurance industry and their conservative allies in Congress.

America's conservatives tend to propose tax breaks (deductions or credits) instead of government programs whenever public opinion forces them to adopt a position on access to health care, housing, and other necessities of life. Thus, for example, when Democrats pushed national health insurance back onto the front burner in the early 1970s, Republicans, the American Medical Association, and what was then called the Health Insurance Association of America supported legislation that would give employers and individuals tax breaks if they purchased health insurance.

The tax credit made a modest comeback in the early 1990s when public pressure for some solution to health-care inflation forced conservatives to propose something resembling a health policy. The Heritage Foundation, one of numerous conservative think tanks, published a tax credit proposal in 1991,[58] but there were, at first, few takers among Republicans. A single event, however, overcame Republican inertia. That was the November 1991 election of Democrat Harris Wofford, who campaigned on national health insurance, to the Pennsylvania Senate seat that Senator John Heinz (R-PA) had occupied before he was killed in a helicopter crash. Wofford was 40 percentage points behind Republican candidate Richard Thornburgh in August 1991, but he won the election with 55 percent of the vote. Post-election surveys showed that half of Pennsylvania's voters said "national health insurance" was one of their top two concerns. Politicians throughout America interpreted Wofford's election to mean Americans wanted Congress to rein in health-care inflation and provide coverage to the uninsured. As George Bush I put it, "One of the messages in Pennsylvania: Try to help people with health care."[59]

The day after Wofford's election, several Senate Republicans introduced a bill to establish refundable tax credits for people who bought health insurance on their own. (A credit is an offset to tax liability that is the same dollar amount for all income-tax payers. A *refundable* credit is one that is available not only to people who pay income taxes but also to people who have incomes too low to owe any taxes.) Three months later, President Bush revealed that he too had a solution to the health-care crisis. He called for tax credits for low-income people and tax deductions for higher-income people. Bush's tax credits were large compared with the credits his son would offer a decade later – $1,250 a year for an individual and $3,750 for a family. He proposed to pay for them with cuts in Medicare and Medicaid.[60]

Late in his 2000 campaign for the presidency, George W. Bush announced he too supported credits. He endorsed refundable tax credits worth up to $1,000 for *individuals* earning up to $15,000 a year and up to $2,000 for *families* earning up to $30,000.* Of course, by the time George W. Bush proposed these credits, health-care inflation made them worth even less than the credits his father proposed in 1992.

George W's proposed tax credit was within the range of credits then being proposed by members of Congress. According to a 2001 report by the Congressional Budget Office, "A number of tax credit proposals were introduced in the 106th Congress. Those proposed credits were typically refundable and ranged from $500 to $1,200 for individual policies and $2,000 to $3,600 for family coverage."[61] Bush reaffirmed his tax credit proposal again in January 2002, at which time he announced he was raising the credit for families to $3,000,[62] and again in January 2004. The Bush administration estimates its tax credit will reduce the ranks of the uninsured by 4 million; Jonathan Gruber of MIT estimates the true number is under 2 million.[63] Whatever the true figure, it is a very small portion of the number of Americans who have no health insurance.†

---

* Under the Bush plan, the value of the credit would begin to drop at $15,000 for individuals and $25,000 for families and disappear completely at $45,000 and $60,000 respectively.

† It is a bit unclear exactly what portion of the uninsured 2 or 4 million is. The most commonly cited number for the number of uninsured in the U.S. is the annual number reported each fall by the Census Bureau. The number for 2003 was 45 million. However, that number is almost certainly not comparable to the 2 and 4 million estimates for Bush's tax credit. Those numbers are probably the number of people who would be insured all year long with the help of the credit, whereas the Census Bureau's number is an estimate of the number of Americans without health insurance at a given point in time (the time at which the survey was taken). According to figures published by the Congressional Budget Office for 1998, the number of those uninsured all year long is about 65 percent of the number of those uninsured at a point in time (Uwe E. Reinhardt, "Is there hope

## Why tax credits are ineffective

Tax credits are milquetoast health policy, to be generous about it. They feed the bloated health insurance industry, and they ask for no sacrifices from the supply side. Only large, very expensive tax credits can reduce the uninsured rate significantly. As the Congressional Budget Office put it, "The amount of a tax credit would have to be fairly large – approaching the full cost of the premium – to induce a large proportion of the uninsured population to buy insurance."[64] The tax credits proposed by Republicans over the last decade have come nowhere near equaling the cost of insurance.

George W. Bush's proposed credit illustrates the problem. Since insurance with reasonably good coverage costs $3,000 to $5,000 for healthy individuals, and $10,000 to $12,000 for healthy families buying policies on their own, and a lot more than that for sick people, it doesn't take a genius to understand why Bush's proposal will do little to reduce the uninsured rate. (Remember, these are credits for people who buy insurance on their own, not through an employer. Premiums for these individuals are much higher than they are for employers.) Dr. Judith Feder, dean of policy studies at Georgetown University, said Bush's plan was like "giving a ten-foot rope to people in a 30-foot hole."[65] Just as a short rope will be useless to someone in a deep hole, so a tax credit worth a fraction of the cost of insurance is useless to low-income people, and even to many middle-income people.

The ineffectiveness of the Bush proposal was illustrated by two studies that demonstrated the difficulty Americans have buying individual policies. A study done by Families USA examined the difficulty *healthy* people have finding insurance that is both adequate and affordable. A study by Georgetown University's Institute for Health Care Research and Policy tested the reaction of health insurance companies to applications by people with mild to severe illnesses.

The study by Families USA analyzed two types of insurance policies in 25 states for healthy 25-year-old and 55-year-old women. The first

for the uninsured?" *Health Affairs* 2003, Web Exclusives, July-December, W3-376-390). If this ratio is accurate, then 29 million Americans were uninsured throughout all of 2003. The Bush tax credits would insure somewhere between 7 and 14 percent of those 29 million people.

type of policy was one that cost $1,000 (the maximum amount of the tax credit for an individual under the Bush proposal); the second was a "standard plan" (which Families USA defined to mean a plan equal in coverage to that in the Blue Cross Blue Shield Preferred Provider Organization plan offered to federal employees). Families USA found serious problems with both plans. Policies costing "only" $1,000 were unavailable in many of the 25 states studied, and where they were available the coverage they offered was terrible. The standard plans were sometimes unavailable and always very expensive.

Tables 10-3 and 10-4 summarize Families USA's findings for both types of plans. Table 10-3 indicates that healthy women cannot get a $1,000 policy in many states (18 of the 25 states did not have $1,000 policies for sale for 55-year-old women). What is not reported in Table 10-3 is that Families USA found that those policies that were for sale did not cover doctor visits, prescription drugs, emergency services, or mental health services in several states. Table 10-4 reports the cost of the *lowest-priced* policies that met the "standard plan" definition in each of the 25 states. You can see that adequate policies were available in 21 of the 25 states for healthy women, but the premiums were far above the maximum $1,000 tax credit proposed by Bush. Remember, the full $1,000 credit would be available only to low-income people. So, to take the worst case shown, a 55-year-old *healthy* Alaska woman, earning $15,000 a year, would have to pay half her annual income – $7,964 – in addition to Bush's $1,000 credit, in order to buy insurance. To take the best case shown, a healthy 25-year-old South Dakota woman, earning $15,000 a year, would have to pay $524 out of her own pocket to buy insurance.

Whereas the Families USA study assumed the applicants were healthy, the study by Georgetown University assumed the applicants suffered from conditions ranging from hay fever to AIDS. The investigators asked 19 health insurance companies across the U.S. to indicate how they would respond to applications for individual health insurance from seven fictitious individuals. According to *American Medical News*:

> The results showed that even the most healthy hypothetical applicant was rejected by some insurers, and all were frequently offered plans with riders barring coverage for their pre-existing health conditions, higher premiums

**Table 10-3: Bush's $1,000 tax credit will buy a policy with shrunken coverage for younger, healthier individuals, and no plan at all for many older and sicker people: Deductibles in, and availability of, insurance policies for healthy women that cost $1,000 a year in 25 states, 2001**

| State | Deductible for healthy, non-smoking female ($) | |
|---|---|---|
| | 25-year-old | 55-year-old |
| Alaska | 1,000 | na* |
| Arizona | 750 | 5,000 |
| Arkansas | 750 | na |
| California | 500 | na |
| Florida | 2,500 | na |
| Illinois | 1,000 | na |
| Iowa | 500 | 5,000 |
| Louisiana | 1,000 | na |
| Maine | na | na |
| Massachusetts | na | na |
| Mississippi | 500 | na |
| Montana | 5,000 | na |
| New Jersey | na | na |
| New Mexico | 5,000 | na |
| New York | na | na |
| North Dakota | 500 | 2,500 |
| Oklahoma | 500 | 5,000 |
| Oregon | 1,000 | 5,000 |
| Pennsylvania | 750 | na |
| South Dakota | 1,000 | na |
| Tennessee | 750 | 2,500 |
| Vermont | na | na |
| West Virginia | na | na |

\* "na" means a $1,000 plan for healthy women was not available.
Source: Families USA, *A Ten-Foot Rope for a 40-Foot Hole*, Families USA Foundation, Washington, DC, September 2001, Table 1, 6.

## Table 10-4: Bush's $1,000 tax credit will contribute only a small fraction of the cost of adequate health insurance for healthy individuals, and an even smaller fraction for sick people: Premiums for "standard plans"[a] for healthy women in 25 states, 2001, ($)

| State | Premium for healthy, non-smoking female 25-year-old | 55-year-old |
|---|---|---|
| Alaska | 3,996 | 8,964 |
| Arizona | 2,340 | 2,892 |
| Arkansas | 2,028 | 4,548 |
| California | 1,375 | 3,096 |
| Florida | 1,776 | 2,488 |
| Illinois | 1,488 | 3,444 |
| Iowa | 1,932 | 3,852 |
| Louisiana | 3,144 | 7,044 |
| Maine | 3,941 | 5,132 |
| Massachusetts | 3,168 | 6,130 |
| Mississippi | 2,256 | 5,052 |
| Montana | 1,788 | 5,448 |
| New Jersey | 4,608 | 4,608 |
| New Mexico | 1,788 | 4,500 |
| New York | na[b] | na |
| North Dakota | na | na |
| Oklahoma | 2,088 | 4,692 |
| Oregon | 1,608 | 3,612 |
| Pennsylvania | 2,412 | 5,388 |
| South Dakota | 1,524 | 3,420 |
| Tennessee | 2,208 | 4,932 |
| Texas | 3,132 | 6,240 |
| Utah | na | na |
| Vermont | na | na |
| West Virginia | 1,703 | 3,924 |

(a) Families USA defined the standard plan as follows: It "could not have a deductible higher than the $250 deductible in the ... BC/BS [Blue Cross Blue Shield] PPO [Preferred Provider Organization, a type of MCP]. In addition, the plan had to be equivalent to the [BCBS PPO] in at least two of the following four measures: (1) co-payments for doctor's office visits of $15 or less; (2) coinsurance for inpatient and outpatient services no higher than 20 percent (the [BCBS PPO] has a lower coinsurance rate of 10 percent); (3) prescription drug coverage with coinsurance no higher than 25 percent or flat co-payments no higher than $12 for generics and $20 for brand name drugs...; or (4) annual out-of-pocket limit of $3,000 or less" (p. 2).

(b) "na" means a "standard policy" for healthy women was not available.

Source: Families USA, *A Ten-Foot Rope for a 40-Foot Hole*, Families USA Foundation, Washington, DC, September 2001, Table 2, 7.

than a completely healthy individual would face, or larger cost-sharing responsibilities than they requested. One character, a man with AIDS, was rejected by all insurers.[66]

I know from personal experience how high insurers can set premiums for even healthy individuals. In 1997 I helped a 58-year-old St. Paul woman write a letter to Cigna after Cigna quoted her an annual premium of $23,692 for health insurance with a $250 deductible and no drug coverage. The premium would have fallen to $18,156 if she had been willing to accept a $2,000 deductible. The woman was going through a divorce and needed to know what her premiums would be in order to negotiate an agreement on alimony with her soon-to-be ex-husband. She wrote Cigna because that was the company that insured her and her husband through 3M, the husband's employer. This woman had been healthy all her life and was still healthy. She said the only medical services she had gotten in recent years was an MRI on her neck to examine a spur, three biopsies on breast tissue that revealed no cancer, and some psychiatric counseling to deal with her grief over the divorce. However, her sister and mother had cancer, a fact she had to report to Cigna's underwriters. Those facts no doubt perturbed the actuaries at Cigna. When I saw Cigna's premiums, I told the woman, "Why doesn't Cigna just come right out and tell you they don't want your business?"

Unlike managed care and high deductibles, tax credits won't harm patients. They will, however, enrich the insurance industry, and they will serve as a fig leaf for politicians who wish to conceal their disinterest in cleaning up the health-care mess.

---

# Endnotes

[1] America's Health Insurance Plans, *Number of HSA Plans Exceeded One Million in March 2005*, http://www.ahipresearch.org/pdfs/HSAExceedMillion050405_full.pdf, accessed July 15, 2005.

[2] Sarah Lueck, "Medicare law reaches the under-65 set, too," *Wall Street Journal*, December 16, 2003, D1, D4.

[3] J. Duncan Moore, Jr., "The father of the HMO mulls quality measures," *Modern Healthcare*, March 22, 1996, 33.

[4] National Center For Policy Analysis, *Who Pays Higher Prices for Prescription Drugs?* Dallas, TX, November 2003, 26.

[5] John C. Goodman and Gerald L. Musgrave, *Patient Power: The Free-Enterprise Alternative to Clinton's Health Plan*, Cato Institute, Washington, DC, 1994, viii.

[6] Ibid., ix.

[7] Senator Phil Gramm, "Why we need medical savings accounts," *New England Journal of Medicine* 1994;330:1752-1753, 1752.

[8] Bernard J. Wolfson, "Medicare fix doubtful this year, experts say," *Orange County Register*, February 22, 2002, http://www.ocregister.com/search, accessed February 24, 2002.

[9] Jeff Goldsmith, "Interview: Politics, technology, and transformation: A conversation with Newt Gingrich," *Health Affairs*, Web Exclusives, July-December 2003, W3-511-520, 515.

[10] Harris Meyer, "GOP reformers push medical IRA plans," *American Medical News*, January 3, 1994, 1.

[11] David E. Rosenbaum, "Tax-free accounts drew yeas from the wary," *New York Times*, November 23, 2003, A23.

[12] Victoria Colliver, "Behind the wheel: New model of health care service gives patients more power but at a price," *San Francisco Chronicle*, June 15, 2001, http://www.sfgate.com/cgi-bin/article.cgi?f=/c/a/2001/06/15/BU100378.DTL, accessed January 21, 2002.

[13] Glenn Howatt, "Definity Health nets major client: Coalition augments revenue, visibility," Minneapolis *Star Tribune*, November 8, 2001, D1.

[14] Milt Freudeinheim, "A new health plan may raise expenses for sickest workers," *New York Times*, December 5, 2001, A1.

[15] Meredith Rosenthal and Arnold Milstein, "Awakening consumer stewardship of health benefits: Prevalence and differentiation of new health plan models," *Health Services Research* 2004;39:1055-1070.

[16] Dwight McNeill, "Do consumer-directed health benefits favor the young and healthy?" *Health Affairs* 2004;23(1):186-193, 191.

[17] U.S. General Accounting Office, *Medical Savings Accounts: Results from Surveys of Insurers*, December 31, 1998, Appendix, 14.

[18] Anthony T. Lo Sasso et al., "Tales from the New Frontier: Pioneers' experiences with consumer-driven health care," *Health Services Research* 2004;39:1071-1089.

[19] Stephen T. Parente et al., "Employee choice of consumer-driven health insurance in a multiplan, multiproduct setting," *Health Services Research* 2004;39:1091-1111.

[20] Mayer, op cit.

[21] Sarah Lueck, "Medicare law reaches the under-65 set, too," *Wall Street Journal*, December 16, 2003, D1.

[22] Mark V. Pauly and John C. Goodman, "Tax credits for health insurance and medical savings accounts," *Health Affairs* 1995;14(1):126-139, 138.

[23] Editorial, *Wall Street Journal*, October 12, 2004, A22.

[24] Susan Lee, "A tax-code cure for ailing health care," *Wall Street Journal*, August 9, 2004, A13.

[25] Michelle Andrews, "Does it pay to manage your own care?" *New York Times*, January 18, 2004, Bu 7.

[26] Goodman and Musgrave, op cit., 107.

[27] Ibid., 88.

[28] Michael Tanner, *Medical Savings Accounts: Answering the Critics*, Cato Institute, May 1995, https://www.cato.org/pubs/pas/pa228.html, accessed July 16, 2005.

[29] Goodman and Musgrave, op cit., 59.

[30] Greg Scandlen, "MSAs can be a windfall for all," National Center for Policy Analysis, November 2, 2001, http://www.ncpa.org/pub/bg/bg157, accessed December 7, 2003.

[31] Sharon Epperson, "Save for your health," *Time*, April 5, 2004, http://www.insurancenewsnet.com/article.asp?a=sa&lnid=83866896, accessed May 9, 2004.

[32] Definity's Web site, http://www.definityhealth.com/marketing/index.html, accessed February 11, 2005

[33] Sharon McIlrath, "Private sector provides no road map for Medicare MSAs," *American Medical News*, August 28, 1995, 1.

[34] Jon B. Christianson et al., "Defined-contribution health insurance products: Development and prospects," *Health Affairs* 2002;21(1):49-64.

[35] David E. Grembowski et al., "Measuring the 'managedness" and covered benefits of health plans," *Health Services Research* 2000;35:707-734, 708.

[36] Personal communication from Molly Hollister, HealthPartners, e-mail, May 31, 2005.

[37] Greg Scandlen, "How consumer-driven health care evolves in a dynamic market," *Health Services Research* 2004;39;1113-1118, 1117.

[38] Pauly and Goodman, op cit., 136.

[39] Regina E. Hertzlinger, "Let's put consumers in charge of health care," *Harvard Business Review*, July 2002, 4-11, 7.

[40] Ibid, 8.

[41] Emmett B. Keeler et al., "Can medical savings accounts for the nonelderly reduce health care costs?" *Journal of the American Medical Association* 1996;275:1666-1671.

[42] Cited in Peter Ferrara, *The Establishment Strikes Back: Medical Savings Accounts and Adverse Selection*, Cato Institute, 1996, http://www.cato.org/pubs/briefs/bp-026.html, accessed November 30, 2002.

[43] *American Health Line*, "MSAs: More competing views on whether they will work," September 27, 1995, 9.

[44] Michael Kendix and James D. Lubitz, "The impact of Medical Savings Accounts on Medicare program costs," *Inquiry* 1999;36:280-290, 287.

[45] Ibid., 289.

[46] Evelyn L. Forget et al., "Medical Savings Accounts: Will they save money?" *Canadian Medical Association Journal* 2002;167:13-147, 146.

[47] Meyer, op cit., 28.

[48] Julie Hudman and Molly O'Malley, *Health Insurance Premiums and Cost-Sharing: Findings from the Research on Low-Income Populations*, Kaiser Commission

on Medicaid and the Uninsured, Washington, DC, March 2003. The first quote is at page 1, the second at page 30.

[49] U.S. Bipartisan Commission on Comprehensive Health Care, *A Call for Action*, September 1990, Washington, DC, 63.

[50] Geetesh Solanki et al., "The direct and indirect effects of cost-sharing on the use of preventive services," *Health Services Research* 2000;34:1331-1350, 1342-43, 1335.

[51] Vanessa Fuhrmans, "A radical prescription," *Wall Street Journal*, May 10, 2004, D1.

[52] Haiden A. Huskamp et al., "The effect of incentive-based formularies on prescription-drug utilization and spending," *New England Journal of Medicine* 2003, 349;23:2224-2232, 2231.

[53] Furhmans, op cit.

[54] Vanessa Fuhrmans, "Higher co-pays may take toll on health," *Wall Street Journal*, May 19, 2004, D1.

[55] Goodman and Musgrave, op cit., 107.

[56] Tanner, op cit.

[57] Karen Davis, "Consumer-directed health care : Will it improve health system performance?" *Health Services Research* 2004;39;1219-1233, 1221.

[58] Stuart M. Butler, "A tax reform strategy to deal with the uninsured," *Journal of the American Medical Association* 1991;265:2541-2544.

[59] Jacob S. Hacker, *The Road to Nowhere: The Genesis of President Clinton's Plan for Health Security*, Princeton University Press, Princeton, NJ, 1997, 39.

[60] "Bush to offer health crisis cure: Medicare, Medicaid curbs would offset his plan's costs," Minneapolis *Star Tribune*, February 3, 1992, 51.

[61] Congressional Budget Office, *Budget Options*, February 2001, http://www.cbo.gov/showdoc.cfm?index=2731&sequence=3, accessed January 22, 2002.

[62] Amy Snow Landa, "White House renews call for health insurance tax credits," *American Medical News*, February 18, 2002, 5.

[63] James D. Reschovsky and Jack Hadley, "The effect of tax credits for nongroup insurance on health spending by the uninsured," *Health Affairs*, Web Exclusives, January-June 2004, W4-113-127.

[64] Congressional Budget Office, op cit.

[65] Henry J. Kaiser Family Foundation, *Health Policy as It Happens, Daily Reports*, October 16, 2000, http://www.kaisernetwork.org/frame/index.cfm?goto=http://www.kaisernetwork.org/healthpolicy_reports/KP001016.5.html, accessed January 22, 2002.

[66] Geri Aston, "Individual market tough for many insurance buyers," *American Medical News*, July 9/16, 2001, 14.

# 11

# Why Medicare for Everyone Is the Best Plan

## Introduction

Our tour of the major issues raised by the health-care reform debate is just about over. We've diagnosed the problem – it is supply-side waste, not overuse – and we've examined in considerable detail the prescriptions recommended by the insurance industry and its allies – managed care and high deductibles. In describing the waste in the system, I've already given you the fundamental arguments for a single-payer system, the third contender in the modern health-care debate. In this chapter I flesh out the arguments for the ideal single-payer or Medicare-for-all system. I say the *ideal* Medicare-for-all system to distinguish my proposed system from some American single-payer proposals (such as legislation pending in California) and facsimiles of single-payer systems in this country (such as Medicare) that incorporate formularies and other bad ideas generated originally by HMOs.

## How a single-payer addresses waste

Table 11-1 lists the information shown in Table 7-5 – the four types of waste and the cost of each type of waste as a percent of total health spending. It also presents the mechanisms a single-payer uses to minimize the waste. As the table indicates, the solution to administrative

## Table 11-1: How a single-payer addresses waste

| Type of waste | Cost as % of spending | Single-payer solution |
|---|---|---|
| Administrative waste Insurance company overhead Provider (doctor and hospital) overhead | 10-15% | One payer |
| Excess capacity | ? | Budgets for hospitals* |
| High fees and prices High fees High drug prices | 10-15% | Price controls |
| Fraud | 3-10% | One payer plus enforcement |

\* For the sake of simplicity, I describe the budgets necessary to reduce excess capacity as "budgets for hospitals." In fact, these budgets will have to extend beyond hospitals to any clinic or entity that makes capital purchases (machines or buildings) in excess of, say, $1 million. Hospitals are the biggest purchasers of capital equipment, but they are not the only ones. Clinics and freestanding imaging centers, for example, buy MRIs, which cost several million dollars per copy.

waste is one payer, the solution to excess capacity is budgets for hospitals, the solution to excessive prices is price controls, and the solution to fraud is one payer and aggressive enforcement of the law.

The solution to high administrative costs, in both the insurer and provider sectors, is one payer that does not use managed-care tactics. When a single-payer with low overhead like Medicare's replaces America's 1,500 or so health insurance companies, system-wide administrative costs will fall substantially, probably by 50 percent. Overhead in the *insurance* sector will drop because the one payer will have much lower overhead costs than any private-sector insurer – be it a managed-care plan (MCP), a pure HSA plan, or, more likely, a hybrid MCP-HSA plan – could ever achieve. Remember, a single public insurer at the national level will need to spend only 1 to 2 percent of its revenues on overhead versus 15 to 35 percent for private insurers. (A state-level single-payer might have overhead just a percentage point or two higher.)

And overhead in the *provider* sector will drop because (a) the public single-payer won't be using managed-care tactics which waste so much of the provider sector's time and money, and (b) providers will have to deal with only one payer, not hundreds or thousands. A system that relies on multiple insurers, be they MCPs or high-deductible plans, can do little to reduce provider overhead.* And, of course, a system of MCPs will do nothing to reduce that portion of provider overhead that is caused by MCPs' managed-care tactics.

The solution to excess capacity is to give the single-payer the authority to approve budgets for hospitals and any other entity that buys expensive equipment such as MRIs (a threshold expenditure could be set at, say, $1 million). Think back to the battle between the two Miami-area hospitals over the Gamma Knife that we discussed in Chapter 6. You recall that a hospital in Coral Gables, Florida, installed one of these expensive machines in October 1993, and a Miami hospital ten miles to the north installed another Gamma Knife five months later. Obviously, the MCP-dominated insurance industry in Florida was powerless to stop this senseless arms race. An insurance industry dominated by large-deductible insurers would have been equally powerless. Only a single-payer, or some other government agency authorized to set budgets for hospitals, could have stopped the madness. Under a single-payer system, both hospitals would have submitted budgets to the single payer, and the single-payer board would have determined how many Gamma Knives the Miami area needed and which hospital or hospitals would be the best place to house them.

The solution to high fees and prices is price controls – limits on what doctors can charge for services, and ceilings on what drug companies can charge for drugs. HSAs, with their deductibles influencing less than 20 percent of total spending, are going to have no influence on the great bulk of health-care spending and, therefore, prices charged

---

* Since the early 1990s, defenders of the current system have often argued that electronic billing (submitting medical bills by computer) will bring about a substantial reduction in administrative costs. Electronic billing is already widespread, so making it even more widespread is not going to save much money relative to total spending. In any case, electronic billing is irrelevant to the question of which type of system is most efficient. Electronic billing is a tool that can be used in any type of health-care system, multiple-payer or single-payer.

for the great bulk of medical goods and services. The current MCP-run system has slowed the growth of physician fees (it hasn't reduced them) and has had no detectable system-wide impact on drug prices. The superior effectiveness of price controls over managed competition and high deductibles is clearest with respect to drug prices. The current MCP-dominated system has proven that MCPs (including HSA plans that use managed-care methods) can only reduce drug prices for themselves (as opposed to all of society), and even this minor victory has been achieved at considerable cost. I discussed one type of cost in Chapter 9 – the damage done to patients by formularies. Another type of cost is the administrative costs associated with formularies. These costs include those that MCPs incur constructing and enforcing formularies, and the costs physicians and pharmacists incur keeping track of, and prescribing according to, the umpteen formularies their various patients have to abide by. For doctors, administrative costs generated by formularies include the cost of arguing with MCP employees about whether the patient can be allowed to use a non-formulary drug.*

There is no perfect solution to fraud, the fourth category of waste. Fraud will afflict any type of insurance system. But the best solution is a single-payer plus an adequate budget for law enforcement. A single-payer will be better at detecting two types of fraud than a multiple-payer system. I'm talking about the second and third of the three types of fraud we discussed in Chapter 7 – billing for services never rendered, and overcharging by double billing (charging two different insurers for the same service). If doctors and other providers have to send their bills

---

* If MCP formularies were based on rigorous scientific evidence about which drugs are the most effective and the safest, we wouldn't have to treat the loss of patient choice as a cost of the MCP system's method of controlling drug expenditures. But MCP formularies are based primarily on the kickbacks MCPs get from drug companies, not on science. Even if some MCPs wanted to give science greater weight than kickbacks, they could do so only rarely because so little research comparing drugs exists. In a 2004 report to Congress, the Medicare Payment Advisory Commission stated, "All plans we interviewed noted that studies that directly compare two or more drugs or classes of drugs in the treatment of a condition are limited and uncommon...." (*Report to Congress: New Approaches to Medicare*, Washington, DC, June 2004, 9). With so little useful information to go on, MCPs wind up making decisions based on anecdotes, which are not conclusive. That leaves only one criterion: cost.

to one payer rather than hundreds of payers, overcharging by double billing becomes very risky because it will be very easy to detect. Billing for services never rendered becomes more difficult as well. It is much easier, for example, for a doctor to claim he worked 36 hours per day last year, or did an unheard-of number of operations last year, and get away with it if he submits his bills to, say, 50 payers rather than one. The one payer's computer could be programmed to warn investigators of any provider who claims to provide an impossibly high number of services. The remaining type of fraud discussed in Chapter 7 – billing for unnecessary services – would not necessarily be any easier to detect under a single-payer than under managed competition or a regime of high-deductible insurers. But this type of fraud will be committed less often in the hospital sector because hospitals will be governed by budgets, not fees per service or per patient.

To sum up, on every one of the four types of waste, a single-payer, armed with the tools described in Table 11-1, will outperform managed competition and high-deductible insurers. Most importantly, a single-payer will not be saving money at the expense of patients. Under managed competition, MCPs save money by denying services to patients, and in the course of doing so, they invade patient privacy.* Under the high-deductible proposal, insurance companies save money by inducing patients to self-ration.

## Research confirms single-payer saves money

Few reliable studies have sought to determine how a single-payer or managed-competition system would affect total health-care spending in the U.S., and none have asked that question about high-deductible proposals. Only a half-dozen peer-reviewed or government-funded studies of system-wide savings achievable by a single-payer system have been published, and none of these attempted to measure the impact of a true single-payer; they measured only the *administrative* savings a single-payer could achieve, and ignored the savings a single-payer would achieve via hospital budgets, ceilings on physician fees and drug prices, and reduced fraud. Even fewer reliable studies have been published on

---

* This occurs because MCPs demand that doctors turn over patient medical records in order for MCPs to assess doctors' decisions to order services.

the effect of managed competition on total expenditures. As we just saw in Chapter 10, the studies that have evaluated the impact of high deductibles on spending have examined only portions of the system (employed people, federal employees, and Medicare beneficiaries), not all Americans.

With one exception, all of the reliable research on the system-wide impact of single-payer and managed-competition systems was done between 1991 and 1993. The exception was research on single-payer savings published by two leaders of Physicians for a National Health Program, David Himmelstein and Steffie Woolhandler, in 1986.[1] The reason that the bulk of the research on single-payer and managed-competition proposals appeared between 1991 and 1993 is that those were the years when single-payer and managed-competition bills were introduced in Congress. The single-payer forces got out of the chute first. Representative Marty Russo (D-IL) introduced a single-payer bill (HR 1300, The Universal Health Care Act of 1991) in March 1991. In 1992, Senator Paul Wellstone introduced the companion to the Russo bill in the Senate (S 2320). In 1993, Representative Jim McDermott (D-WA) and Senator Wellstone introduced slightly different versions of the Russo bill (HR 1300 and S 491). Managed-competition bills were introduced in 1992 by Representative Jim Cooper (D-TN), and by Cooper, President Clinton and others in 1993.

Research on these bills generated headlines – headlines that were exhilarating for single-payer advocates and discouraging for managed-competition buffs. Check out these headlines about research by the U.S. General Accounting Office and the Congressional Budget Office:

- "GAO backs health care based on Canadian plan."[2]
- "Single-payer plan saves most: CBO report says proposal also would serve most people."[3]
- "Budget office study says single-payer health plan would be least expensive."[4]
- "Budget chief sees no health cost cuts in 'managed care.'"[5]
- "CBO puts high price on managed competition."[6]

These are not selective samplings of the headlines. *All* the research, and *all* the headlines about the research, say the same thing: Single-payer is far less expensive than managed competition. The reverse has never happened. No headline has ever appeared describing research that said managed competition would cost less than a single-payer system.

One of the most damaging studies was a CBO study comparing Representative Russo's 1992 single-payer bill and Representative Cooper's 1992 managed-competition bill. The CBO reported that Russo's bill would have cut national spending by 9 percent seven years after enactment, whereas Cooper's managed-competition bill would have increased spending by 1 percent seven years later. As if that weren't bad enough, the CBO reported that Russo's single-payer bill would have reduced the uninsured rate in the U.S. to zero whereas Cooper's bill would have reduced the number of uninsured only by one-third.[7]

Research by the GAO comparing the administrative costs of the U.S. and Canadian systems was typical of the research done on single-payer systems back then. It examined only the administrative savings achievable by a single-payer; it made no effort to determine the extent to which a single-payer could reduce excess capacity, high fees and prices, and fraud. The GAO's findings are shown in Table 11-2. The GAO concluded that if

---

## Table 11-2: The administrative savings from a single-payer would be enough to cover the uninsured and underinsured: Estimates of the percentage change in total health-care spending due to single-payer savings in administrative costs, 1991

|  | Insurers | Physicians | Hospitals | Total |
|---|---|---|---|---|
| Administrative savings | -4.8% | -2.1% | -2.6% | -9.5% |
| Cost of additional insurance |  |  |  | 9.0% |
| Newly insured |  |  |  | 2.6% |
| Currently insured |  |  |  | 6.5% |
| Net change |  |  |  | -0.5% |

Source: The author's calculations using the dollar figures reported in U.S. General Accounting Office, *Canadian Health Insurance: Lessons for the United States*, Washington, DC, 1991, 63, Table 5.1.

---

the U.S. had administrative costs as low as Canada's that U.S. total spending would fall by 9.5 percent. Roughly half of that savings would come from reduced overhead in the U.S. insurer sector, and the other half from reduced overhead for doctors and hospitals. The GAO also estimated how much it would increase U.S. total spending to guarantee first-dollar coverage (which means no out-of-pocket costs for covered services) to all Americans, including the uninsured. The GAO concluded that would increase total spending by 9.0 percent. In other words, the GAO found that the administrative savings alone under a single-payer would be so extensive we could cover not only the uninsured for what we're paying now, but could eliminate deductibles and co-payments for the insured, and still cut total spending by half a percentage point.

The savings in administrative costs from a single-payer may be even higher than the GAO estimated. Although the market share held by the MCP wing of the health insurance industry was around 95 percent by 1991 (the year the GAO study was published) and could not, therefore, have risen much further, hospitals and clinics were still adapting to the spread of managed care, and the market share of *HMOs* continued to rise throughout the 1990s. Those factors probably caused insurer administrative costs to rise even further during the 1990s. If that happened, it is reasonable to conclude that the administrative costs generated by managed care have risen since 1991 and that the reduction in total spending due to a cut in administrative costs under a single-payer today would be higher than the 9.5 percent reduction estimated by the GAO. The potential savings today are probably somewhere between 10 and 15 percent.

Of course, administrative waste is not the only type of waste a single-payer can reduce. Imagine how much more we could save if we were to give an American single-payer the authority to set hospital budgets and limits on physician fees and drug prices. Back in Chapter 7, I refrained from guesstimating the savings a single-payer could achieve by cutting back on excess capacity (with hospital budgets) because the evidence on this issue is so poor. But I did estimate that price controls on physician fees and drug prices could cut another 10 to 15 percent off total spending. If administrative savings amount to 10 percent of the national bill, and price controls take off another 10 percent, the total savings comes to 20 percent, and we haven't even subtracted any savings achieved in the realm of excess capacity or fraud.

Depending on how comprehensive the coverage is, a 20-percent cut in national spending would be more than enough, or just about enough, to pay for universal coverage. If our goal is to extend coverage typically held by employed Americans (that is, coverage with deductibles and co-payments) to the uninsured, we would need to free up only about 3 percent of total expenditures. If we want to provide *all* Americans with *first-dollar* insurance, we'd have to free up a total of about 9 percent of all health-care expenditures, according to the GAO report we just reviewed. Given the uncertainties associated with such an estimate, let's round off to 10 percent.* If we include long-term care in our definition of universal coverage, we'd have to free up perhaps another 10 percent

---

* The GAO study on Canada presented in Table 11-2 concluded that insuring the uninsured with typical American coverage (that is, coverage with typical deductibles and co-pays) would cost 2.6 percent of total health-care spending. Other studies derive a similar estimate. For example, a 1997 study, which assumed the uninsured would get coverage with typical deductibles and co-payments, estimated a range of 2 to 3 percent (Pamela Farley Short et al., "The effect of universal coverage on health expenditures for the uninsured," *Medical Care* 1997;35:95-113).

These two estimates – 2-3 percent to extend first-dollar coverage only to the uninsured, and 9 percent for universal first-dollar coverage – do not take into account the effect that eliminating managed care will have on utilization rates, nor the effect of improved quality due to (1) insuring the uninsured, (2) eliminating managed care, and (3) eliminating the need for insured people to switch insurers. Switching insurers often causes delays in getting care, and often forces patients to switch doctors, and both events are associated with diminished quality of care (Peter Franks et al., "On being new to an insurance plan: Health care use associated with the first years in a health insurance plan," *Annals of Family Medicine* 2003;1:156-161). Higher utilization rates will increase costs, but improved health may reduce costs. Because solid data on both factors are scarce, it is difficult to know whether the net effect will be an increase or decrease in total spending. I have seen several studies that attempted to determine the reduction in utilization caused by managed care; I have seen no system-wide studies of the effect universal insurance will have on the health of the uninsured and on the health of the insured who switch plans and, therefore, on total spending. In the absence of good data, I assume the net effect of these factors on the cost of universal coverage is zero. The remainder of this footnote gives you some idea of what might happen to cost if my assumptions are wrong, that is, if the increase in utilization due to the elimination of managed care is not offset by a reduction in costs due to improved health.

of current health-care expenditures.* To sum up, if we want universal coverage with deductibles and co-payments, plus coverage for long-term care services, we'd need the equivalent of roughly 10 percent of current health-care spending.  If we want universal *first-dollar* coverage plus coverage for long-term care, we would need the equivalent of about 20 percent of total spending.  But 20 percent is a conservative estimate of what an American single-payer could save.

---

In my vision of single-payer, managed-care tactics would be outlawed. However, some single-payer proposals permit HMOs to continue to exist.  But because few people would enroll in an HMO if they could get free care or nearly free care from non-HMO doctors, it is safe to assume that utilization of medical services will increase almost as much under a single-payer proposal that permits HMOs as one that does not.  The increase in costs due to higher utilization in a managed-care-free environment will be relatively small compared to the savings a single-payer will achieve.  According to the Congressional Budget Office, HMOs – generally the tightest form of managed care plans – reduce utilization rates below levels seen in traditional, unmanaged fee-for-service insurance companies by 8 percent (Congressional Budget Office, *The Effects of Managed Care and Managed Competition*, Washington, DC, 1995).  But since only 25 percent of Americans are enrolled in HMOs, the reversal of this 8-percent reduction caused by eliminating HMOs isn't going to affect the entire population.  System-wide, eliminating managed-care insurers would mean only a 3 percent increase in utilization (1.08 times .25 equals 2.7 percent).

If we take the most conservative assumption – that improved health in the uninsured and the currently insured will have no cost-reducing effect – then the total cost of eliminating managed care and extending first-dollar coverage to all Americans will be 12-13 percent (9-10 percent due to the elimination of out-of-pocket payments plus 3 percent due to the elimination of managed care).

* I derive this estimate using the only good proposal for a national long-term care plan I know of – the proposal laid out by the Pepper Commission in 1990.  This commission, officially known as the U.S. Bipartisan Commission on Comprehensive Health Care, made proposals to solve the crisis in both the health-care sector, as it is traditionally defined, and the long-term care sector (The Pepper Commission, *A Call to Action*, U.S. Government Printing Office, Washington, DC, 1990).  Its proposal to make nursing-home and home health care affordable to everyone was pretty good.  The commission estimated that this program would have raised total spending on long-term care by as much as $43 billion had it been implemented in 1990 (see page 130), which amounted to just under 7 percent of the $647 billion the commission estimated the U.S. would spend on health care that year (see page 65).  To be on the safe side, I'm estimating a good national long-term care insurance program would cost about 10 percent of total spending today.

## Privacy and democracy: Two other reasons to support single-payer

A single-payer system has two other advantages over the current MCP-run system: (1) By eliminating MCPs that use utilization review, a single-payer system will enhance patient privacy; and (2) by reducing the health insurance industry to a shadow of its former self, and by reducing the incentive for providers and drug companies to get big, a single-payer system will augment the influence of public opinion on health policy at the expense of the gigantic MCPs, hospital chains, clinics and drug companies that dominate the health-policy debate today.

Patient privacy has been virtually destroyed by MCPs, in particular, by their use of utilization review. Under the traditional insurance system, patient privacy was violated, but only to the extent necessary to prevent fraud. Traditional insurers did not demand that doctors send them patient files in order to argue with doctors about their decisions. Before MCPs took over, doctors and hospitals submitted claim forms to insurers listing a few publicly available facts about the patient (name, sex, and address) plus the patient's age and a few codes to indicate what services were rendered. Thus, an insurance company employee receiving the claim form would know that Dr. X performed an angiogram on Jane Doe. But the insurance company employee would not learn other facts that would typically appear in a patient's file, for example, that the angiogram was ordered because Ms. Doe had been experiencing chest pain with exertion for the past six months, and that the angiogram found 90-percent occlusion in one of her coronary arteries. To take another example: The employee of a traditional insurance company could learn from a typical claim form that John Doe underwent treatment for depression; the employee would *not* learn that John Doe was physically abused as a child, has nightmares about aggressive animals, and often thinks about committing suicide.

Between the formation of the traditional health insurance industry in 1929 and its demise at the hands of MCPs in the 1990s, Americans came to accept the minimal invasion of patient privacy required by traditional insurers. Traditional insurers would demand information from patients at two points – when people applied for insurance, and after they received medical care and filed a claim. For large groups (typically employees in firms with more than 50 to 100 employees), traditional insurers would ask only for a few bits of information such as name, address, age, and sex. For individuals and for most small groups, traditional insurers would also "underwrite," that is they would ask for information about the applicants' health history and use that information to decide whether to insure the person or group and what premium to charge if the insurer accepted the application. When patients got medical care, someone (the patient or the doctor) would submit a claim form. The claim form did not include data from medical records. Except in rare cases when the traditional insurers felt fraud was being committed against them, insurers paid the claim without asking for data from patient medical records.

The MCP industry changed the rules. It continued to extract health history data from individual and small-group applicants the way the traditional insurers had, but it vastly expanded the amount of medical data it extracted from doctors (usually without patients knowing it), before, during, and after treatment. Utilization review and appeals contesting drug formularies require doctors to deliver to MCPs information about patients typically found only in medical records. According to industry observer Jon Gabel, utilization review spread like wildfire during the 1980s and early 1990s. "Such techniques were so rare in 1977," says Gabel, "that few references to them exist in the literature. By 1988 nearly 70 percent of workers with job-based health coverage were enrolled in a plan with preadmission review, and about one-fifth were in a plan with a primary care gatekeeper. By 1998 prospective utilization review techniques were so widespread that the major national surveys ceased to ask about their presence."[8] MCPs can be brazen in their demands for information. For example, a psychiatrist told me Blue Cross and Blue Shield of Minnesota demanded that he turn over his notes on one of his depressed patients so Blue Cross could determine whether the patient really was depressed.

A system built around sellers of large-deductible policies may well turn out to be just as invasive of patient privacy as the current system. High-deductible insurers will unquestionably want to continue the time-honored practice of cherry-picking, which means they'll have to continue underwriting as aggressively as the MCPs do. And the early evidence indicates large-deductible insurers intend to keep managing care.

A single-payer system would not underwrite, that is, it would not ask Americans numerous questions about their health history before insuring them, and it would not manage care. Nor would an ideal single-payer peruse patient medical records for the purpose of publishing report cards. For these reasons, a single-payer system would be much less invasive of patient privacy than one based on either MCPs or large-deductible insurers.

In addition to lower cost, better quality, and improved privacy, a single-payer system will give ordinary people greater influence over health policy than is possible under either an MCP or large-deductible regime. There are two reasons for this. First, social control of industry pricing decisions is formalized under a single-payer system. No longer will Americans be expected to influence industry decisions as *consumers* "shopping" in dysfunctional health-care markets. Instead, we will be influencing health policy decisions as *voters*. Second, the power of the various players in the health-care industry will be reduced by a single-payer system.

The main loss of industry power will occur in the insurance industry. Its power will be reduced to a tiny fraction of its current level. Under all single-payer proposals, non-HMO health insurers will be allowed to sell only a small number of non-essential health and health-related services.* Under some single-payer proposals, health insurance companies would be allowed to process claims, as they do now for Medicare, if they can demonstrate that they can do so more efficiently than the government can. In either case, the insurance industry will have a much reduced revenue stream from which to skim money to finance lobbyists, advertisements, and other activities designed to influence the public and members of Congress.

---

* Some single-payer bills permit HMOs to exist. That is not a good idea. HMOs drive up costs and damage quality. On a truly level playing field, HMOs would disappear under a single-payer system because people would not enroll in them if unmanaged doctors were available at no cost or at the same cost. But HMOs have demonstrated their ability to tilt the playing field. They have persuaded Congress to take money out of Medicare's traditional fee-for-service program in order to overpay them to insure Medicare patients. In view of this history, it is reasonable to anticipate HMOs and their allies will seek to starve the public, fee-for-service segment of a single-payer program in order to fatten the privatized, HMO sector of the program.

A single-payer system will also appreciably reduce the political power of specialists and drug companies by reducing their incomes. A single-payer will probably reduce the power of hospitals and drug companies by prohibiting reimbursements for lobbying and limiting reimbursements for advertising. I say "probably" because no one can guarantee that the new regulators will take steps to stop these industries from lobbying. I am constantly amazed that so-called "regulated" utilities have oodles of money to advertise and lobby legislators and regulators.

## The argument for building on Medicare

If you agree with me that a single-payer system scores better than a managed-care or large-deductible system on cost, quality, privacy, and democracy, then you're ready to think about the politics of establishing a single-payer. How should we go about enacting a single-payer system? Should we introduce a bill to establish the complete single-payer system, or should we establish a single-payer in phases? If we phase a single-payer in, should we use Medicare as a cornerstone around which to build a complete single-payer? Should we concentrate on the federal or state level?

There is no reason why we can't employ all strategies simultaneously. There is no reason why we couldn't simultaneously introduce single-payer bills and bills that enact components of a single-payer, and there's no reason why we couldn't simultaneously introduce both types of single-payer bills in Congress and state legislatures. But if I were restricted to one strategy, I would endorse a phased-in federal strategy using Medicare as the cornerstone. The reason I prefer to build in stages is that it avoids rousing all the enemies of a full-blown single-payer bill at once. The complete Russo-McDermott-Wellstone single-payer bills, and the single-payer bills introduced in many state legislatures during the 1990s, infuriated every powerful interest at once – the health insurance industry (which didn't want to be drastically reduced), the doctor organizations, hospitals, drug companies, and equipment manufacturers (which hated the thought of lost income from budgets and price controls), many employers (who disliked the payroll taxes virtually all single-payer bills relied on to some degree), and conservatives (who disliked tax increases to pay for the uninsured). If we were to take on, for example, just the issue of price controls on drugs, we would have "only" the powerful drug industry fighting us tooth and claw. Conservative groups that are not players in the health-care industry would join the drug industry (the Chamber of Commerce, for example, can always be counted on to take the wrong side in any aspect of the health reform debate), but these groups would not fight with the ferocity of someone whose interests are being attacked directly.

I prefer to build on Medicare rather than start from scratch because Medicare is a known commodity, it is very popular, it has already demonstrated its efficiency, and, of course, it resembles a single-payer. Medicare's single-payer features have allowed Medicare to outperform the private sector. Medicare's greater efficiency is not obvious if you merely compare the growth rates in *total* spending by Medicare and the private-sector, something Republican members of Congress did during the 1992-1996 inflation lull and for a few years thereafter, to justify their claim that Medicare needed to be turned over to the allegedly efficient health insurance industry. If we compare growth in *total* spending by Medicare with growth in *total* spending by the nation's health insurance industry during the 1992-1996 period, the insurance industry appeared to be more efficient than Medicare. During that time, growth in premiums, and in the nation's total health-care bill, slowed considerably, but Medicare's growth rate did not. Consequently, during those years Medicare's annual growth in total expenditures was higher than the private sector's. As I have already explained, the slowdown in private-sector spending during the inflation lull was caused primarily by swings in the insurance industry's "underwriting cycle" and the merger avalanche that ripped through the industry beginning in 1992. Medicare, thankfully, was not part of the industry and was not influenced by the underwriting cycle, and was spared the upheaval and the need to low-ball prices created by merger fever in the private sector. Republicans, nevertheless, used the private-sector's brief period of apparent superiority over Medicare as an excuse to call for the privatization of Medicare. Although Republicans continued to press for the privatization of Medicare after private-sector inflation came back with a vengeance, we have heard no more nonsense from Republicans about the private sector's allegedly lower inflation rate since the late 1990s.

But a comparison of year-to-year changes in *total* expenditures by Medicare and the insurance industry tells us little about the relative efficiency of Medicare and the health insurance industry because enrollment in Medicare is usually growing faster than enrollment in private-sector plans. The only useful comparison is one which compares growth rates in *per person* spending, not total spending. On this basis, Medicare wins. Between 1969 and 1997, the annual average increase in per capita spending by the insurance industry was 11.4 percent versus 10.4 percent for Medicare.[9] The difference would have been even greater if the period of comparison had been limited to the post-1983 period. Medicare did not have authority to control spending on hospitals until 1983, and didn't have authority to impose price controls on doctors until 1992. All Medicare could do before these dates was reimburse hospitals according to the costs hospitals claimed they incurred, and reimburse doctors according to their "usual and customary" fee.

Even per-person-expenditure comparisons, however, are not perfectly comparable. Medicare's numbers include payment for limited coverage of long-term care that few private policies cover. On the other hand, Medicare's numbers (prior to 2006) do not include payments for drugs consumed outside a hospital, which most private policies do cover. But when Medicare and private plans are compared on spending on comparable services (which means that long-term care and drug expenditures are removed from expenditure totals), Medicare continues to outperform the private sector. Measured this way, per capita spending by Medicare grew 9.6 percent annually between 1970 and 2000 versus 11.1 percent for the private sector during that period.[10]

Medicare has achieved greater efficiency than the private sector has with low overhead costs and the ability to set limits on what it pays doctors and hospitals. Medicare has always outperformed the private sector in the insurer overhead department because Medicare doesn't spend money on all the administrative functions private-sector insurers do. We went over this in Chapter 6. Table 11-3 makes the point again in a slightly different and perhaps more memorable way. It compares the number of employees, number of insured, and the employee-to-insured ratio of the larger U.S. MCPs, two Canadian provincial health programs, and Medicare.

Let's focus first on the MCPs and Medicare. The first thing you notice about Table 11-3 is that Medicare's enrollment is huge compared with that of the MCPs, yet Medicare has far fewer staff (about 4,000) than all of the MCPs listed except tiny Oxford.* Aetna, the largest U.S. health insurer in 2001, insured less than half the number of people Medicare did, yet Aetna needed almost nine times the number of staff to do it. The Medicare figure of 9,277 people insured per employee is 20 times more than the Aetna figure of 458.

But this comparison between Medicare and MCPs is unfair to the MCPs because Congress requires Medicare to hire private-sector firms to process its claims. An apples-to-apples comparison would have to attribute at least some of those private-sector claims processors to Medicare. (The cost of these private-sector claims processors *is* included in the 2 percent Medicare overhead figure.) But even that adjustment would not appreciably alter Medicare's tremendous efficiency advantage over the MCPs. Table 11-3 indicates that the single-payers for the Canadian provinces of Saskatchewan and Ontario (which do not outsource claims processing) insure 7,000 to 8,000 people per employee, far above the 400 to 500 typical of American MCPs. Because Medicare is so much larger than any Canadian provincial plan, its economies of scale might very well mean that its insured-per-employee ratio is as high or higher than those of the Canadian provinces, even after adjusting Medicare's staff total upward to reflect the fact that private-sector employees process claims for Medicare.

The other advantage Medicare has had over the private sector has been its ability to set relatively low payment rates to hospitals and doctors. Since the late 1980s, Medicare has been paying doctors and hospitals 70 to 85 percent of the rate private insurers pay.†

---

* Since 1977, when HCFA (now the Centers for Medicare and Medicaid Services) was created, HCFA's total number of employees has always hovered around 4,000. This fact was stated in an open letter to Congress from 14 well known health policy experts published in the January/February 1999 edition of *Health Affairs*. "When HCFA was created in 1977," they wrote, "Medicare spending totaled $21.5 billion, the number of beneficiaries served was 26 million, and the agency had a staff of about 4,000 full-time-equivalent workers. By 1997 Medicare spending had increased almost tenfold to $207 billion, the number of beneficiaries served had grown to 39 million, but the agency's workforce was actually smaller than it had been two decades earlier" (Stuart Butler et al., "Crisis facing HCFA and million of Americans," *Health Affairs* 1999;18(1):8-11, 9).

† The ratio of Medicare's payments to private-sector payments varies over time. In 1990, Medicare paid *doctors* 70 percent of the private-sector rate; in 1996, Medicare paid doctors 71 percent of the private rate (Physician Payment

## Table 11-3: Managed care plans are much less efficient than Canadian provincial health insurance programs and Medicare: Number of enrollees and employees of selected U.S. plans and Canadian provincial programs, 2001, and Medicare, 1999

| Insurer name | No. of insured | No. of employees | No. of insured per employee |
|---|---|---|---|
| US Plans | | | |
| Aetna | 17,170,000 | 37,500 | 458 |
| Anthem | 7,883,000 | 14,800 | 533 |
| Cigna | 14,300,000 | 44,600 | 321 |
| Humana | 6,435,800 | 14,500 | 444 |
| Oxford | 1,490,600 | 3,400 | 438 |
| Pacificare | 3,388,100 | 8,200 | 413 |
| United Healthcare | 8,540,000 | 30,000 | 284 |
| WellPoint | 10,146,945 | 13,900 | 730 |
| Canadian Programs | | | |
| Saskatchewan Health Plan | 1,021,288 | 145 | 7,043 |
| Ontario Health Insurance Plan | 11,742,672 | 1,433 | 8,194 |
| U.S. Medicare (1999) | 39,140,386 | 4,219 | 9,277 |

Sources: Steffie Woolhandler et al., "Costs of health care administration in the United States and Canada," *New England Journal of Medicine* 2003;349:768-775, for all data but Medicare data and insured-per-employee data. Medicare enrollment data are from Centers for Medicare and Medicaid Services, http://www.cms.hhs.gov/statistics/enrollment/natltrends/hi_smi.asp, accessed May 12, 2004. Medicare employees figure is from William T. Gormley, Jr. and Cristine Boccuti, "HCFA and the states: Politics and intergovernmental leverage," *Journal of Health Politics, Policy, and Law* 2001;26(3):557-580. The insured-per-employee figures were calculated by the author.

Medicare is more efficient than the private sector even though Medicare has long labored under the disadvantage of having to pay MCPs that enroll Medicare beneficiaries far more, somewhere in the range of 15 to 35 percent more, than it would cost Medicare's traditional program to insure those beneficiaries. As of 2005, 13 percent of Medicare's beneficiaries were enrolled in the so-called Medicare Advantage program (the latest name for the Medicare HMO program), and nearly all of that 13 percent were enrolled in HMOs. The Medicare Prescription Drug, Improvement and Modernization Act of 2003 increased the HMO subsidies by 11 percent,[11] so the range of estimated overpayment since 2004 has been on the order of 25 to 45 percent.

Congress did not intentionally authorize the pre-2003 subsidies. In fact, in 1982 when Congress changed the way Medicare paid HMOs in order to encourage more HMOs to participate in Medicare, Congress deliberately instructed Medicare to pay Medicare HMOs only 95 percent of what Medicare paid clinics and hospitals which served traditional fee-for-service (FFS) Medicare enrollees. For example, if the average cost of insuring a senior in the traditional Medicare program was $6,000, Medicare had to pay Medicare HMOs $5,700 (.95 times $6,000) for each senior they enrolled. Congress did this because it was under the illusion that HMOs were more efficient than FFS insurers, including traditional Medicare, and that paying HMOs 95 percent of the per capita cost of insuring the average FFS Medicare enrollee would give HMOs a sufficient incentive to participate in Medicare while at the same time saving Medicare some money. The 95-percent rate took effect in 1985.

What Congress didn't anticipate was that Medicare HMOs would enroll disproportionately healthy seniors. As we saw in Chapter 9, the seniors Medicare HMOs enrolled were so much healthier than the

---

Review Commission, *Annual Report to Congress 1996*, Washington, DC, 1996). That percent stood at 81 in 2002 (Medicare Payment Advisory Commission, *Report to the Congress*, March 2004, 112). In 1990, Medicare paid *hospitals* at a rate equal to 70 percent of the private-sector rate (my calculations based on figures presented in Congressional Budget Office, *Single-Payer and All-Payer Health Insurance Systems Using Medicare's Payment Rates*, Washington, DC, 7). In 2003, the *New York Times* reported on a study that found Medicare pays "providers" 85 percent of the private rate (Robert Pear, "Critics say proposal for Medicare could increase costs," May 6, 2003).

average FFS Medicare seniors that they cost the HMOs only 55 to 80 percent of what it cost FFS Medicare to insure an average Medicare FFS enrollee. That means that Congress should have authorized Medicare to pay HMOs far less than 95 percent of the FFS per capita cost; the appropriate rate was probably in the range of 60 to 80 percent. By paying HMOs 95 percent instead of 60 to 80 percent, Medicare in effect gave the average HMO a subsidy on the order of 15 to 35 percent.* Despite this handicap, Medicare (the HMO and FFS portions of Medicare combined) has contained costs more effectively than private-sector insurers have.

Medicare is not simply cheaper than the private sector. It is more efficient, which means its lower costs are not due to lower quality. Like studies comparing the quality of national health-care systems, studies comparing the quality of the entire Medicare program with the quality of the entire private-sector insurance industry are extremely rare. The one such study I am familiar with compared the attitudes of privately insured adults age 19 to 64 with those of Medicare beneficiaries age 65 and older. Because the survey did not segregate the responses of elderly people enrolled in Medicare's traditional program from those enrolled in Medicare HMOs, the study's comparison of private-sector insurers with Medicare was biased in favor of the private sector because Medicare beneficiaries in HMOs are much more likely to experience denial of medical services than are beneficiaries in the traditional Medicare program. Nevertheless, Medicare outperformed the private insurance industry. The authors reported the results in two forms: adjusted and unadjusted for differences in health, income, and insurance coverage.

Table 11-4 presents the unadjusted results. Medicare beneficiaries rated Medicare more highly in ten out of 12 measures than the nonelderly rated their private-sector plans. The two measures Medicare performed worse on were both measures of out-of-pocket costs. Medicare's superior performance is significant because the elderly Medicare beneficiaries were three times as likely to rate their health as fair or poor,

---

* In the Balanced Budget Act of 1997, Congress authorized Medicare to ratchet the 95-percent rate down to 92.2 percent over the period 1998 to 2002. For a variety of reasons, this legislation failed. By the early 2000s, the rate had risen above 100 percent. Nevertheless, the MCP industry continues to lobby for even larger subsidies.

were more than twice as likely to have incomes below 200 percent of the federal poverty level, and had worse coverage for a higher premium on average than the nonelderly privately insured. Why is this important? Because research demonstrates that people who are sick are less likely to be satisfied with their provider, and common sense tells us people who are poor and getting worse coverage for their premium dollar should be less satisfied with their insurer. (The authors did not attempt to quantify how much worse Medicare coverage was. Citing previous research, they merely observed that "Medicare beneficiaries have less comprehensive benefits and often pay higher out-of-pocket premiums than those covered by employer plans pay, and their Part B premiums exceed premiums paid directly by employees for employer coverage.")[12] Yet, despite these enormous advantages for the private sector – the people it insured were much healthier, much wealthier, and had better coverage that often cost them less – the private sector lost on all but two of the measures of quality shown in Table 11-4.

For example, 64 percent of Medicare beneficiaries rated their insurance "excellent" versus 54 percent of the privately-insured nonelderly. Perhaps most amazingly, Medicare elderly were slightly less likely to report going without care because of cost. Even though they had lower incomes, worse coverage, and higher out-of-pocket expenditures, the percent of Medicare elderly who went without care because of costs (18 percent) was below the analogous figure for those insured by the private sector (22 percent). The private sector managed to win only on the last two measures which indicated the Medicare-insured were likely to pay more out of pocket than the privately insured. Obviously, these two measures were heavily influenced by the worse financial condition of Medicare beneficiaries. Arguably, these last two measures were so biased in favor of the private sector they shouldn't have been treated as useful quality measures.

When the authors of this study adjusted ten of the 12 scores for differences in income, health status, and presence or absence of drug coverage (the Medicare elderly were less likely to have drug coverage), the private sector performance looked even worse relative to Medicare's than it looks in Table 11-4. Table 11-5 presents these results in terms of odds ratios. Medicare walloped the private sector on all eight of the measures for which score differences were statistically significant (which

## Table 11-4: Medicare provides higher quality coverage than private-sector insurers do: Experiences with insurance and medical care under private-sector and Medicare coverage, unadjusted for income, health status, or drug coverage, 2001

|  | Private insurance (age 19-64) | Medicare elderly (age 65 and older) |
|---|---|---|
| Insurance is excellent or very good | 54% | 64% |
| Negative insurance experiences[a] | 61% | 43% |
| Paid a lot out of pocket for Rx or dental | 37% | 31% |
| Had difficulty getting referral to specialist | 9% | 2% |
| Very satisfied with care | 51% | 62% |
| Rated physician as excellent | 37% | 39% |
| Very confident of future ability to get care | 37% | 50% |
| Went without needed care in past year due to costs[b] | 22% | 18% |
| Did not go to dentist in past year due to costs | 18% | 8% |
| Had problems with medical bills in past year[c] | 25% | 16% |
| Total out-of-pocket costs >$500 | 39% | 47% |
| Total out-of-pocket costs > 5% of income | 10% | 29% |

(a) Percents represent respondents who said yes to one of these three statements: "Plan did not pay anything for care respondent thought was covered;" "Plan covered only a part of service"; and, "Reached limit on what plan paid for specific illness/injury." Private-sector insurers lost by large margins on all three of these statements.

(b) Percents represent respondents who said yes to one of these four statements: "Did not fill prescription"; "Did not get needed specialist care"; "Skipped recommended test or follow-up"; and, "Had a medical problem, did not visit doctor or clinic." Private-sector insurers lost to Medicare by small margins on the last three statements, and tied with Medicare on the first one.

(c) Percents represent respondents who said yes to one of these three statements: "Not able to pay bills;" "Contacted by a collection agency for bills;" and, "Had to change way of life to pay bills."

Source: Karen Davis et al., "Medicare versus private insurance: Rhetoric and reality," *Health Affairs*, Web Exclusives, 2002, W311-324, Exhibit 2.

**Table 11-5: Medicare provides higher quality coverage than private-sector insurers do: Experiences with insurance and medical care under private-sector and Medicare coverage expressed as odds ratios (Medicare score divided by private-sector score), adjusted for income, health status, and drug coverage, 2001**

|  | Odds ratio |
|---|---|
| Insurance is excellent | 2.66* |
| Negative insurance experiences[a] | 0.32* |
| Paid a lot out of pocket for Rx or dental | 0.43* |
| Very satisfied with care | 1.70* |
| Rated physician as excellent | 1.37* |
| Very confident of future ability to get care | 2.04* |
| Went without needed care in past year due to costs[b] | 0.33* |
| Had problems with medical bills in past year[c] | 0.25* |
| Total out-of-pocket costs >$500 | 0.82 |
| Total out-of-pocket costs > 5% of income | 1.15 |

* Statistically significant

(a) Percents represent respondents who said yes to one of these three statements: "Plan did not pay anything for care respondent thought was covered;" "Plan covered only a part of service"; and, "Reached limit on what plan paid for specific illness/injury." Private-sector insurers lost by large margins on all three of these three statements.

(b) Percents represent respondents who said yes to one of these four statements: "Did not fill prescription"; "Did not get needed specialist care"; "Skipped recommended test or follow-up"; and, "Had a medical problem, did not visit doctor or clinic." Private-sector insurers lost to Medicare by small margins on the last three statements, and tied with Medicare on the first one.

(c) Percents represent respondents who said yes to one of these three statements: "Not able to pay bills;" "Contacted by a collection agency for bills;" and, "Had to change way of life to pay bills."

Source: Karen Davis et al., "Medicare versus private insurance: Rhetoric and reality," *Health Affairs*, Web Exclusives, 2002 W311-324, Exhibits 3-5.

means the differences in scores were subjected to a test to ensure that they weren't a fluke). Only on the last measure – "total out-of-pocket costs > 5% of income" – did the private sector win, and this difference wasn't statistically significant. The first line in Table 11-5 indicates, for example, that elderly Medicare recipients were 2.66 times as likely as private-sector insured to say they think their insurance is excellent. The second line indicates that Medicare recipients were only a third as likely as the privately insured to say they had had a negative experience with their insurer in the past year. The second-largest difference appeared in response to a question about the respondents' confidence in their "future ability to get care"; Medicare respondents were twice as likely to say they were confident about that.

The authors suggested that the Medicare benefiaries' more positive evaluation of their insurance and access to care could reflect their more stable coverage. Ninety-nine percent of the Medicare respondents said they had been insured the entire preceding year while only 92 percent of the privately insured said that (not shown in their tables nor in Tables 11-4 and 11-5). The authors noted, moreover, that a substantial portion of these 92 percent (they didn't say what portion) had changed plans during the preceding year, which often means changing physicians. I would add that the much greater discontinuity in insurance and physician care might have affected responses on the quality-of-care questions as well as the responses to the insurance and access questions, and that the absence of managed care in the main Medicare program (the FFS program) also played a role in the much higher satisfaction rates of Medicare beneficiaries.

In short, Medicare resembles a single-payer system in the most important respect – it is more efficient than private-sector insurers of any type. Its overhead costs are much lower, its provider reimbursements are lower, and the quality of its coverage and medical care is better than the private sector's.

Medicare differs, however, from an ideal version of a single-payer system in three ways. The most glaring difference is that Medicare cannot set budgets for hospitals. The reason for that is, of course, that Medicare only insures the 42 million elderly and disabled Medicare beneficiaries, not the entire U.S. population. Because Medicare insures only one-seventh of the U.S. population, Congress has never debated, much less acted on, a proposal to let Medicare control hospital spending for the entire population. Medicare has had to settle for what I call "mini-budgets" – payments that cover all costs associated with each hospitalized patient. For example, Medicare has a set payment for patients who are hospitalized for hip fracture surgery. If the patient is particularly healthy and the surgery produces no complications and, therefore, the Medicare payment exceeds the hospital's actual costs, the hospital keeps the difference. Conversely, if the surgery causes complications and the patient ends up costing the hospital more than its Medicare payment, the hospital has to absorb the loss. Because this mini-budget method requires that doctors and hospitals fill out many more forms than would be necessary if hospital spending were controlled by annual budgets negotiated with a single-payer, this method is more expensive to administer than an annual budget would be.

Another difference between Medicare and an ideal single-payer program is that Medicare allows HMOs to insure Medicare beneficiaries. Thanks to huge overpayments from Medicare, most HMOs can afford to add coverage for drugs and other goods and services not covered by traditional Medicare (for little or no additional premium), and this added benefit has caused millions of seniors to enroll in HMOs. Even if HMOs were saving the taxpayer money, they should be booted from the Medicare program because of the damage they've done to quality of care and patient privacy. But they don't save Medicare money – they are costing Medicare money. They should be kicked out of Medicare immediately.*

A third discrepancy between an ideal single-payer and Medicare is that Medicare's coverage has significant holes in it. The biggest hole is long-term care, and the next biggest is drugs (the drug coverage which takes effect in 2006 will reduce but not eliminate this hole). The out-of-pocket costs that seniors have to pay for hospital and physician services constitute smaller, but still obnoxious, gaps in Medicare's coverage.

Based on complaints from doctors who are sympathetic to a single-payer system, I suspect that Medicare has recently begun to impose too

---

* A similar question is whether Medicare should reduce the role of insurers as claims administrators. Throughout its history, Medicare has contracted for claims-processing services with the nation's big insurers. Congress should order a study of whether Medicare would save money processing claims itself. I have little doubt that it would.

many documentation requirements on doctors. These requirements may be no worse than those private-sector insurers impose, but that's no excuse.* Medicare's paperwork may be excessive, and if so, it should be cut back.

We also need to explore ways to enhance citizen participation in Medicare's decision-making processes. Currently, the average citizen has very little involvement in the making of Medicare policy. Congress functions as Medicare's board of directors, and the public does have much more influence over Medicare than we have over the boards of the big MCPs. But that's not good enough. In drafting legislation to create a national Medicare-for-all program, we should consider creating regional, state, and local citizen boards that would have advisory, and for some issues, decision-making authority. For example, the decision about how many emergency rooms a state or metropolitan area should have, and where those ERs should be, should have extensive input from residents of the area affected. The decision about the number of ERs would have to be made within limits set by national and state citizen boards on hospital spending. However, the decision about where those ERs should be located should be entirely up to local residents and should not require national oversight unless the local board violates basic principles of fairness (by, for example, depriving some communities of access to timely emergency services). On the other hand, larger questions affecting the whole nation, such as what services will be covered and how much physicians should be paid, should be made by a national board. We should apply the same principle to state-level single-payers – decision-making and advisory authority should be pushed as close to the local level as possible.

Despite its defects, Medicare is the most efficient insurer in the country, and is unquestionably the most popular. It enjoys these advantages over all other insurers because it's the closest thing America has to a single-payer. We should build a single-payer system for all Americans around Medicare. Specifically, we should fill the coverage gaps in Medicare, drop Medicare's eligibility age from 65 to zero, give Medicare the authority to set hospital budgets and drug price controls,

---

* According to an early 1990s survey of physicians by the American Medical Association, it took doctors equal amounts of time to file Medicare and Blue Shield claims.

kick the HMOs out of the program, and reduce Medicare's paperwork. We could then legitimately claim to have the world's best health-care system.

## Getting from here to there: Defending traditional Medicare

Unfortunately, the first step we must take in creating a Medicare-for-all program is a defensive one. If we're going to have a Medicare program we want to build on, we must stop the Republicans and their cheerleaders in the health policy community from privatizing Medicare. Since 1995, Republicans have campaigned to convert Medicare from a traditional fee-for-service insurance program into a voucher plan that would force low- and middle-income seniors into MCPs. In its essentials, the plan is nothing more or less than managed competition for Medicare enrollees. Republicans began their campaign by announcing that Medicare will face a financial "crisis" when the baby boomers begin to retire in 2010. Rather than address the obvious problem – the need for more revenue, and revenue from a source other than the regressive payroll tax – Republicans chose to attack Medicare as inefficient and in need of "modernization," code for "lets make the elderly suffer managed-care medicine as the nonelderly have for the last two decades."

The "crisis" talk is scare talk. One could say, with as much logic, that the nation's elementary schools faced a "crisis" in the 1950s when the first baby boomers entered elementary school, or that the Pentagon faced financial crises during the wars in Afghanistan and Iraq. There was of course no financial "crisis" in public education in the 1950s, and the Pentagon never came close to "bankruptcy" in the months after September 11, 2001. America found the money to give elementary education to the baby boomers, and America found the money to overthrow the Taliban and Saddam Hussein. Yes, the retirement of the baby boomers will mean Medicare needs more money. But, absent more evidence, one may not leap from that simple conclusion to the conclusion that the existing Medicare program is inefficient and suffering a "crisis."

Despite evidence that MCPs do not save money for the nonelderly and in fact raise the cost of the Medicare program, Republicans have pressed ahead with their privatization, managed-competition scheme.

The complete Republican plan was not formally unveiled until 1999. However, on October 24, 1995, the public got a sneak preview of what Republicans had in mind for Medicare when Newt Gingrich was caught explaining the plan to a private meeting of Blue Cross Blue Shield executives. According to news accounts as well as a videotape of Gingrich's speech later released by the AFL-CIO, Gingrich said the traditional Medicare program "would wither on the vine" under the Republican proposal as seniors were induced to leave it and enroll with private-sector insurers.

Republicans began their campaign to privatize Medicare with legislation that would make it easier for MCPs of all stripes (not just HMOs and MSA insurers) to qualify as Medicare insurers and to induce seniors to leave traditional Medicare. This legislation, which folded the existing Medicare HMO program into a new program called "Medicare+Choice" (pronounced "Medicare plus choice") within Medicare, became law in 1997 as part of the 1997 Balanced Budget Act (the same law that set up the pilot MSA project within Medicare). Medicare+Choice was a bust. Medicare+Choice remained almost exclusively the province of HMOs (MSA insurers and non-HMO MCPs stayed away from the program), and these HMOs found they couldn't make a buck off America's elderly despite their huge subsidies from the taxpayer, and began pulling out of the Medicare program all over the country in 1998.

Republicans, however, persisted. Their solution was to throw more money at the HMOs in the hope that they wouldn't leave Medicare. They were supported in this effort by most health policy experts. As one member of the health policy establishment put it in 2001, "Remarkably, the policy community's faith in the competitive model has persisted despite the acutely disappointing performance of Medicare+Choice."[13] Republicans succeeded in including an 11-percent increase in Medicare's overpayments to MCPs in the Medicare Prescription Drug, Improvement and Modernization Act of 2003. That law also changed the name of the program one more time, from Medicare+Choice to Medicare Advantage.

When they enacted Medicare+Choice in 1997, Republicans were well aware that Medicare+Choice alone was not going to get them what they wanted. They knew the 1997 law left out a key ingredient of managed competition – financial pressure to induce people to leave their fee-for-service insurer (in this case, traditional Medicare) and enroll in MCPs. Republicans revealed their solution to this "problem" early in 1999 at the final meetings of a temporary commission known as the National Bipartisan Commission on the Future of Medicare. At these meetings, they announced their support for a proposal to strip seniors of their right to whatever care they needed under Medicare and to replace that right with a voucher that seniors would have to use to buy health insurance. This voucher could be used to pay the premium for either a private-sector policy or for access to the traditional Medicare program. You heard me correctly: Republicans want to force the traditional Medicare program to charge a premium. The voucher would have been worth just enough to buy an MCP policy but nowhere near enough to pay traditional Medicare's premium. Why would traditional Medicare be more expensive under managed competition? I answered that question back in Chapter 9 when I explained how MCPs were able to keep their premiums below those of traditional insurers. MCPs enroll healthier people than traditional insurers do (including FFS Medicare), and MCPs ration care and cost shift in ways that simply aren't available to traditional insurers.

Republicans on the Bipartisan Commission failed to line up the requisite super-majority (11 of 17 votes) required to endorse their voucher scheme, and the idea sank from public view when the commission disbanded in March 1999. But 18 months later, George W. Bush revived this awful idea. He endorsed the voucher scheme in September 2000 during his campaign for the presidency. Bush, like other Republicans, doesn't use the word "voucher" to explain his proposal. He claims, rather, that he is merely attempting to give seniors "more choice," as if seniors have been clamoring for something other than Medicare to insure them. He does not mention, and at times explicitly denies, the financial compulsion that lies at the heart of his proposal. "You can choose to keep your current Medicare benefit, exactly the way it is, or … you can add to it and you can improve it," he said when he endorsed the Republican voucher scheme on September 5, 2000. "It's your choice." On July 13, 2001, he said, "No change, no threats, no problems," by way of explaining his plan to "modernize" Medicare.

Just as there has never been substantial public support for managed competition, so there is now very little public support for the right wing's

Medicare voucher scheme. "[T]he public has not entirely warmed up to a ... voucher plan for Medicare," reported the Kaiser Family Foundation in 1996 in a press release explaining a poll it cosponsored with Harvard University. "[O]nly 32 percent favor mandatory vouchers that would be used to purchase private health insurance, while 64 percent favor keeping Medicare as it is today."[14] But neither the absence of public support nor the dismal performance of MCPs has embarrassed Republicans and health policy experts into abandoning their fantasy that vouchers and competition will improve Medicare. Bruce Vladeck, who administered Medicare early in the Clinton years, offered these acid remarks about the experts' support for the voucher plan: "There is a consensus among the policy elite, the think-tank folks, the academics, but if you tried these ideas with the public, they'd think you were insane. If you listen to beneficiaries, it's not 'choice' they're asking for – they want additional benefits."[15] John Palazzari, an 80-year-old retiree from Los Gatos, California, expressed the prevailing sentiment among Medicare beneficiaries this way: "The biggest thing the government could do for the seniors is keep Medicare like it is, and add a prescription drug benefit."[16] This gap between public and Republican opinion on whether to turn Medicare into a managed-competition showcase is huge. This gap is an asset for those of us working for a Medicare-for-all program. It is the most important reason why Republicans will fail in their campaign to privatize Medicare.

The most immediate task before those of us who want to preserve traditional Medicare is to prevent Republicans from giving even more money to Medicare HMOs. Over the longer haul, we must roll back the gigantic overpayments to HMOs. If Medicare HMOs cannot afford to offer drug coverage for little or no premium, seniors won't enroll in them, and Medicare Advantage will, to use Newt Gingrich's words, "wither on the vine." If, on the other hand, Republicans succeed in increasing the size of the HMO welfare check, more seniors will give up traditional Medicare and enroll in HMOs. Republicans will use the increased enrollment in MCPs to confuse the public into thinking HMOs are more efficient than traditional Medicare.*

---

* My call for an end to overpayments to Medicare HMOs applies as well to the drug-only plans, the so-called Pharmacy Benefit Managers (PBMs), which, along with Medicare HMOs, will start selling the scrawny Medicare drug coverage that takes effect on January 1, 2006.

## Getting there from here: Phasing in Medicare-for-all

I became a proponent of phasing in a single-payer system around 1995, and was open to the idea before that. By 1995, the national single-payer movement had failed to get a single-payer bill out of either house of Congress, and had succeeded in getting single-payer legislation passed out of just one house in only five state legislatures. In California in 1994, proponents of Proposition 186, a single-payer initiative, were outspent by opponents by a ratio of three to one, and the initiative lost three to one – 73 to 27 percent. In Minnesota, COACT and the Health Care Campaign of Minnesota had been granted only two hearings in the Democratic-controlled state legislature on our single-payer bill, and one of these was a meaningless "informational" hearing held in front of just four members of the committee. At the one bona fide hearing we were given, our chief author did not ask for a vote because we knew we would have lost it by a large margin. I concluded in 1995, and still believe today, that until the distribution of power between the proponents and opponents of single-payer changes dramatically, we will not get a single-payer system all at once.*

Fortunately for those of us who think the phased-in approach makes sense, there is nothing inherent in the way single-payer systems work that requires that they be enacted all at once. Canada, for example, began phasing in its single-payer system by establishing single-payer, hospital-only insurance, province by province. Once all provinces had set up hospital insurance programs, Canada began phasing in physician insurance, again province by province. Still later, Canada phased in price controls on brand-name drugs. Once you realize that the components of a Medicare-for-all system, or any other ideal single-payer system, can be enacted separately, you can begin to think about alternatives to a strategy of enacting the whole enchilada at once.

Here are the main components of an ideal single-payer:

---

\* Of all the events that could significantly enhance the power of the single-payer movement, the most likely to occur in the near term is the entry of the labor movement into the ranks of the single-payer movement. The AFL-CIO does not support single-payer and shows no signs of doing so any time soon. But the rising cost of health insurance has worried union leaders for a decade. The double-digit inflation of the early 2000s is causing some union leaders to think seriously about a single-payer system.

- extending coverage to the uninsured (all at once or in stages);
- replacing the insurance industry with one payer;
- giving the one payer or some other government agency the authority to regulate hospital charges (either by setting limits on charges for individual procedures, or by setting budgets for hospitals);
- giving the one payer or some other government agency the authority to set limits on doctor fees; and
- giving the one payer or some other government agency the authority to set limits on drug prices.

These five components could be implemented separately or together, and, if separately, in any order. We could, for example, take on first the task of subjecting drug companies to price controls. Obviously, in such a scenario we haven't created a single-payer yet, so some entity other than the not-yet-created single-payer would have to administer the drug price controls. Since I'm suggesting we build on Medicare, Medicare would be the obvious federal agency to take on the task of administering drug price controls. Similarly, we could pass legislation giving Medicare, or some government agency other than the future single-payer, the authority to set limits on physician fees (after negotiating with physician groups) and hospital charges (after holding hearings at which hospitals present evidence in support of their proposed charges). Once we've done that, we could make Medicare the nation's single-payer by lowering Medicare's eligibility age from 65 to zero, and outlawing the sale of health insurance for any service already covered by Medicare. If we wanted to, we could solve the uninsured problem at the same time by setting up a tax system to replace the current system of voluntarily buying insurance, or we could postpone solving the uninsured problem and deal with it separately.* Once Medicare was responsible for insuring all or most Americans, we could give Medicare the authority to

---

* If we decided to postpone solving the uninsured problem, this phase of installing a single-payer could be accomplished one of two ways. We could simply authorize Medicare to begin selling insurance to the nonelderly. Because Medicare is so much more efficient than the private sector, Medicare would

set budgets for hospitals, not merely control what hospitals charge for particular services.

Or we could do everything in reverse order. We could insure the uninsured first (by enrolling them either in Medicare or Medicaid), make Medicare the sole payer, and then give Medicare the authority to set hospital budgets, physician fees, and drug prices. Moral of story: The components of a single-payer system need not be installed in any particular order. In my view, the only order that makes sense is one that maximizes the likelihood of victory.

Because the issue of drug prices is so hot now, and will remain so until price controls are enacted, it seems logical to attack the problem of drug prices first. Because the elderly account for most drug purchases, and because Medicare will begin to provide limited but very expensive drug coverage to seniors in 2006, the opening battle for drug price controls will almost certainly be fought as part of the war to give Medicare the authority to negotiate with drug companies over the price of drugs covered by Medicare. The 2003 law creating drug coverage for Medicare beneficiaries expressly forbids Medicare from extracting discounts from drug manufacturers. Once Medicare has the authority to set limits on what drug companies can charge seniors for drugs, we can undertake a campaign to extend that authority to drugs purchased by the nonelderly.

When we get to the point of insuring everyone, we'll have to deal with the issue of how to finance universal coverage. The basic financing issues raised by universal coverage are quite simple. The major tax questions raised by any new government program – health-related or

---

probably be able to undersell the private sector and, to quote Newt Gingrich one more time, the private sector would "wither on the vine." But this is not a certain outcome in the current U.S. market where cherry-picking is so rampant. It's possible that Medicare would get stuck with sicker nonelderly Americans, just as traditional Medicare now gets stuck with the sicker seniors that Medicare HMOs don't want or can't attract. To prevent that outcome, this scenario would also require other reforms, including community rating and laws requiring insurers to accept all applications. A second way to achieve the conversion to a single-payer would be to outlaw the sale of insurance which duplicates Medicare's coverage, and require that Medicare be the sole seller of health insurance to the nonelderly. People wouldn't have to buy health insurance, but if they wanted to, they'd have to buy it from Medicare. This slightly less voluntary version of single-payer would reduce the risk that Medicare would end up insuring only the sick nonelderly.

otherwise – relate to the *fairness* and *sufficiency* of the taxes, and those
fairness and sufficiency issues must be addressed regardless of whether
we make coverage universal under a single-payer, managed competition,
high-deductible, or any other system. I believe, and the people I've
worked with in Minnesota believe, that universal coverage under any
system, including a single-payer system, should be paid for with progressive taxes, which means taxes that take a rising proportion of income as
the taxpayer's income rises. The only progressive taxes in America, at
the local, state or federal level, are the personal income and estate taxes.
But estate taxes raise far too little money to function as the primary
source of funding for a universal health insurance program. That leaves
the income tax as the only tax that qualifies as both progressive and
capable of raising sufficient income to finance universal coverage.

## Dealing with Canada-bashing

In Chapter 1, I described a debate between an advocate of managed
competition, an advocate of MSAs, and me, advocating single-payer,
that took place in October 1996. Single-payer won the votes of eight
of the 14 participating citizens, managed competition got three votes,
and MSAs got zero. Not once during the three-and-a-half hours of
discussion did I use the word "Canadian-style system" to describe the
single-payer system I was proposing. But when the Minneapolis *Star
Tribune* reported on this forum nine days later, the headline read,
"Canadian-style care starting to look more attractive to panelists."[17]

Regardless of our strategy – introducing legislation that establishes
a complete single-payer system, or introducing several bills that phase in
a single-payer system – our opponents and, to a lesser extent, the media
will convey to the public the impression that our proposed American
single-payer looks exactly like Canada's system. It is quite misleading
to describe the single-payer proposals put forth by American single-
payer advocates as "Canadian-style" or "Canadian-anything" plans. For
that reason, I avoid terminology that suggests American single-payer
advocates want to install "the Canadian system" in America. Canada's
system is, of course, an example of a single-payer system, and, as we
saw in Chapter 5, Canada's health-care system may be slightly superior
to ours. But there is a huge difference between Canada's single-payer
and the system proposed by American single-payer advocates: American

single-payer advocates are proposing that America continue to outspend Canada and the rest of the world by almost the same huge margins that prevail today. In Table 3-3, we saw that the U.S. spent $4,887 per person in 2001, far more than second-place Switzerland ($3,322) or fifth-place Canada ($2,792). The CBO found that the single-payer bill introduced by Representative Russo in 1991 would have cut total U.S. health expenditures by 9 percent. A 9-percent cut in spending levels in 2001 would have reduced U.S. per capita spending from $4,887 to $4,448. The latter number is still a whole lot more – 59 percent more – than Canada's $2,792. Neither I nor any other American single-payer advocate is proposing a net reduction in excess of 10 percent.

The difference between Canada's spending level and the spending levels proposed by American single-payer advocates is very important. If the public understands that American single-payer proponents want America to continue to spend 60 percent more than Canada, they are not likely to give credibility to claims by single-payer opponents that every alleged problem in the Canadian system will inevitably be reproduced in an American single-payer. But this difference in spending levels is easily obscured by phrases like "Canadian-style plan." Opponents of an American single-payer plan will compare any American single-payer bill to Canada's system, and will peddle exaggerations and falsehoods about Canada's system, no matter what proponents say or do. But that doesn't mean single-payer proponents should make it easy for opponents to get away with obfuscations and lies. But that's what we do by claiming, or letting the media claim, that we want a "Canadian-style" system in America. The first solution to Canada-bashing, then, is not to describe the Medicare-for-all plan as a "Canadian" plan.

That doesn't mean we can or must avoid talking about the health systems of Canada and other nations in the course of explaining why a single-payer system is a good system. In fact, some pro-single-payer arguments presented in this book cannot be made without resort to data from other nations. The experience of other countries is particularly useful in documenting four assertions: that the U.S. health-care system is very expensive; that the quality of the U.S. system can't explain it's high cost (recall, for example, the statistic presented in Chapter 5 that the U.S. ranked 24th out of 26 countries in infant mortality rates); that U.S. doctors and hospitals have high administrative costs (the only way to know whether a single payer reduces overhead costs for providers is to compare the overhead costs of U.S. providers to providers in a single-payer system such as Canada's); and that physician fees and drug prices are very high in the U.S. Information from other countries, even though it is limited to these four subjects, may lead even sympathetic listeners to the mistaken conclusion that American single-payer advocates want to bring an exact replica of Canada's system to the U.S. But if single-payer advocates cite data from other countries, it's important that they make it clear that we support an *American* single-payer system – a Medicare-for-all system – that will continue to spend at levels even with or slightly below the current U.S. spending level.

But even if we make this clear, single-payer opponents will still engage in Canada-bashing. So I will close this chapter on why a single-payer system is the best solution to the health-care crisis with an analysis of the allegations most commonly made against Canada's system. The allegation I've heard most often over the years is that medical care is rationed in Canada. A second common allegation is that Canadians must wait for most medical services and, as a result, many go to the U.S. for health care. A less common myth is that doctors are leaving Canada "in droves" and coming to the U.S. A fourth myth is that those Canadians who get medical care receive inferior care.

My short answer to all of these allegations, as I've just indicated, is that even if they are true they are not relevant because I'm not proposing to bring Canada's system down to the U.S. in a box next week. I'm proposing, rather, an American plan that retains America's whopping expenditure levels. If I have time for a longer answer, I'll offer a few statistics comparing the U.S. and Canadian systems. I have assembled a few of the more telling statistics, some of which we discussed in Chapter 5, in Table 11-6 below. Then I conclude, "Can you imagine what a fantastic system Canada would have if Canada were spending $4,887 per person instead of $2,792? That's the system we'll have under an American single-payer."

The claim that Canadians are denied health care, that Canadian patients and doctors come to the U.S. in large numbers, and that Canadian medical care is inferior are all nonsense. We saw in Table 4-5 that Americans are far more likely to say they are denied medical care than Canadians are. We saw in Table 4-7 that Canadians see their doctors more often than Americans do, which suggests Canada's supply of doctors is not suffering from the alleged hemorrhaging of doctors south to The Land of HMOs. Several studies of cross-border patient traffic have concluded that border-crossing is miniscule and goes both ways. For example, the GAO reported:

> Recent data show, however, that there is very little border-jumping. The Pepper Commission [the bipartisan commission which issued a report on the American system in 1990] and the American Medical Association recently conducted informal surveys of American hospital administrators expecting high numbers of Canadian patients. Both groups concluded that few Canadians seek care at American medical centers. Canadians accounted for less than 1 percent of total admissions in each of the nine border hospitals surveyed by the Association. The Pepper Commission identified Buffalo General hospital, with about 3 percent Canadian admissions, as having the largest share of Canadian patients.[18]

Other estimates report even lower percentages of U.S. hospital admissions attributable to Canadians. According to an article written by two Americans and a Canadian, "[T]he largest hospital network in the [Detroit] region reported that only about 35 of its 35,000 annual admissions were for Canadian residents for 1992-1994."[19] Detroit, like Buffalo, is right on the U.S.-Canadian border, and its hospitals, therefore, are as convenient for many Canadians as some Canadian hospitals. Yet only 35 of 35,000 admissions – a tenth of one percent – were for Canadians. And of the tiny percent of Canadians who seek treatment in America, most do so because it is convenient or medically necessary to do so. In other words, they either live near a U.S. facility such as Buffalo General, or they are traveling in the U.S. when they get sick.

The only criticism of Canada with any truth to it is the one about waiting lines. For a very small fraction of non-urgent medical services, waiting lines have developed in Canada. Only on very rare occasions (possibly fewer per capita than in the U.S.) are the wait times health-threatening. The province of Ontario recently had to send a tiny frac-

---

## Table 11-6: The quality of Canada's system is as good if not better than the quality of the U.S. system: Comparisons of the U.S. and Canadian health-care systems

* Canada's uninsured rate has been zero since 1971; America's has ranged from about 11 to 16 percent.

* A 1995 survey of Americans and Canadians revealed that 12 percent of Americans and 8 percent of Canadians were unable "to get needed medical care," that 30 percent of Americans and 16 percent of Canadians said they "postponed needed medical care," and that Americans spent an average of $993 out of their own pockets for health care compared to $302 for Canadians (Donelan et al., *Health Affairs,* 1996).

* In 2003, our infant mortality rate was 7.0 per 1,000 births while Canada's was 5.4. In 2003, life expectancy at birth for males in America was 74.5 years versus 77.2 in Canada, and life expectancy for females was 77.2 in America versus 82.1 in Canada (Organization for Economic Cooperation and Development, 2005).

* American adults are much more likely to report their health is poor than are Canadians (Kaplan et al., *Journal of Epidemiology and Community Health,* 2004).

* A study conducted by Canadians and Americans found that Canadian mortality rates were lower for eight of ten types of surgery, slightly higher for open prostatectomy, and almost identical for hip fracture repair (Roos et al., *Health Affairs,* 1992).

* A study conducted by the U.S. General Accounting Office reported that Canadians are 5 percent more likely to survive lung cancer than Americans, 4 percent less likely to survive breast cancer, and equally likely to survive colon cancer and Hodgkin's disease (Gorey et al., *American Journal of Public Health,* 1997).

(Table 11-6 continued)

* Quebec adults who suffer a heart attack are as likely to die within one year as Americans who suffer heart attacks (Pilkote et al., *Medical Care*, 2003).

* A study of the quality of care of patients with end-stage renal disease concluded, "Manitoba patients were more than twice as likely to receive kidney transplants as U.S. ... patients. No patients in Manitoba used reprocessed dialyzers, compared with 57 percent of U.S. ... patients. After adjustment for all case mix and treatment variables, the mortality rate was 47 percent higher in the United States" (Hornberger et al., *Medical Care*, 1997).

* The average leukemia patient waits nine months for a bone marrow transplant in America versus ten months in Canada (Silberman et al., *New England Journal of Medicine*, 1994), and Americans wait five weeks for a knee-replacement surgery while Canadians wait 12 weeks (Coyte et al, *New England Journal of Medicine*, 1994).

* A study of the quality of care for diabetics in the U.S. and Canada concluded "those with diabetes in the U.S. have a greater chance of not receiving recommended care" (Klarenbach and Jacobs, *Diabetes Care*, 2003).

---

tion of its cancer patients to the U.S. for radiation therapy because of a temporary shortage of radiation therapists. This shortage was not life-threatening, but nevertheless it should not have happened. It is difficult to imagine how the U.S. could suffer from a similar shortage due to the implementation of a single-payer system if the U.S. health expenditure levels remain as high as they are now.

## Endnotes

[1] David U. Himmelstein and Steffie Woolhandler, "Cost without benefit: Administrative waste in U.S. health care," *New England Journal of Medicine* 1986;314:441-445.

[2] "GAO backs health care based on Canadian plan," Minneapolis *Star Tribune*, June 4, 1991, 8A.

[3] Sharon McIlrath, "Single-payer plan saves most: CBO report says proposal also would serve most people," *American Medical News*, August 9, 1993, 2.

[4] "Budget Office study says single-payer health plan would be least expensive," Minneapolis *Star Tribune*, December 22, 1993, 12A.

[5] Robert Pear, "Budget chief sees no health cost cuts in 'managed care,'" *St. Paul Pioneer Press*, February 3, 1993, 7A, published originally in the *New York Times*.

[6] Tom Hamburger, "CBO puts high price on managed competition," Minneapolis *Star Tribune*, May 5, 1994, 7A.

[7] Congressional Budget Office, *Estimates of Health Care Proposals from the 102nd Congress*, Washington, DC, 1993.

[8] Jon R. Gabel, "Job-based health insurance, 1977-1998: The accidental system under scrutiny," *Health Affairs* 1999;18(6):62-74, 70.

[9] Katharine Levit et al., "National health expenditures in 1997: More slow growth," *Health Affairs* 1998;17(6):99-110.

[10] Cristina Boccuti and Marilyn Moon, "Comparing Medicare and private insurers: Growth rates in spending over three decades," *Health Affairs* 2003; 22(2):230-237.

[11] "Insurers to get more from Medicare," Minneapolis *Star Tribune*, January 20, 2004, A3.

[12] Karen Davis et al., "Medicare versus private insurance: Rhetoric and reality," *Health Affairs*, Web Exclusives, October 9, 2002, http://www.healthaffairs.org/WebExclusives/Davis_Web_Excl_100902.htm, 4.

[13] Marsha Gold, "Medicare+Choice: An interim report card," *Health Affairs* 2001;20(4):120-138.

[14] Kaiser-Harvard Program on the Public and Health, "Public not following battles in Washington over Kassebaum/Kennedy and medical savings accounts," press release, July 30, 1996.

[15] Robin Toner, "Major battle looms over Medicare," *New York Times*, February 11, 2001, Section 1, 28.

[16] Barbara Feder Ostrov and Lisa M. Krieger, "Skeptical response to plan for Medicare: Some of Bush ideas have failed in past," San Jose *Mercury News*, March 5, 2003, http://rd.yahoo.com/dailynews/fc/us/health_care_debate/news_stories/*http://www.bayarea.com/mld/mercurynews/news/5319563.htm, accessed May 17, 2004.

[17] Glenn Howatt, "Canadian-style care starting to look more attractive to panelists," Minneapolis *Star Tribune*, October 9, 1996, A15.

[18] U.S. General Accounting Office, *Canadian Health Insurance: Lessons for the United States*, Washington, DC, June 1991, 60.

[19] Steven J. Katz et al., "Canadians' use of US medical services," *Health Affairs* 1998;17(1):225-235, footnote 22, 235.

# 12

# Predictions

We've come to the end of our grand tour of the U.S. health-care reform debate. We've seen how our jerrybuilt health-care system took shape after the Great Depression, and how it fell apart. The first sign that all was not well was the rapid growth in the number of uninsured beginning in the late 1970s. The second unmistakable sign was the double-digit inflation of the late 1980s. The merger madness of the early 1990s and the HMO backlash of the late 1990s were also symptoms of a health-care system suffering from a fundamental disease. The return of double-digit inflation around 2000 was the equivalent of a two-by-four over the head. Even formerly ardent managed-care advocates got the message: The American experiment with managed care has been a bust.

We've examined and rejected the bad advice from the experts about how to get out of this mess. We've seen that the experts' favorite explanation – that Americans get too many medical services – is not supported by the evidence, and that the only fair statement to make about the evidence is that it indicates underuse is more prevalent than overuse. And even if the overuse excuse were correct, we've seen that the experts' solutions to overuse – managed competition and high-deductible policies – are incapable of cutting health-care inflation but are quite capable of damaging quality of care. Managed competition and high-deductible policies are incapable of cutting health-care inflation because they address the wrong problem – volume of services – not the most fundamental problem – the *price* at which health-care services are sold and the administrative waste, excess capacity, and fraud that force prices up.

If the U.S. had money to burn and no problems other than a sick health-care system to worry about, a single-payer system would not be imperative. We could just raise taxes to whatever level is necessary to ensure that all Americans have health insurance at the outlandish price at which insurance is sold today. But, of course, our resources are finite, and we have numerous other problems demanding their share of our national resources. Given this reality, it is fair to say that a single-payer system is the best solution to the health-care crisis, morally and financially.

The problem is, the single-payer movement is not yet strong enough to overcome the opposition of the insurance industry and the right wing. But that's going to change. At the end of Chapter 2, I predicted the U.S. would eventually adopt price controls and would probably also adopt a single-payer financing mechanism, but only after muddling through a phase, lasting a decade or two, in which we experiment with high-deductible plans and tax credits. I doubt a single-payer will be adopted in one act of Congress. I predict that a combination of forces will push Congress, and some state legislatures, to enact a single-payer system in stages. The most important of these forces will be the outcome of the national debate about campaign finance reform, American public opinion about health policy, and the inability of the health-care system to contain cost. I think of the last force – relentless health-care inflation – as a gigantic tectonic plate that is slowly and with great force ramming up against the tectonic plate of public opinion. Sooner or later the pressure created by these two massive plates grinding into one another will create an earthquake or, more likely, a series of quakes, leading to a fundamental restructuring of our health-care financing system.

The corrupting influence of money on politics will affect the timing of the earthquake. But big money won't stop the quake, it will only delay it. The health-care system, left to its own devices, is incapable of preventing itself from wasting money and driving health costs up inexorably. But American public opinion is not going to change either.

Americans have been furious about health-care costs for some time, and are only going to become more so. Moreover, a big majority of the American public has long believed that health care is a right, or if not a right, then a necessity of life that all Americans should have access to in order to participate in our economy and democracy. In 1995, pollster Daniel Yankelovich wrote, "A 1938 Gallup poll reported that 81 percent of adults nationwide believed that 'government should be responsible for medical care for people who can't afford it.' Fifty-three years later the number was 80 percent – a remarkably stable conviction."[1] Public opinion will not permit the health insurance industry to solve the inflation problem by inflicting further damage on access and quality, either with a return to the aggressive managed-care tactics of the 1990s or by pushing substantial numbers of low-income and sick people into HSAs.

The only question is when the tension between rising costs and public opinion will erupt into political action, and whether the upheaval that resolves this tension will occur all at once or in a series of smaller quakes. If true campaign finance reform is enacted, the tension will be resolved sooner rather than later. With or without campaign finance reform, the likeliest scenario is a series of reforms that culminate first in expenditure controls (wielded over a multiple-payer system), and then, finally, a true Medicare-for-all program.

For the next few years, the fight over cost containment will focus on Medicare. With the exception of prescription drug costs, politicians will shy away from doing anything significant to reduce costs for the nonelderly. It is relatively easy for politicians to take positions in favor of price controls for the elderly because Medicare's price controls are already established, Medicare is a popular program, and the elderly are a powerful constituency. It is much more difficult for politicians to advocate price controls for the benefit of the nonelderly. This is not to say that politicians will ignore the nonelderly. Some will recommend programs that require the taxpayer to pay more to reduce the number of uninsured, either with tax credits or expansion of existing government programs like Medicaid. But with the exception of drugs, they will, in the short term, do little to reduce costs for the nonelderly.

In the immediate future, the biggest battle will be over the Republican campaign to privatize Medicare, a campaign that reached peak intensity during the 2003 debate over the extension of Medicare's coverage to drugs. House Republicans introduced legislation that added drug coverage to Medicare and privatized Medicare with a voucher scheme like the one proposed by Republican members of the National Bipartisan Commission on the Future of Medicare in 1999. House Republicans didn't get full-fledged privatization, but the final Medicare drug bill did include a provision requiring a privatization experiment in six cities beginning in 2010. Rep. Bill Thomas (R-CA), leader of the House Medicare privatizers, and other conservative Republicans were so upset over the conference committee's failure to adopt full-blown privatization that they nearly sank the entire drug bill. These Republicans will continue to press for greater privatization, if not with explicit legislation requiring it, then with legislation increasing the overpayments to Medicare HMOs so that HMOs can increase their Medicare enrollment.

Democrats have also shown they are eager to continue the 2003 debate over the drug bill. They were so upset by the bill that, within two months of its signing, they had introduced legislation to repeal its prohibition on Medicare negotiating limits on drug prices and the increased HMO welfare payments. The Democrats' long-overdue interest in reducing the HMO overpayments could spell the end of the Republican campaign to privatize Medicare. If Republicans cannot guarantee a steady stream of overpayments to the HMO industry, HMOs will withdraw from the Medicare program. The news that Medicare vastly overpays HMOs will eventually seep out, and that fact and the unattractiveness of HMOs and HSAs (which conservatives are also promoting as the solution for Medicare inflation) will doom the privatization campaign. But the privatization campaign may well stagger along for another decade before it peters out.

Beyond this battle over Medicare privatization, my crystal ball gets cloudier. I see two possible developments. I see a few state legislatures enacting single-payer systems, and many state legislatures enacting components of single-payer systems (drug price controls or large drug-buying coalitions which negotiate low prices with drug companies being the most likely), all of which will further legitimize the single-payer proposal. And I see a gradual consolidation of America's purchasers of health insurance into fewer and bigger buyers, including an expansion of Medicare by lowering the age at which Americans become eligible, an expansion of Medicaid by raising the income below which Americans become eligible, and perhaps a consolidation of employers into large buying groups. If buyers of health insurance become bigger and fewer, the notion that we're better off with just one buyer will gain credibility.

Citizens and citizen organizations can play a significant role in hastening real reform by keeping the suffering the current system causes before the public eye, and by helping the public, legislators, and the media understand what the real issues are. The media and some newcomers to the health-care reform debate often approach the debate with tunnel vision and become preoccupied with secondary issues. If they're looking at the problem (as opposed to solutions), they focus on horror stories – this uninsured person died, that HMO patient was kicked out of the hospital too soon, etc. If they're looking at reform proposals, they tend to ask whether a particular type of medical service will be covered under this or that "reform" bill, or whether this or that bill is "politically feasible." These are legitimate issues, but they are not the most fundamental issues. The most fundamental questions are, What are the causes of health-care inflation, and how do we address those causes? If you've read this book, you know the answer to those questions. I urge you to get involved in the fight for a Medicare-for-all program.

## Endnotes

[1] Daniel Yankelovich, "The debate that wasn't: The public and the Clinton plan," *Health Affairs* 1995;14(1):7-23, 12.

# Appendix A
## Three Examples of Patients Harmed by Managed-Care Plans Who Could Not Sue

### Introduction

In Chapter 9, I argued that legislation granting patients the right to sue managed care plans (MCPs) will not make a substantial reduction in the rate at which MCPs deny care or provide inferior care to patients. I referred the reader to this appendix for evidence of how difficult it is for people who have been abused by an MCP to sue. In this appendix, I describe the battles of three patients I worked with that illustrate how easy it is for MCPs to get away with shoddy care.

### Kate versus United Behavioral Systems

The first of three malpractice victims I will discuss was a thin, shy and fastidiously polite woman in her thirties whom I will call Kate because she was deathly afraid of anyone ever finding out the depth of her mental health problems. She was given up for adoption by her mother when she was born because her mother was in poor health, but she never developed a close relationship with her adoptive parents. By the time she was 20, Kate suffered from severe depression. By the time she was 30, she was suffering from bronchitis, sinusitis, and an eating disorder (she would alternate between starving herself and going on eating binges).

In 1992, this vulnerable woman was clobbered with two heavy-duty stressors. She discovered, after a long search, who her birth mother was and, to her dismay, that her birth mother had died in a car crash when Kate was two. On November 4 of that same year, her younger brother Jim (the son of her adoptive parents) attempted to kill his girlfriend, and then himself (he was successful at neither). As it turned out, November 4 was also the date of Kate's first appointment at the Metrodome Square Clinic in Minneapolis, a mental health clinic run by what was then called United Behavioral Systems (UBS), a subsidiary of United HealthCare, at that time the nation's second-largest private-sector health insurer after Aetna. Kate was supposed to show up at 11:00 a.m. to take several tests to see what types of services she qualified for (God forbid she should have met a real live therapist right off the bat). But when she woke up on the morning of November 4, she found a message from the girlfriend of her brother Jim on her answering machine saying Jim had attempted to kill her and had been taken by ambulance to a hospital because "he wasn't breathing."

Kate was distraught, not just for Jim's sake but for the sake of Jim's two small children. Reasonably enough, Kate wondered whether that day might be the wrong day to take tests designed to assess her emotional state. She phoned a social worker with whom she had long been in therapy and asked for her advice. The social worker told her she should keep her appointment but to inform staff at the clinic of what she was going through and let the clinic decide whether she should take the tests that day. But, in part because she was so shy and in large part because the clinic staff had no time for her, she was unable to get any Metrodome Square Clinic staff to discuss this question with her. She took the tests, but even after turning her answer sheets in she could not get anyone at the clinic to talk to her about the distress she was going through at that moment. A receptionist gave her another appointment and told her to come back. Kate left the clinic in tears.

This brusque treatment characterized the remainder of Kate's encounters with UBS and the Metrodome Clinic. The clinic's various personnel refused to diagnose her with depression even though Kate scored 37 on the Beck Depression Inventory, a score which indicated "extremely severe depression," and even though seven other mental health therapists (three of whom Kate saw after being rejected by the clinic) stated in writing that she was severely depressed. The clinic insisted that Kate suffered an eating disorder only, and claimed that group therapy on Saturdays was sufficient to treat this disorder. Kate had a hard enough time developing relationships with therapists in one-on-one settings. She was petrified at the thought of group therapy. Although she protested, UBS and the clinic refused to diagnose depression and refused to authorize individual therapy for treatment of any condition.

If you believe the AMA-Chamber-of-Commerce rhetoric about malpractice suits, you're no doubt thinking Kate merely needed to call an attorney and she'd be in court suing the clinic in no time. But, for two reasons, a lawsuit was out of the question. First, Kate could not have expected a large jury award had she sued. She did not commit suicide, and was not disfigured or maimed as a result of UBS's failure to diagnose her accurately. For this reason, and because proving that Kate was depressed and that UBS failed to diagnose depression would require Kate's attorney to pay several psychiatrists or psychologists to testify on Kate's behalf, no attorney would have wanted to take Kate's case. But there was an even more basic reason why Kate never sued. She, like so many other mental health patients in America, could not imagine testifying to a judge or, worse, to a judge and a jury, about her mental state and the pain and humiliation UBS put her through. For this reason, Kate never gave a lawsuit a moment's thought.

## Barbara Herold versus Allina

The subject of my second horror story had a reaction similar to Kate's. Her name (her real name) was Barbara Herold. Her father, 80-year-old Joseph K, who was insured by Allina, Minnesota's largest HMO at the time, was carelessly misdiagnosed by his Allina doctor after he fell and he died shortly after his fall. (Barb asked me not to reveal her father's last name in order to ensure that her mother's identity was never exposed.) Joseph's injury occurred on Sunday, December 1, 1996. That morning, he slipped on the ice on the sidewalk leading up to his house in Minneapolis while he was feeding the birds in his yard. Joseph was accustomed to physical activity; he played golf in the summer and drove himself anywhere he needed to go. But this active man died the next Friday, December 6. According to the Hennepin County Medical Examiner's Office, Joseph's death was due to "cardiopulmonary complications" caused by his fall.

Joseph's injuries that Sunday morning hardly suggested his fall would prove to be fatal. A fractured rib, diagnosed that morning in a hospital emergency room, was the extent of his injuries. Fractured ribs can be very painful, so painful you don't want to breath, but they are ordinarily not life-threatening. The main risk you run with a rib fracture is that lack of ventilation in the lung, caused by shallow breathing, will permit an infection of the lung to set in. Joseph was told by the doctor at the hospital to see his primary care doctor on Monday. But on Monday, when he went to his Allina clinic to see his doctor, the doctor was not in. A substitute doctor did nothing more than listen to Joseph's lungs to see if they were clear. Although Joseph told the doctor that he had severe chest pain and weakness in his legs, the substitute doctor did not take his temperature or his blood pressure.

Joseph's regular doctor could not see him until about noon on Thursday, about 18 hours before Joseph would die. By then, Joseph was manifesting obvious signs of a severe infection. He was hoarse, had a temperature, was vomiting, and suffered explosive diarrhea that his wife had to clean up because he was too weak to move unassisted. But Joseph's regular doctor took no action when Joseph visited him in a wheel chair on Thursday. He sent Joseph home with instructions (as he put it in Joseph's medical record) to "call or return to the office if not improving." Joseph's wife Jerry was flabbergasted at the doctor's inaction, and phoned Barb to tell her she intended to take Joseph to an emergency room. Knowing that HMOs would force patients to eat the costs of emergency room visits that the HMO later determines were not warranted, Barb urged Jerry not to do that until she, Barb, had spoken to Joseph's doctor herself.

Barb reached Joseph's doctor at about 2:30 Thursday afternoon. She reminded the doctor of the terrible symptoms Joseph was suffering and asked why the doctor had done nothing. "He might have the flu," the doctor replied. Realizing this doctor was not about to hospitalize her father, Barb now switched strategies and sought to get the doctor to admit her father to a nursing home. The doctor casually replied that he would send a "nurse evaluator" to see Joseph the next morning. Barb, who lived in Rochester, a two-hour drive south of Minneapolis, spent the remainder of the day making calls to nursing homes near her parents' home so that Joseph could move immediately into a home once the Allina nurse authorized nursing home care. Barb did not trust Allina to find her father a decent nursing home that would be near enough that his wife could visit him regularly.

The next morning, Barb drove through a snowstorm to Minneapolis. She checked out the nursing home she had investigated by phone the previous day, then drove over to her parents' house. She arrived at 9:00 a.m. and walked in. Neither parent was in sight. Her mother emerged from the kitchen.

"Where's Pop?" Barb asked.

"He's gone. He's dead," replied her mother. "They've already taken him away."

Joseph had died at about 6:30 that morning. Barb called the Allina nurse to tell her it was too late to do any evaluating. The nurse must have passed the word on to Joseph's doctor, because he called that afternoon. He said he was "shocked." Oddly, the doctor left the country several months after Barb requested her father's medical records. Neither Barb nor her mother ever received an apology from Allina.

Two physicians who examined Joseph's records at my request concluded that Joseph probably died of an infection that got out of control. Both thought Joseph's care had been substandard. As I've already mentioned, the county medical examiner found Joseph died from complications of his fall.

Barb and I discussed a malpractice suit at some length. Barb and her three siblings were interested enough in a lawsuit that I spoke to two attorneys about Joseph's case. One turned me down, and the other hinted he might turn me down after he got more familiar with the case. The attorneys said they were unlikely to take the case because of Joseph's age. They said a large portion of the damages awarded to patients are damages for lost years of employment, and that they could not risk sinking $20,000 to $40,000 in developing the suit because the award might not cover their costs. Remember, attorneys usually take negligence cases (malpractice is negligence committed by doctors) on a "contingency basis," which means they get nothing if the plaintiff loses and one-third of the award of the plaintiff wins.

I could tell from the lawyers' questions that they were also concerned by the fact that the physicians who had reviewed Joseph's file were not certain about the immediate cause of death; they could only say Joseph *probably* died from an infection. The county medical examiner's statement that Joseph died as a result of his fall was not the equivalent of a statement that he died because of medical treatment he didn't get after his fall. The attorneys gave me the impression that they reasoned as follows: They multiplied a relatively small award times an unknown risk of being unable to prove that Joseph died of an infection due to lack of medical care, and concluded the case was not worth taking.

But Barb faced an even more intractable problem in the form of her mother's fear of having to testify. Jerry was so traumatized by the sudden loss of her husband that she was often unable to discuss Joseph's death even with Barb, even in the privacy of her own home. Barb said her mother would sometimes respond to Barb's questions about her father's last days with dead silence, as if her gears had just frozen up inside. Barb knew there was no point in asking her mother how she would feel about testifying; she wouldn't do it. Because Jerry was the only witness, other than Joseph's negligent doctor, who observed Joseph's awful symptoms, her testimony would have been essential. Barb and her siblings never sued.

## Linda Harris versus Park Nicollet Clinic

On March 5, 1998, Linda Harris, a Minneapolis resident in her thirties, noticed painful swelling in her right cheek. During the first three weeks of this infection, she was unable to get either her primary care doctor or her ear-nose-and-throat doctor at Park Nicollet Clinic (Minnesota's second-largest clinic after the Mayo Clinic) to do anything to diagnose or treat her infection. This was no minor infection. Three weeks after it began, the infection had grown to the size of a chicken egg, and Linda had stopped sleeping. Four weeks after it began, the entire right side of her face was swollen and she had stopped eating because she couldn't get her jaws to open wide enough to admit food into her mouth. At this point the swelling was so severe her lower jaw was jutting leftward. On March 30, a Park Nicollet nurse rejected Linda's request to see an ENT doctor immediately and scheduled an appointment for her for the next day with Linda's regular ENT doctor. On March 31, this doctor initially refused to take any action. After Linda badgered him "to do something," the doctor ordered a CT scan, which showed (upon analysis the next day) that Linda had severe infection in the salivary duct in her right cheek, possibly caused by a stone in the duct.

But Linda's ENT doctor still refused to hospitalize her. Amazingly, he insisted her primary care doctor should do that. On April 2, Linda vomited violently through a slit between her teeth, and was finally admitted to a hospital where she was placed on intravenous antibiotics for four days. The refusal of Linda's doctors to order any test to determine the nature of her infection until March 31, and her ENT doctor's refusal to admit her to a hospital right away, extended Linda's terrible pain for perhaps a week. Linda gradually recovered fully.

I knew even before talking to an attorney that the likelihood of a lawyer wanting to sue for Linda was low. She had suffered outrageous pain for an inexcusably long time, but she had suffered no lasting harm, which means damages would be too low to sustain an attorney's interest in a lawsuit. The two attorneys I spoke to about Barb Herold's case expressed even less interest in taking Linda's case, for precisely the reasons I anticipated.

## Conclusions

The three cases I've just reviewed reveal why it is so easy for MCPs to harm patients and get away with it. Enormous obstacles stand between victims of malpractice and initiation of a lawsuit. In two of these cases, the primary obstacle was the unwillingness of the victims to proceed. I realize this picture of shy and scared Americans expressing horror at having to testify contradicts the image of the voracious American patient who sues at the drop of a hat. But precisely because shy and traumatized people like Kate and Jerry don't appear in courtrooms, the public never hears about them.

In all three cases, "insufficient" damage to the patient constituted another significant barrier to the courtroom. None of the three patients suffered enough damage to make a suit worthwhile. Kate suffered "mere" emotional pain and prolongation of the damage done by her eating disorder. Joseph K. suffered the ultimate loss, but his suffering was, mercifully, short, and he was 80 years old, which means he didn't lose a penny in foregone wages. Linda suffered "mere" excruciating pain, her pain was over in a matter of weeks, and she suffered no lasting damage.

A third significant obstacle is the difficulty victims often have in proving (a) that the physician violated the standard of care (this is difficult because American law requires that the standard be proven with the testimony of one or several physicians, which is expensive, and physicians in the same community are often reluctant to testify against one another), and (b) that the violation of the standard of care resulted in harm to the patient. The standard of care that applied to the three cases I've reported would not have been easy to articulate, and the violation of these standards was not as obvious as it is, for example, in cases where the wrong leg is cut off or a sponge is left in an abdomen after surgery. The issues in the cases of Kate, Joseph, and Linda were much more complex. Did Kate have the symptoms of depression in addition to an eating disorder, and if so, what should UBS have done for her? Were Joseph's symptoms of infection obvious enough that his doctor should have known Joseph had to be hospitalized immediately? Were Linda's symptoms of infection serious enough that her doctors should have ordered tests sooner and admitted her to the hospital sooner? I'm somewhat confident that with enough money these three patients could have proven violation of the standard of care, and resulting harm. But that's the rub. Resources for any lawsuit are not infinite, and attorneys have to make judgments about whether they can prove certain assertions to a judge or jury within the constraints of a budget determined by the damages they think they can get.

My personal knowledge of these three cases strengthens my belief that the California and Harvard studies discussed in Chapter 5, which showed that 4 and 2 percent of malpractice victims, respectively, sue, were sound studies. Large numbers of people who are harmed by malpractice never sue. There is, however, an opposite problem: Too many people with no grounds to sue do sue. These legally groundless claims are often brought by people who suffered an injury while being treated, but the injury was not caused by physician negligence. Accidents do happen, and sometimes no one is to blame. This problem of groundless lawsuits is less common than the problem of true victims not suing, but that is no consolation to the doctors who suffer the emotional and financial pain of being sued. Taken together, these problems – victims of negligence not suing, and people suing who were not hurt or who were hurt through no fault of the doctor – mean our malpractice system is not good at identifying and compensating real victims of malpractice. I support wholeheartedly further research about how to improve the malpractice system.

# Appendix B
## Evidence That Insurance Industry Overhead Averages 15 to 35 Percent

**Background**

In order for Americans to evaluate the benefits of replacing the current multiple-payer, managed-care health insurance system with a single-payer, nonmanaged-care system, we need (among other data) a reasonably good estimate of the difference in the cost of administering the two types of systems. To do that, we need a good estimate of administrative spending in the insurance and provider sectors under the current system, and a good estimate of administrative spending by the single insurer in a single-payer system and by providers under a single-payer system. In this appendix, I discuss just one of these figures: administrative costs for private-sector insurers. I said in the text that I estimate that the average overhead of U.S. private-sector health plans is in the range of 15-to-35 percent of revenues (or expenditures). In this appendix, I discuss the sources for that estimate and their limitations.

To orient you, let me begin with an overview of the entire health-insurance system. Table B-1 shows the proportions of Americans who have insurance and the proportion who don't, and, for those with insurance, their primary source of insurance. (I've included two states, Minnesota and Texas, to give you some idea of the variation among states.) You can see that 54 percent of Americans had employer-sponsored insurance

## Table B-1: Health insurance status of Americans, Minnesotans, and Texans, percent of total population, 2003

|                       | US   | Minnesota | Texas |
|-----------------------|------|-----------|-------|
| Employer-sponsored    | 54%  | 65%       | 48%   |
| Individually purchased| 5    | 6         | 4     |
| Medicaid              | 13   | 10        | 13    |
| Medicare              | 12   | 10        | 9     |
| Uninsured             | 16   | 8         | 25    |
| Total                 | 100  | 100*      | 100*  |

* Total does not come to 100 due to rounding.

Source: Census Bureau, reported in Kaiser Family Foundation, Statehealthfacts.org, http://www. state health facts.org/cgi-bin/healthfacts.cgi?action=compare&category=Health+Coverage+%26+Uninsured& subcategory=Insurance+Status&topic=Distribution+by+Insurance+Status, accessed July 21, 2005.

in 2003, another 5 percent had insurance they purchased on their own (that is, as individuals, not part of a group), 13 percent were insured by Medicaid, and 12 percent by Medicare. Accurate overhead costs for Medicaid (5 percent of revenues) and Medicare (2 percent) have long been available. That's not the case for privately-financed insurance. There are three reasons why: there is no one national agency that monitors all insurers; health policy researchers in America have little interest in the issue; and health insurers come in a variety of forms.

I have already commented on two of these factors – state regulation and disinterest on the part of the health policy community. I noted in Chapter 6 that just estimating the number of health insurers operating in the U.S. is difficult because there is no national agency in charge of regulating health insurance companies; that job is left to the 50 states. Some states do not have a single source of data on health insurance, and states may not even know how many insurers are operating within their borders. Minnesota illustrates both problems. Until recently, Minnesota gave its Department of Health sole authority to regulate HMOs and the Department of Commerce sole authority to regulate all other health insurers. Minnesota's Department of Commerce does not know how many health insurance companies actually sell insurance in Minnesota; it knows only how many are *licensed* to do so. (There were 843 licensed as of February 2004. The Department guessed the number actually marketing policies at that time was 250). A second factor that makes estimating insurer administrative costs difficult, which I have previously noted, is that health policy analysts in the U.S. have little interest in studying administrative spending despite the enormous bite (about one-third) that administrative costs take out of our health-care dollar.

A third factor is the variety of health insurance companies. Insurers vary by nonprofit/for-profit status, how tightly managed they are, whether they sell primarily to employers or to individuals, and whether they offer merely "third party administrator" services (e.g., claims processing and managing care) to self-insured firms as opposed to "full service insurance" including bearing risk. The variety of insurers, coupled with the absence of a single regulator with a single set of rules for classifying expenditures, guarantees confusion.

The few studies that have attempted to sketch out the administrative costs of the different sectors of the insurance industry tend to break the industry down into for-profit traditional indemnity insurers, for-profit managed-care insurers, nonprofit Blue Cross Blue Shields, nonprofit HMOs, and self-insured firms. I will do likewise.

## Synthesizing the evidence

The first successful traditional insurance company – the program started in 1929 at Baylor University Hospital which later became a Blue Cross company – must have had very low administrative costs in its infancy. Because the coverage offered by the program was quite simple, claims processing was relatively easy and inexpensive. The insurance covered a few hospital-based services (for example, operating room and anesthesia services) during the first 21 days of hospitalization per year, and excluded hospitalization for a few diseases (such as smallpox, tuberculosis, and chronic mental illness). In its first few years, the hospital's marketing costs consisted mainly of phone calls to employers in the Dallas area urging them to enroll their employees in the program. (Dallas schools, the Republic National Bank, and the *Times Herald* were the first employers to sign up.)[1]  Because the hospital's insurance program faced no competition from other insurers in its early years, advertising was not as important as it would be later.  For many years, the hospital program and its successor Blue Cross company did no underwriting, that is, it did not gather information on the health status of applicants to set premiums higher for sicker applicants and lower for healthier applicants.  In the early years, the hospital did not hire lobbyists to persuade the Texas Legislature and Congress to do favors for its insurance program, nor did the hospital pay for huge salaries and expensive perks for the people who ran its insurance program.  And prior to the spread of managed care, the hospital did not spend money on utilization review, incentives for doctors, and the data collection these activities require.

All that changed radically over the next three decades.  The number of medical services covered grew substantially, making claims processing more complex.  Competitors of Blue Cross formed, and most of them priced their policies lower for healthier people and higher for sicker people, and this forced all insurers to spend more money on marketing and underwriting.  The for-profit insurers, of course, also devoted a portion of their revenues to profit.  As health insurance became big business, health insurance companies did what other large American corporations do – they spent money on lobbyists, trade associations, and big salaries and expensive perks for managers.  All of these activities drove up the insurance industry's overhead costs.  The widespread adoption of managed-care tactics, especially utilization review, in the 1980s added yet another layer of overhead costs.  On the other hand, the advent of computers and consolidation within the insurance industry may have lowered overhead costs.

The net effect of these changes was great inflation in the overhead costs of insurers from the low levels of the first Blues.  Research indicates that by the 1980s these costs consumed approximately 30 percent of the revenues of the typical for-profit indemnity insurer.  A study of for-profit insurers based on data from the Health Insurance Association of America concluded overhead ate up 26 percent of the revenues of plans selling to *groups* and 41 percent of the revenues of plans selling to *individuals* in 1985.[2]  An analysis of the premiums paid and benefits received by 3,765 nonelderly Americans insured through employers in

1987 concluded the average premium paid was $1,741 and the average benefit paid was $1,145, which means the insurers spent 34 percent of premium revenue on overhead. This same study, which was conducted by a federal agency, found that overhead for insurance purchased individually by 386 nonelderly individuals was 43 percent.[3]

A study on the overhead costs of the non-HMO wing of the insurance industry as of 1988 indicated that the overhead for those insurers, not counting profit, was 27 percent (see Table B-2). This study examined what its authors called the "commercial" health insurers, defined as those insurers that were for-profit and not HMOs. (Because all the Blues were still nonprofit at that time, the Blues were excluded from this study along with all HMOs.) The five largest of these insurers, measured in terms of premium revenues, were Prudential, Aetna, Metropolitan Life, Travelers Insurance, and Principal Mutual. Because profit in the health insurance industry averages roughly 5 percent,* total administrative costs probably exceeded 30 percent on average in these traditional for-profit insurers in the 1980s. In other words, for every dollar of revenues those insurers took in, they spent about 30 cents on marketing, underwriting, lobbying, profit, etc., and 70 cents on medical care.

All of the studies I've just reviewed examined traditional for-profit insurers in the 1980s. These studies excluded two large players in the insurance industry – the budding HMO industry and the five-dozen or so Blue Cross Blue Shield plans. What were their administrative costs? Let's start with the HMOs.

The spread of managed care made the task of measuring insurer administrative costs much more difficult. Prior to the advent of managed care, there was no controversy about the proper classification of insurer expenditures; checks an insurer cut for providers were classified as medical care, and everything else was overhead. But when HMOs began to multiply, and when traditional insurers began to adopt managed-care tactics, some insurers, particularly nonprofits, felt it was appropriate to classify some of the costs of "managing care" as medical costs.

---

* *Fortune* reports that profit as a percent of sales for the life and health insurance industry was 6.4 percent in 2001, 2.9 percent in 2002, and 8.0 percent in 2003 (April 15, 2002, April 14, 2003, and April 5, 2004 editions of *Fortune*). The Centers for Medicare and Medicaid Services estimated for-profit health insurers made a profit of 4 percent in 2002 (see Table B-4).

## Table B-2: Administrative costs of for-profit health insurance companies,* 1988

|                               | Dollars (billions) | As % of premium revenues |
|-------------------------------|--------------------|--------------------------|
| Commissions                   | $6.9               | 12.5%                    |
| Salaries, wages and benefits  | 4.5                | 10.2                     |
| Rent and other expenditures   | 2.2                | 4.0                      |
| Printing, postage and phone   | 0.9                | 2.1                      |
| Advertising                   | 0.3                | 0.5                      |
| Total                         | 14.9               | 26.7                     |

* The source used the term "commercial" insurance companies, defined to mean all for-profit insurers (which, at that time, excluded all Blue Cross Blue Shield companies) that were not HMOs.

Source: Robert Brandon et al., "Premiums without benefits: Waste and inefficiency in the commercial health insurance industry," *International Journal of Health Services* 1991;21:265-283, Table 2.

HMOs claimed to have an average overhead of 14 percent in 2002, and as low as 11 percent in 1997.[4] The nation's largest nonprofit HMO, Kaiser Permanente, has long reported very low overhead costs relative to other private insurers. In 2002 Kaiser claimed its overhead was 7.5 percent of expenditures.[5] Kaiser treats a substantial portion of its management costs as medical care costs, according to Doug Sherlock who monitors industry expenditures.[6] So too do other nonprofit HMOs. In a debate about whether for-profit or nonprofit managed care plans are more efficient, representatives of Group Health Cooperative of Puget Sound, a nonprofit HMO, claimed their administrative costs ranged between 7 and 9 percent of revenues over a five-year period.[7] The CEO of a for-profit MCP countered with the argument that nonprofit HMOs define some of their "claims processing, provider relations, provider contracting, and membership services [as] medical expenses."[8]

Medica, currently Minnesota's largest HMO, has been counting administrative costs as medical costs for more than a decade. That's why it was able to report overheads in the low teens in the 1990s and a 9.0 percent rate for 2002.[9] In 1993, the Citizens League, a corporation-funded good government group, reported:

> Medica made an important change in its 1992 annual statement to the Department of Health.... In previous years, Medica reported all of the management fee paid to United HealthCare [the national insurance company that Medica hired to "manage" Medica] as an administrative expense. For 1992, Medica allocated a portion of the management fee to medical services. It argued that fees for quality assurance, nurses, and related medical management services provided by United were medical, rather than administrative, costs.[10]

Medica's bookkeeping games inspired other Minnesota HMOs, all nonprofit by law, to do likewise. Allan Baumgarten, who wrote the Citizens League report and now publishes analyses of the insurance industries of several states in his own name, wrote in his 1994 report about Minnesota's HMOs:

> Frankly, ... some HMOs keep changing their allocation of costs to administration and medical care, and it is hard to be confident that the figures in the state filings portray an accurate picture.... Other HMOs have apparently picked up on [Medica's accounting] change and have also reallocated portions of their management fees paid for utilization review, medical management or sometimes provider relations, to medical costs. This year Group Health [one of two HMOs that merged to form HealthPartners] took note of what others were doing and moved $9 million in clinic operating costs from administrative to medical costs. The result: Its administrative costs per commercial member per month went from $15.71 in 1992 to $10.98 in 1993.[11]

As this last statistic on Group Health suggests, MCPs can drastically reduce their reported overhead costs with bookkeeping games.

Other evidence indicates Medica's real overhead is a lot higher than the 9 to 13 percent it has been reporting to the Minnesota Department of Health over the last decade. In 2001, Minnesota's Attorney General Mike Hatch revealed that Medica's overhead was "at least" 18 percent in 1998, 19 percent in 1999, and 19 percent in 2000.[12] The Attorney General's estimates are consistent with a document Medica sent to my former employer, Minnesota COACT, in the mid-1990s announcing that Medica customers could expect to get back, on average, 82 percent of the premiums they paid in the form of health-care payments, which means 18 percent was retained by Medica for non-health payments. These 18- and 19-percent figures are much higher than the 10-percent overhead Allina reported to Minnesota's Department of Health for the years 1998, 1999 and 2000.[13]

Another study indicates that Medica's overhead may be higher than 19 percent. However, because this study was not based on an audit, it is not as reliable as the Attorney General's report. This study was done by a retired accountant for the Minnesota Physician Patient Alliance (MPPA). (I used to sit on MPPA's board.) The accountant went to the Minnesota Department of Health (the agency that used to regulate HMOs) and asked to see the annual expenditure reports filed by Medica and Minnesota's second- and third-largest HMOs – HealthPartners and Blue Plus. On the basis of these reports, the accountant concluded the administrative costs of these three HMOs averaged somewhere between 12 and 31 percent. The range was this broad because the accountant was unable to determine whether all of the expenditures in a category called "other professional services" should have been treated as medical expenses. This category, per Department of Health instructions, mixes up health-care *professionals* (such as dentists, psychologists, and nurses) with *administrative* employees (janitors, "quality assurance analysts, administrative supervisors, secretaries ... , and medical records clerks"). This kitchen-sink category accounted for 19 percent of the three HMOs' expenditures. That's why the upper and lower bounds of the accountant's estimate spanned 19 percentage points.[14]

I have no similar evidence that would lead me to believe national for-profit MCPs play the bookkeeping games some nonprofit HMOs play to minimize their overhead costs. The administrative costs of the larger for-profits in the 1990s were in the 20-to-30-percent range, much higher than those reported by Kaiser and the Minnesota HMOs and close to the 30-percent level reported by traditional insurers in the 1980s. Four large MCPs (all for-profits) reported in documents they filed with the Securities Exchange Commission overheads ranging from 18 to 33 percent for 1999 (see Table B-3). According to a 2003 report by the Centers for Medicare and Medicaid Services (CMS), for-profit health insurers incurred expenditures on non-medical costs that equaled 24 percent of their expenditures in 2002[15] (see Table B-4). A study based on a survey of dental HMOs asking about 1995 expenditures reported administrative expenses as a percent of all expenditures ranging from a low of 27 percent to a high of 47 percent.[16] Reports on particular insurers indicate some insurers have overhead way beyond the 30-percent range. For example, the Fort Lauderdale *Sun-Sentinel* reported that some Florida Medicaid HMOs "spend nearly half their budgets on administrative and other non-medical costs."[17]

The differences between the for-profits and the nonprofit HMOs cannot be attributed to differences in profit (or surplus or net income, in the case of the nonprofits). Profits earned by the average for-profit and the surplus earned by the average nonprofit are not available, but

---

## Table B-3: The four largest health insurance companies as of 2002 and their overhead as of 1999

| Company | Number of people insured | Overhead* |
|---|---|---|
| United Health Group | 16.2 million | 18% |
| Aetna | 14.4 million | 25% |
| Cigna | 13.3 million | 33% |
| Wellpoint | 13.1 million | 25% |
| Total | 57.0 million | |

\* Overhead is defined as the percent of revenues not spent on medical care.

Sources: Enrollment data from Milt Freudenheim, "Cigna to feel major loss in customers," *New York Times*, October 29, 2002, C4; overhead figures from Steffie Woolhandler and David U. Himmelstein with Ida Hellander, *Bleeding the Patient: The Consequences of Corporate Health Care*, Common Courage Press, Monroe, ME, 2001, 109.

---

---

## Table B-4: Expenditures by for-profit health insurance companies, as a percent of total expenditures, 2002

| | |
|---|---|
| Medical care costs | 76.0% |
| Sales, general, and administrative | 16.0% |
| Other net expenses[a] | 3.3% |
| Profit: | 4.4% |
| Total | 100.0%[b] |

(a) Includes "depreciation, amortization, net interest, and taxes."
(b) Total does not come exactly to 100 percent due to rounding.
Source: Centers for Medicare and Medicaid Services, *Health Care Industry Market Update: Managed Care*, March 2003, http://www.cms.hhs.gov/reports/ hcimu/hcimu_03242003.pdf, accessed July 22, 2005.

---

they appear to be similar; both appear to be in the 3-to-6 percent range. Whatever small differences in net income exist, they can't explain the large difference between the overheads of Kaiser and Minnesota's HMOs and, say, Aetna's 25 percent overhead. I suspect the explanation for the difference is that nonprofits have an incentive to shift administrative expenditures into the medical expenditure category that the for-profits do not have. Nonprofits want to appear to their regulators and the communities they serve to be behaving in a manner consistent with their nonprofit status and deserving of the reduced tax load nonprofit status confers. The bookkeeping games that Minnesota's HMOs began to play in the early 1990s may also have been motivated by the criticisms of their overhead costs by the Health Care Campaign of Minnesota, the single-payer coalition I used to work for.

Blue Cross Blue Shield plans have long claimed their overhead is on the order of 15 percent. According to CMS, the Blues reported a 13 percent overhead for the first half of 2002. In the first few decades, the Blues' overhead may well have been at or below 15 percent. In their history of the Blues plans, the Cunninghams report that the three Blue Cross plans operating in Pennsylvania in 1957 had an average overhead of 7 percent.[18] But 15 percent might be low today.

CMS speculated that the Blues have lower overhead costs than the for-profits because the Blues don't have to advertise as heavily as the for-profits because their name is so well established. I suspect bookkeeping games with administrative costs associated with "managing care," and the incentive of nonprofits to minimize their overhead, also play a role. We get some hint of that if we compare the overhead of Wellpoint, a former nonprofit Blues company, with the 15-percent figure claimed by the nonprofit Blues. From 1993 until 1996, Wellpoint was a for-profit subsidiary of nonprofit Blue Cross of California (Wellpoint was the latter company's managed-care plan). In 1996 Blue Cross of California converted from a nonprofit to a for-profit, and the roles of Wellpoint and Blue Cross of California were reversed – Wellpoint became the parent company. By 1999, Wellpoint's overhead was 25 percent (see Table B-3) and, by 2002, Blue Cross of California's overhead was 24 percent.[19] Nonprofit plans would claim the higher overhead of for-profit insurers is proof that nonprofits are more efficient than for-profits and/or that nonprofits put less emphasis on profit. This may be true in some sectors of the economy, but I have seen no evidence that nonprofit status significantly affects spending priorities in the health insurance sector. I suspect that Wellpoint's and Blue Cross of California's overheads are high relative to those of the nonprofit Blues because the latter declare some administrative costs to be medical costs.

Insurance companies that sell primarily to individuals have much higher overhead costs than insurers that sell to groups, but because only 5 percent of Americans are insured through individually purchased insurance, the higher administrative costs incurred by plans selling individually purchased insurance don't have a substantial effect on the average.

To sum up, the data suggest that the typical for-profit MCP operates at 20 to 35 percent overhead, the typical nonprofit HMO operates at 15 to 25 percent, and the typical Blues plan at 15 percent and probably higher. Because nonprofit HMOs insure only about 10 percent of the nonelderly insured today,[20] their overheads have relatively little weight on the average for the entire industry. It's the overheads of the for-profit MCPs and the Blues, who together control nearly all of the other 90 percent, that have the dominant influence on the industry average. Because estimates of market share don't break down the industry cleanly into the categories I've been using, it's difficult to say with precision how much of the nonelderly market belongs to the Blues and how much to the for-profit MCPs, but 35 percent for the Blues and 50 percent for the for-profit MCPs is a good guess. Given this distribution, we may estimate that the average industry overhead is somewhere in the 15-to-35-percent range.

## An apparent discrepancy

In its annual report on U.S. health spending, CMS breaks spending down into five categories, one of which is insurance overhead. The actual title for this category is, "Government administration and net cost of private health insurance." "Government administration" refers to the administrative costs of government programs (these costs are dominated by the overheads of Medicare and Medicaid), while "net cost of private health insurance" refers to the overhead of private-sector plans. Over the 1998-2003 period, the expenditures on overhead by all private-sector insurers reported by CMS ranged from 11 to 14 percent of total spending by all private insurers.[21] For those who don't know how CMS calculates this figure, the CMS figures seem to contradict the 15-to-35-percent estimate I have reported in this appendix. Two facts help us reconcile these apparently contradictory numbers.

First, CMS gets its numbers on HMOs from the state agencies that regulate HMOs, and because these agencies don't have the funds to audit HMO reports, these data effectively come straight from the HMOs. Likewise, CMS gets its numbers on Blue Cross Blue Shield Plans directly from those plans.[22] CMS does not subject these HMO and Blues reports to audits, so if the nonprofit HMOs and the nonprofit Blues are playing bookkeeping games to deflate their overheads, CMS cannot detect it and cannot prevent these games from influencing what CMS reports in its "net cost" category.

The second factor that pulls CMS's "net cost" figures down is the inclusion in CMS's figure of not just *plan* overhead but the overheads of self-insured employers as well. CMS breaks self-insured employers into two categories: those that are completely self-insured (they "accept risk" *and* process their own claims), and those that only "accept risk" (they set aside their own money to cover their employees' medical bills, but they hire an insurance company to process claims and, perhaps, manage care). Both types of self-insured firms have much lower overhead costs than do MCPs. Together they account for about 40 percent of all privately insured Americans. CMS estimates that completely self-insured employers have an overhead of 1 percent. Because completely self-insured employers are effectively small single-payers, I would expect their overheads to be low, but 1 percent is below even gigantic Medicare's overhead and therefore seems too low. The CMS analyst I spoke with said this estimate was based on a 1980 survey; she agreed the survey was probably out of date. (CMS derives the overheads of those self-insured employers that contract out the claims-processing function from a survey of "third party administrators" available at businessinsurance.com.)[23]

## A last harrumph

If the nation's health policy experts had put as much time and energy into estimating overhead costs as they have into estimating overuse and managed care's impact on it, we would now be in a position to make a much more accurate estimate of the cost of insurance industry overhead. But that didn't happen. The data we do have are, however, good enough to support my conclusion that the industry overhead average is somewhere between 15 and 35 percent of revenues. Whatever the true average is – 15 percent, 25 percent, 35 percent – it is far, far above Medicare's overhead of 2 percent.

## Endnotes

[1] Robert Cunningham III and Robert M. Cunningham, Jr., *The Blues: A History of the Blue Cross and Blue Shield System*, Northern Illinois University Press, DeKalb, IL, 1997, 6.

[2] Mark V. Pauly and Allison M. Percy, "Cost and performance: A comparison of the individual and group health insurance markets," *Journal of Health Politics, Policy and Law* 2000;25;9-26, Table 7, 19.

[3] Ibid., Table 9, 20.

[4] Kaiser Family Foundation, *Trends and Indicators in the Changing Health Care Marketplace 2005*, Exhibit 6.10, http://www.kff.org/insurance/7031/ti2004-6-10.cfm, accessed July 22, 2005.

[5] Centers for Medicare and op cit., March 2003, http://www.cms.hhs.gov/reports/hcimu/hcimu_03242003.pdf, accessed July 20, 2005.

[6] Douglas Sherlock, personal communication, May 27, 2004.

[7] Phillip M. Nudelman and Linda M. Andrews, "The 'value added' of not-for-profit health plans," *New England Journal of Medicine* 1996;334:1057-1059.

[8] Malki M. Hasan, "Let's end the nonprofit charade," *New England Journal of Medicine* 1996;334:1055-1057.

[9] Minnesota Department of Health, *Administrative Costs at Minnesota Health Plans in 2002*, St. Paul, MN, November 2003.

[10] Citizens League, *Minnesota Managed Care Review, 1993*, Minneapolis, MN (no publication date listed), 30.

[11] Allan Baumgarten, *Minnesota Managed Care Review, 1994*, Minneapolis, MN, 1994.

[12] Mike Hatch, Attorney General, State of Minnesota, *Memorandum of Understanding with Allina Health Systems, Inc. ("Allina") and with Medica Health Plans ("Medica") based on its Compliance Review: Administrative Expenses*, http://www.ag.state.mn.us/consumer/PDF/Allina/Allina_AdminExp. PDF, accessed March 14, 2002.

[13] Ibid.

[14] Minnesota Physician Patient Alliance, *Managed Care Costs: Where Do Minnesota HMOs Spend Our Money?* Minneapolis, MN, 1998.

[15] Centers for Medicare and Medicaid Services, *Health Care Industry Market Update: Managed Care.*

[16] James B. Bramson and Marye E. Feldman, "A review of dental HMO expenses: Where do the dental premium dollars really go?" *Journal of the American Dental Association* 1996;127:118-122.

[17] Fort Lauderdale *Sun-Sentinel*, December 11, 1944, reported in *American Health Line*, December 13, 1994, 3.

[18] Cunningham and Cunningham, op cit., 104.

[19] Laurence Darmiento, "Blue Cross chafes at high ranking on 'political list,'" *Los Angeles Business Journal*, April 22, 2002, http://www.findarticles. com/p/articles/mi_m5072/is_16_24/ai_91091125, accessed July 22, 2005.

[20] Kaiser Family Foundation, op cit., Exhibit 5.10.

[21] Author's calculations based on data in Centers for Medicare and Medicaid Services, "Table 3: National Health Expenditures, by Source of Funds and Type of Expenditure: Selected Calendar Years 1998-2003," http://www.cms.hhs.gov/ statistics/nhe/historical/t3.asp?, accessed July 22, 2005.

[22] Cathy Cowan, Centers for Medicare and Medicaid Services, personal communication, June 3, 2004.

[23] Ibid.

# About the Author

Kip Sullivan has been teaching and writing about the American health-care crisis since 1986. His articles on this subject, which now number over 100, have appeared in the *New York Times*, the *Los Angeles Times*, *The Nation*, the *Washington Monthly*, the *New England Journal of Medicine*, and *Health Affairs*.

Mr. Sullivan is a graduate of Pomona College and Harvard Law School. With the exception of a three-year stint with the New York Legal Aid Society, he has spent his entire adult life working for citizen organizations. From 1980 to 2000, he was an organizer, researcher and lobbyist for Minnesota Citizen Organizations Acting Together (COACT), an organization that teaches citizens how to work together for social justice. In 1986, COACT endorsed universal health insurance and appointed Mr. Sullivan as the campaign director for that issue. This assignment required Mr. Sullivan to develop a thorough understanding of the health-care crisis – not just its obvious symptoms, but its origins and the various proposals to solve it – and to explain the crisis to the average person. Since 1986, Mr. Sullivan has explained the health-care crisis and the debate about it to thousands of people, including members of religious organizations, unions, farm groups, political organizations, and legislators.

Mr. Sullivan's background makes him unique among those who write about health policy. Unlike most health policy experts, he has had to explain health policy to everyday people as opposed to other health policy experts or students interested in becoming health policy experts. Unlike most health policy experts, Mr. Sullivan has no financial connection to the health-care industry. He has been completely free to seek a solution to the health-care crisis that will benefit the average person as opposed to health insurance companies, pharmaceutical manufacturers, and other powerful interest groups that dominate the debate about how to solve the health-care mess.

Printed in the United States
52074LVS00004BA/1-75